Case-based Reviews in
PEDIATRIC INFECTIOUS DISEASES

AF068044

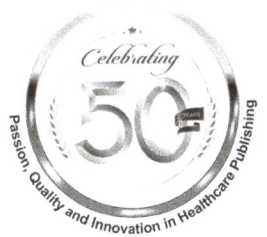

Case-based Reviews in
PEDIATRIC INFECTIOUS DISEASES

Editors

Ajay Kalra
MD DCH MNAMS FIAP
Erstwhile Professor
Department of Pediatrics
SN Medical College
Agra, Uttar Pradesh, India

Vipin M Vashishtha
MD FIAP
Director and Consultant Pediatrician
Mangla Hospital and Research Center
Bijnor, Uttar Pradesh, India

Foreword
YK Amdekar

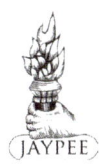

JAYPEE BROTHERS MEDICAL PUBLISHERS
The Health Sciences Publisher
New Delhi | London

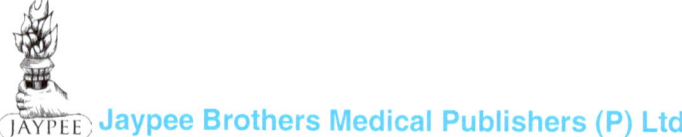 **Jaypee Brothers Medical Publishers (P) Ltd**

Headquarters
Jaypee Brothers Medical Publishers (P) Ltd
4838/24, Ansari Road, Daryaganj
New Delhi 110 002, India
Phone: +91-11-43574357
Fax: +91-11-43574314
Email: jaypee@jaypeebrothers.com

Overseas Office
J.P. Medical Ltd
83, Victoria Street, London
SW1H 0HW (UK)
Phone: +44 20 3170 8910
Fax: +44 (0)20 3008 6180
E-mail: info@jpmedpub.com

Website: www.jaypeebrothers.com
Website: www.jaypeedigital.com

© 2021, Jaypee Brothers Medical Publishers

The views and opinions expressed in this book are solely those of the original contributor(s)/author(s) and do not necessarily represent those of editor(s) of the book.

All rights reserved. No part of this publication may be reproduced, stored or transmitted in any form or by any means, electronic, mechanical, photocopying, recording or otherwise, without the prior permission in writing of the publishers.

All brand names and product names used in this book are trade names, service marks, trademarks or registered trademarks of their respective owners. The publisher is not associated with any product or vendor mentioned in this book.

Medical knowledge and practice change constantly. This book is designed to provide accurate, authoritative information about the subject matter in question. However, readers are advised to check the most current information available on procedures included and check information from the manufacturer of each product to be administered, to verify the recommended dose, formula, method and duration of administration, adverse effects and contraindications. It is the responsibility of the practitioner to take all appropriate safety precautions. Neither the publisher nor the author(s)/editor(s) assume any liability for any injury and/or damage to persons or property arising from or related to use of material in this book.

This book is sold on the understanding that the publisher is not engaged in providing professional medical services. If such advice or services are required, the services of a competent medical professional should be sought.

Every effort has been made where necessary to contact holders of copyright to obtain permission to reproduce copyright material. If any have been inadvertently overlooked, the publisher will be pleased to make the necessary arrangements at the first opportunity. The **CD/DVD-ROM** (if any) provided in the sealed envelope with this book is complimentary and free of cost. **Not meant for sale.**

Inquiries for bulk sales may be solicited at: jaypee@jaypeebrothers.com

Case-based Reviews in Pediatric Infectious Diseases

First Edition: **2021**
ISBN: 978-93-5270-673-0

Contributors

AJ Chitkara MD FIAP
Director and Head
Department of Pediatrics
Max Superspecialty Hospital
New Delhi, India

Ajay Gaur
MD PhD FIAP FICMCH Dip FW Child Dev
Cert IYCF (UK)
Professor and Head
Department of Pediatrics
GR Medical College
Gwalior, Madhya Pradesh, India

Ajay Kalra MD DCH MNAMS FIAP
Erstwhile Professor
Department of Pediatrics
SN Medical College
Agra, Uttar Pradesh, India

AK Patwari MD DCH
Professor and Head
Department of Pediatrics
Hamdard Institute of Medical
Sciences and Research
New Delhi, India

Alka Agrawal MD FIAP
Professor and Head
Department of Pediatrics
Santosh Medical College
Ghaziabad, Uttar Pradesh, India

Amit Agarwal MD (Ped) FIPNA FISPN
Consultant Pediatric Nephrologist
Madhukar Rainbow Children Hospital
New Delhi, India

Ankita Bhandari MBBS DCH
Senior Resident (NICU)
Department of Pediatrics
DY Patil Medical College
Navi Mumbai, Maharashtra, India

Anupam Sachdeva MD
Incharge
Pediatric Hemato-Oncology Unit
Department of Pediatrics
Center of Child Health
Sir Ganga Ram Hospital
New Delhi, India

Arun Shah
MD DCH FRCP (London) FIAP
FNNF FIAMS
Consultant Pediatrician
Head
Department of Pediatrics
Prasad Hospital
Muzaffarpur, Bihar, India

Ashok Banga MD
Director and Consultant
Department of Pediatrics
Chirayu and Astha Hospitals
Gwalior, Madhya Pradesh, India

Atul Kulkarni MD
Assistant Professor
Venkatesh Hospital
Ashwini Rural Medical College,
Hospital and Research Centre
Solapur, Maharashtra, India

Bharat Mehra MBBS MD (Pediatrics)
Associate Consultant
Department of Pediatrics
Max Superspecialty Hospital
New Delhi, India
Fellowship in Pediatric Emergency and
Critical Care (SGRH)

Dhanya Dharmapalan MBBS MD
Consultant in Pediatric Infectious
Diseases
Apollo Hospitals
Navi Mumbai, Maharashtra, India

Dipti Agarwal MD MAMS
Associate Professor
Department of Pediatrics
Dr Ram Manohar Lohia Institute of
Medical Sciences
Lucknow, Uttar Pradesh, India

Kheya Ghosh Uttam DCH DNB FIAP
Associate Professor and NICU-In-Charge
Institute of Child Health
Kolkata, West Bengal, India

Mallar Mukherjee MD
Assistant Professor
Institute of Child Health
Kolkata, West Bengal, India

Monjori Mitra DCH DNB
Associate Professor
Institute of Child Health
Kolkata, West Bengal, India

Nimisha Arora MD (Pediatrics)
Assistant Professor
Department of Pediatrics
Santosh Medical College
Ghaziabad, Uttar Pradesh, India

Pallavi Gahlowt MD
Assistant Professor
Department of Community Medicine
DY Patil Medical College
Navi Mumbai, Maharashtra, India

Prabhas Prasun Giri MD MRCPCH (UK)
Associate Professor
Institute of Child Health
Kolkata, West Bengal, India

Prakash Petchimuthu MD
Senior Resident
Department of Pediatrics
GR Medical College
Gwalior, Madhya Pradesh, India

Pranjali Saxena MD
Assistant Professor
Department of Pediatrics and
Neonatology
Era's Lucknow Medical College and
Hospital
Lucknow, Uttar Pradesh, India

RK Sabharwal MD DM (Neurology)
Chief
Division of Pediatric Neurology and
Epilepsy
Institute of Child Health
Sir Ganga Ram Hospital
New Delhi, India

Rajesh Rai MD
Head
Department of Pediatrics and
Neonatology
DY Patil Medical College
Navi Mumbai, Maharashtra, India

(Col) Rekha Mittal MD
Additional Director
Pediatric Neurology
Madhukar Rainbow Children's Hospital
New Delhi, India

Ridhimaa Jain MBBS DCH DNB
Senior Resident
Department of Pediatrics
Child Development Center
Maulana Azad Medical College
New Delhi, India

Rohit Bannerji MD
Assistant Professor
Institute of Child Health
Kolkata, West Bengal, India

Sanjay Verma MD
Professor (Pediatrics)
Infectious Disease Unit
Department of Pediatrics
Advanced Pediatric Centre (APC)
Postgraduate Institute of Medical
Education and Research (PGIMER)
Chandigarh, India

Shrish Bhatnagar
MD (Ped) SR (Ped Gastro, SGPGIMS) MIAP
MISG
Professor and Head
Department of Pediatrics
Era's Lucknow Medical College and
Hospital
Lucknow, Uttar Pradesh, India

Vikram Hirekerur MD
Associate Professor
Ashwini Rural Medical College,
Hospital and Research Centre
Solapur, Maharashtra, India

Vimlesh Soni
Assistant Professor
Department of Pediatrics
Maharishi Markandeshwar Institute of
Medical Sciences and Research
Ambala, Haryana, India

Vineet Saxena MD FIAP
Head
Department of Pediatrics and
Neonatology
Anand Hospital
Meerut, Uttar Pradesh, India

Vinod Gunasekaran MD FNB FIAP
Consultant and Head
Pediatric Hemato-Oncology Unit
Kauvery Hospital
Trichy, Tamil Nadu, India

Vipin M Vashishtha MD FIAP
Director and Consultant Pediatrician
Mangla Hospital and Research Center
Bijnor, Uttar Pradesh, India

Vivek Saxena MD
Consultant Pediatrician
Vatsalya Hospital
Kanpur, Uttar Pradesh, India

Yashwant Rao MD
Professor and Head
Department of Pediatrics
GSVM Medical College
Kanpur, Uttar Pradesh, India

YK Amdekar MD
Erstwhile Professor of Pediatrics
Grant Medical College and
JJ Group of Hospitals, Mumbai
Consultant Pediatrician
Jaslok and Breach Candy Hospital
Mumbai, Maharashtra, India
President of IAP (1995)

Foreword

I am happy to write a foreword to *Case-based Reviews in Pediatric Infectious Diseases*. Choice of infectious diseases is most apt as not only infectious diseases from major part of pediatric practice but they often pose challenges in terms of diagnosis and rational treatment. Case-based learning helps to develop skills for analytical thinking and reflective judgment by reading discussion on real-life situations faced in practice. Reviews offer insight into a thought process of arriving at a probable diagnosis, choosing appropriate tests and instituting rational treatment. This book is different than a textbook in that it combines basic knowledge and analytical skills that together pave the way for rational practice. Readers would identify similar situations that they may have faced in office practice and compare author's views with their own. In effect, it becomes an interactive self-learning exercise. It is the best way of continuing medical education.

Clinical medicine presents with different types of challenges and this book deals with all of them with representative case scenarios. Patient usually reports to a pediatrician with symptoms that must be properly analyzed with detailed history and focussed physical examination to arrive at a probable diagnosis. Broad diagnosis such as pneumonia is often possible but specific etiology is not easy to judge and needs rational thinking. Even when specific etiological diagnosis is made, complications may prove a hurdle in successful outcome. Non-specific physical findings such as hepatosplenomegaly may indicate an infectious disease that demands rational consideration because it may as well be a non-infectious disease. Positive infection-specific antibodies may indicate recent or old infection, carrier state or even cross-reacting antibodies to another infection, and hence interpretation of such tests need caution. Imaging modalities denote pathology more than etiology as in case of ring enhancing lesion on CT brain scan that may suggest tuberculosis, cysticercosis or transient disappearing benign lesion. Such are the challenges of infectious diseases and reader will find in this book, all such practical issues presented with case-based discussions. Immunization is the integral part of prevention of infectious diseases and is rightly addressed in this book.

It is an irony that every sick child is presumed to be suffering from infection and unfortunately prescribed an antibiotic at the first contact. Abuse of antibiotics have thus led to increasing drug resistance. It is possible to make reasonably correct decisions about presence or absence of infection and whether infection is bacterial or otherwise. With varied types of case-scenarios, I am sure, reader will be stimulated to think rationally that will pave the way for ideal clinical practice. It is time that we all join this crusade against infections and I wish every reader gets sensitized after studying this excellent book.

YK Amdekar MD
Erstwhile Professor of Pediatrics
Grant Medical College and JJ Group of Hospitals, Mumbai
Consultant Pediatrician
Jaslok and Breach Candy Hospital
Mumbai, Maharashtra, India
President of IAP (1995)

Preface

Come fever and the first thing that strikes our mind is Infection!! Which indeed, is the case most of the times. Yet infections may not always be associated with fever (as happens in congenitally acquired infections) and not all fevers are due to infections. There can be no better way to bring out these fine nuances than by studying the case-based scenarios, which is what this book intends to do.

The most essential part of a student's instruction is obtained ....not in the lecture-room, but at the bedside.
–Oliver Wendell Holmes

The authors have unfolded the mystery behind each case, step by step, working on them as if they were detectives.

Methods of physicians are like those of a detective, one seeking to explain a disease, other a crime.
–Anonymous

We have purposely placed these case studies randomly and have not grouped them under any class, so that the readers have an element of surprise and wonder whether it is a case of infection or a mimic.

Observation is not merely the power of seeing, looking or matching. It should evolve and proceed through a carefully directed analytic exercise to shed new light, provide meaningful insight, propose creative solutions or arrive at novel conclusions.
–Sir William Osler

We hope the readers will find this collection interesting and of help in evolving the art of rationally analyzing the cases in hand.

Ajay Kalra
Vipin M Vashishtha

Acknowledgments

We are thankful to Shri Jitendar P Vij (Group Chairman), Mr Ankit Vij (Managing Director), Mr MS Mani (Group President), Ms Chetna Malhotra Vohra (Associate Director—Content Strategy), Ms Pooja Bhandari (Production Head), Dr Rajul Jain (Development Editor) and entire team of M/s Jaypee Brothers Medical Publishers (P) Ltd, New Delhi, India, for giving the go-ahead at the very beginning and helping us in every way possible to bring out this book.

Contents

1. A Child with Fever for Three Months 1
   YK Amdekar

2. Approach to a Child Having Fever with Coma 10
   Vipin M Vashishtha

3. A Child with Recurrent Fever 35
   Yashwant Rao

4. Fever with Positive Tuberculin Skin Test 45
   Ajay Gaur, Prakash Petchimuthu

5. Fever Beyond One Week 50
   Arun Shah

6. Typhoid Fever with Jaundice 56
   Kheya Ghosh Uttam, Prabhas Prasun Giri

7. Children with Pyrexia and Unilateral Pleural Effusion............. 62
   Rohit Bannerji, Mallar Mukherjee, Monjori Mitra

8. Prolonged and Confusing Fevers in Children............................ 76
   Rajesh Rai, Ankita Bhandari

9. Fever with Splenomegaly 88
   Dipti Agarwal

10. An Infant with Deep Jaundice and Acholic Stools 97
    Alka Agarwal, Nimisha Arora

11. Child with Unusual Infections 108
    Vinod Gunasekaran, Anupam Sachdeva

12. An Infant with Cataract and Positive IgM Rubella................... 117
    Bharat Mehra, AJ Chitkara

13. A Child with Prolonged Diarrhea 122
    AK Patwari

14. An Infant with Microcephaly with Recurrent Seizures 129
    Rekha Mittal, Ridhimaa Jain

15. Neurocysticercosis in Children 140
    RK Sabharwal

16. A Child with Recurrent or Nonresolving Pneumonia 151
    Vimlesh Soni, Sanjay Verma

17. A Case of Recurrent Jaundice 161
    Shrish Bhatnagar

18. Case-based Scenarios in Rickettsial Infection 168
    Atul Kulkarni, Vikram Hirekerur

19. Case Scenarios on Rational Antibiotic Usage 177
    Dhanya Dharmapalan

20. Approach to a Case of Matted Lymphadenopathy 185
    Vineet Saxena, Pranjali Saxena

21. A Two-month-old Child with Acute Kidney Injury 191
    Amit Agarwal

22. Pediatric Septic Shock 198
    Vivek Saxena

23. Unusual Skin Manifestations of Pediatric Tuberculosis 210
    Rajesh Rai, Pallavi Gahlowt

24. Adolescent Immunization 216
    Ashok Banga

Index *231*

Chapter 1

A Child with Fever for Three Months

YK Amdekar

INTRODUCTION

In the year 1961, Petersdorf and Beeson defined pyrexia of unknown origin (PUO) as persistent fever for more than 3 weeks or in spite of investigations in the hospital for more than 1 week. PUO is now defined as persistent fever at the end of three outpatient visits or 3 days in the hospital without finding a cause or in spite of 1 week of relevant investigations. The common causes of PUO include bacterial infections [tuberculosis (TB), subacute bacterial endocarditis, and brucellosis], viral infections [EB virus (Epstein–Barr virus) and CMV (cytomegalovirus)], fungal and parasitic infections (kala-azar), noninfective illnesses (rheumatic diseases and malignancy), and rarely central fever due to hypothalamic disturbances, hyperthyroidism, heat fever, and drug fever. Analysis of detailed history and focused physical examination are the prerequisites of a rational approach to diagnosis which is then confirmed by relevant tests.

CASE 1

A 6-year-old child presented with fever for the last 3 months. The child was well prior to the onset of present illness when he started with high fever. After few days of symptomatic therapy, he was treated with multiple antibiotics such as amoxicillin, gentamycin, and ceftriaxone but fever persisted to varying degree. He had poor appetite and lost 4 kg weight. There were no other symptoms. There was no history of recent travel or contact with animals. There was no significant family history. The physical examination showed chronically sick child, with weight 17 kg, height 109 cm, moderate pallor, enlarged liver with 10-cm span, firm in consistency, not tender, spleen 4 cm, no jaundice, ascites, significant pallor, lymphadenopathy, skin rash, and joint involvement. Other systems were normal.

Q1. What is differential diagnosis?

Ans. This child has progressive inflammatory disease as suggested by prolonged fever with loss of weight over 3 months. Hepatosplenomegaly is the only positive finding in this child. Absence of jaundice rules out hepatocyte disease and absence of ascites rules out portal hypertension. So, hepatosplenomegaly in this child is likely due to reticuloepithelial cell involvement secondary to infection or noninfective disorder such as systemic inflammatory disease or malignancy. Systemic inflammatory disorder would have manifested with skin rash, arthritis, mouth ulcers, or other organ involvement over few weeks and so is unlikely. Absence of severe anemia, purpura, or lymphadenopathy rules out hematological malignancy though histiocytosis including hemophagocytic lymphohistiocytosis (HLH) is a possibility as anemia and thrombocytopenia may be subclinical. Slowly progressive chronic infections include tuberculosis, brucellosis, CMV, malaria, and kala-azar besides fungal infection. Malaria and kala-azar would have severe pallor and large splenomegaly while CMV would have localized in some organs causing dysfunction such as jaundice in hepatitis. Fungal infection presents in an immunocompromised host and so unlikely in this child. Primary streptococcal infection may present with prolonged fever due to toxins produced by bacteria but fever may not last so long for 3 months and hence unlikely in this child. So, differential diagnosis in this child would include infections such as tuberculosis and brucellosis, though histiocytosis including HLH secondary to infection is not obvious.

Q2. What investigations would you consider?

Ans. Complete blood count (CBC), peripheral smear, and erythrocyte sedimentation rate (ESR)—neutrophilic leukocytosis may favor brucellosis, anemia, and thrombocytopenia may suggest HLH. High ESR is expected in all three conditions:
1. Abdominal ultrasonography (USG)—may reveal liver and spleen echostructure that may offer clue to diagnosis
2. Chest X-ray—to look for tuberculosis focus
3. Results of these tests should decide further tests.

Laboratory Test Results
- *CBC*: Showed moderate neutrophilic leukocytosis with thrombocytosis and moderate anemia—normocytic normochromic with ESR 108 mm
- *Chest X-ray*: Normal
- *Abdominal USG*: Showed multiple small abscesses in liver and spleen.

Q3. What further tests would you order?

Ans. Multiple small abscesses may suggest brucellosis or abscesses may be mistaken for granulomas. So one must order serological tests for brucellosis; it is a noninvasive test and if the antibody test is positive, diagnosis can be reasonably confirmed. Computed tomography (CT) scan of abdomen is done to confirm abscesses in liver and spleen as granulomas may be mistaken for abscesses on USG.

Blood culture and pus culture from USG-guided drainage are performed to rule out common bacterial infections. As common bacterial infection is not likely and it is not easy to culture *Brucella* organism, this test may not help. PCR may be the most specific test for diagnosis of infections but often it is not available.

Laboratory Test Result
Brucella antibody test was positive though this antibody is known to cross-react with many other bacteria and so is not confirmative.

Final Diagnosis
Diagnosis of brucellosis was made on circumstantial evidence of prolonged fever resistant to commonly used antibiotics and presenting with multiple abscesses in liver and spleen. Child was treated with oral tetracycline and improved.

Q4. Why did this child not respond to multiple antibiotics?

Ans. Antibiotics of choice for brucellosis are tetracycline, rifampicin, and aminoglycosides. As *Brucella* bacteria multiply inside the cells, antibiotic needs to be continued for 4-6 weeks. Empirical antibiotic use is usually restricted to few days and in case of no response, antibiotic is changed. This explains why gentamycin did not work in this child.

Take Home Message

Prolonged fever may be due to infection or noninfective disorder. If it is due to infection, it may be chronic infection, partially treated infection, or infection-induced immunological or toxin-mediated disorder. Partially treated infection often localizes to kidneys, lungs, or brain and usually provides some clues. Partially treated typhoid fever may present without localization, but fever does not last for 3 months. Toxin produced by bacterial infection such as streptococci may prolong fever but not for 3 months. Noninfective cause must be ruled out in a child with fever for 3 months and include evolving systemic inflammatory disorder or malignancy, often hematological.

CASE 2

A 10-year-old child presented with fever for last 3 months. He was well prior to onset of present illness. It started with low-grade fever that has varied in intensity over time in spite of various drugs used including antibiotics. He has poor appetite and has lost some weight. Over the last one month, he seems to get tired with accustomed exertion and is reluctant to go out to play. There are no other symptoms. Physical examination showed mild fever in a child who looked chronically sick. His pulse rate was 120/min and respiratory rate 25/min. He had moderate hepatomegaly firm in consistency with span of 10 cm, mildly tender, spleen not palpable, engorged neck veins and absent hepatojugular reflux (HJR), no murmur or cardiomegaly, chest was clear, and other systems normal.

Q1. What is differential diagnosis?

Ans. This child has presented with subacute onset of slowly progressive disease with exertional tiredness, disproportionate tachycardia (heart rate faster than that expected with fever), and mildly tender hepatomegaly without jaundice. It suggests cardiac and liver involvement of long duration. Mild hepatic tenderness indicates either mild inflammation or congestion. Bacterial or amoebic liver abscess is unlikely as there would have been severe tenderness with fast progression. Chronic hepatitis should have presented with jaundice. However, mild jaundice may not be visible clinically and may be picked up by blood test. If not inflammation, then it may be congested liver and engorged neck veins and disproportionate tachycardia support such a possibility. However, it is not cardiac failure as there is no cardiomegaly and HJR is absent. Engorged neck veins without HJR suggest obstruction to superior vena cava and congested liver is due to obstructed inferior vena cava. So diagnosis is constrictive pericarditis. Fever of long duration is in favor of chronic infection, most likely to be tuberculosis. Restrictive cardiomegaly would be another possibility as it also presents with gradually progressive cardiac disease without cardiomegaly. So, differential diagnosis in this child stands to be constrictive pericarditis due to tuberculosis and restrictive cardiomyopathy must be ruled out.

Q2. What investigations would you consider?

Ans.
- *CBC*: May not be directly helpful except to pick up comorbid deficiency anemia
- *ESR*: Significantly high ESR may favor infection
- *Chest X-ray*: Expected to show normal size heart without signs of cardiac failure, to look for focus of tuberculosis
- *2D echocardiogram*: Expected to reveal diminished filling of cardiac chambers and may show thickened pericardium
- *CT chest*: May not add any more information
- *Mantoux test*: Positive test does not help to diagnose tuberculosis while negative test at the age of 10 years may be taken against diagnosis of tuberculosis
- *Gastric aspirate for AFB (acid-fast bacilli)*: It may be worth it though in absence of obvious lung lesion, test may be negative
- *Biopsy*: It is too invasive test and better avoided.

Laboratory Test Results
- CBC was within normal limits
- ESR was 85 mm/end of 1 hour
- 2D echocardiogram showed thickened pericardium
- Gastric aspirate did not show AFB.

Final Diagnosis
- Constrictive pericarditis due to TB
- Diagnosis is based on circumstantial evidence of prolonged fever due to subacute onset of chronic infection resulting in constrictive pericarditis

and tuberculosis being the most common cause of such presentation in local epidemiology.
- Child was treated with anti-TB treatment and improved.

Take Home Message

Diagnosis in a child presenting with prolonged fever evolves over time as physical signs appear as disease progresses. Periodic physical examination often offers a clue to diagnosis more than randomly ordered laboratory tests. Physical finding of enlarged liver demands observation for engorged neck veins, if any that may suggest not a primary liver disease but evidence of venous congestion or obstruction. Empirical antibiotic therapy should be avoided and minimum relevant laboratory tests must be ordered prior to antibiotic therapy. Partially treated bacterial infections pose a challenge to diagnosis and usually end up with increased morbidity. Noninfective diseases should always be kept in mind.

CASE 3

A 5-year-old child presented with fever off and on for last 3 months. He was well prior to present illness. It started as mild-to-moderate fever that increased over next few days to higher degree. Fever would spike 3–4 times a day at the interval of 6–8 hours and reduce in severity after antipyretic drugs. Fever pattern hardly changed over last 3 months though there were periods of low-grade fever interspersed with high fever. There were no other significant accompanying symptoms. Few antibiotics were tried in succession for a period varying from 4–7 days without any sustained improvement. Several tests were done that included CBC (repeated several times), blood and urine cultures (often done after antibiotic therapy), cerebrospinal fluid (CSF) examination and culture, serology for various infections, imaging studies, rheumatological tests, and bone marrow examination. Except persistent neutrophilic leukocytosis with thrombocytosis, there were no significant abnormalities in other test results. Considering systemic inflammatory disease, steroids were tried but stopped after few days as the child seemed to deteriorate. This child was referred for further evaluation. Physical examination at the end of 3 months revealed the following:
- Weight 14 kg (had lost 5 kg)
- Height 104 cm
- Temperature 100°F
- Pulse 140/min
- Respiration 25/min
- Blood pressure 90/55 mm
- Mild pallor
- No other significant findings on general examination
- Systemic examination was normal.

Q1. What is differential diagnosis?

Ans. This child is progressively deteriorating as evident by loss of 5 kg over last 3 months in a previously healthy child. Mild-to-moderate fever gradually increasing in severity over next few days may suggest initial bacteremia that settled in some organ resulting in higher degree of fever. However, organ in which it may have settled has not manifested with specific symptoms. This is what happens typically in a typhoid fever. However, it would have usually responded to several antibiotics, unless this bacterial strain was partially resistant. Thus, nonlocalizing partially treated bacterial infection is probable in this child. Other infections including tuberculosis, chronic viral, fungal, or parasitic infections are unlikely as they would have been localized by now. Fever of long duration may also be systemic onset of inflammatory disorder but would have by now developed joint involvement, skin rash, or organ affection. Common malignant disorders in children are hematological and by now would have manifested with symptoms such as pallor, or bleeding. Thus, this child is probably suffering from bacterial infection that is not properly treated. The only significant physical finding in this child is disproportionate tachycardia for age, degree of fever, and anemia while respiratory rate and blood pressure are within normal limits. This suggests cardiac involvement without any evidence of structural defect or it is an acquired disease and fever denotes inflammation, mostly infective as there are no other signs of systemic inflammatory disorder. As this is a chronic progressive infection, it favors diagnosis of subacute bacterial endocarditis.

Q2. What investigations would you consider?

Ans. Specific investigation would be echocardiogram for evidence of endocarditis and any structural defect.
- Chest X-ray for cardiomegaly and status of pulmonary circulation
- Electrocardiogram (ECG) for any rhythm disturbance
- Blood culture is done for etiological diagnosis. Multiple blood samples would enhance bacterial yield
- CBC is done for evidence of acute bacterial infection
- Abdominal USG is done to assess spread of infection in other organs such as liver, spleen, or kidneys even in absence of clinical findings.

Laboratory Test Results
- 2D echocardiogram showed vegetation on mitral valve. There was no structural defect in the heart
- Chest X-ray revealed mild cardiomegaly
- ECG was within normal limits
- Blood culture grew *Streptococcus viridans* sensitive to penicillin
- WBC 18,000/mm^3, P 72, L 26, M 2, E 0, Hb 10 g%, Pl 3.2 lakhs
- Abdominal USG normal.

Final Diagnosis
Subacute bacterial endocarditis without any valvular defect is diagnosed. Diagnosis is based on vegetation seen on echocardiogram and blood culture

showing growth of *S. viridans*. This type of infection is commonly seen in damaged valve while infection in normal valve presents more acutely. This child presented with subacute illness due to partial treatment with antibiotics. As antibiotics in such a case need to be continued for at least 4 weeks, early discontinuation or change of antibiotics must have caused acute illness behave like subacute disease.

The child was treated initially with intravenous penicillin and gentamycin but after blood culture report suggested sensitivity to penicillin, gentamycin was omitted. Therapy has to be continued for 4-6 weeks till vegetation disappear and so also reversal of all other laboratory and clinical parameters. Supportive treatment includes symptom relief and nutritional rehabilitation.

Take Home Message

Bacterial endocarditis is often subacute or chronic infection because heart valves have no dedicated blood supply and so when bacteria get attached to the valve to form vegetation, antibiotics do not reach the site of disease. It is also the reason why antibiotics need to be administered intravenously for 4-6 weeks to ensure control of infection. Thus this is one of the bacterial infections that may continue to manifest for many weeks, and hence referred to as subacute bacterial endocarditis. Thus, this is one example of chronic active bacterial infection.

CASE 4

An 8-year-old child presented with fever for last 3 months. He was apparently well prior to onset of present illness that started with an erratic fever pattern. At times, he would get severe rigors with high fever ending with sweating and normal temperature while at other times, fever would be continuous, low grade for several hours. He had no other significant accompanying symptoms. However over the last 3 months, he had poor appetite and had lost considerable amount of weight and became severely cachectic. Several tests were done without any clue to diagnosis though tests revealed severe anemia for which he received packed red blood cell transfusion and so also few courses of antibiotics and antimalarial drugs were tried without benefit.

On physical examination, the child looked wasted and chronically sick with severe pallor.

Weight 16 kg, height 120 cm, pulse rate 134/min, RR 36/min, no lymphadenopathy, bone and joints normal, no edema.

Abdomen distended, more in upper part, liver 5 cm below costal margin, firm, not tender, liver span 12 cm, spleen 8 cm firm, no ascites, soft systolic murmur over precordium and other systems were normal.

Q1. What is differential diagnosis?

Ans. This child has severe progressive disease as suggested by development of cachexia and had also resulted in severe anemia requiring transfusion.

It indicates a probable hematological disorder. Long-duration fever may favor diagnosis of malaria; however, it would have been easy to prove by simple tests and moreover this child did not respond to trial with antimalarial drugs. Severe anemia requiring transfusion at this age is not likely to be deficiency anemia. There has been no history of blood loss or evidence of hemolysis in the form of jaundice. Hence, anemia in this child must have resulted from bone marrow disorder. Bone marrow aplasia is ruled out as hepatosplenomegaly is not a feature and it would have presented with bleeding manifestations in the form of purpura or ecchymosis. Acute lymphatic leukemia is less likely as disease often manifests over short time and cachexia is not a feature. Chronic myeloid leukemia mostly presents without significant anemia. Bone marrow infiltration is often a slow progression and those with prolonged fever may be due to myelofibrosis or HLH; both are commonly secondary to infection that may go unnoticed. Another possibility is a chronic infection itself such as kala-azar (leishmaniasis). In fact cachexia due to disease, as often seen in malignant disorders in adults, is rare in children but untreated kala-azar does present in similar way.

Q2. What investigations would you consider?
Ans.
- CBC, peripheral smear, and ESR
- Reticulocyte count
- Bone marrow examination
- Depending upon bone marrow examination result, further tests need to be planned to rule out either HLH or kala-azar.

Laboratory Test Results
- Hb 4 g% microcytic hypochromic anemia
- WBC 16500, P 63, L 30, M 4, E 3, Platelet 0.35 lakh, ESR 120 mm
- Corrected reticulocyte count 3%
- Bone marrow examination showed *Leishmania donovani (LD)* bodies
- No further tests were carried out as diagnosis is confirmed. Serological tests are not dependable.

Final Diagnosis
Bone marrow showing LD bodies is the gold standard of diagnosis of kala-azar. He was treated with amphotericin B. Liposomal preparation is most preferred but costly. Antimony compounds are also used in the treatment of kala-azar such as sodium stibogluconate. Child recovered completely.

Take Home Message

Severe anemia as a significant feature often suggests hematological disease, either primary or secondary. Anemia with hepatosplenomegaly is a feature of either hemolytic anemia or bone marrow infiltration. A chronically sick and febrile child almost favors bone marrow infiltrative disorders. Diagnosis is confirmed only on bone marrow examination and at times marrow aspiration fails and marrow biopsy may be necessary. Similarly in case of strong clinical suspicion of bone marrow involvement, single bone marrow examination may not pick up the diagnosis and repeat examination may be necessary. This is because many diseases evolve over time to offer classical laboratory results.

SUGGESTED READING

1. Bennett JE, Dolin R, Blaser MJ. Mandell, Douglas, and Bennett's Principles and Practice of Infectious Diseases. Elsevier Inc., 2014. 3697 p.
2. Longo DL, Fauci AS, Kasper DL, Hauser SL, Jameson J, Loscalzo J (Eds). Harrison's Principles of Internal Medicine, 18th edn. New York, NY: McGraw-Hill; 2012.
3. Parthasarthy A. IAP Textbook of Pediatrics, 7th edn. India: Jaypee Brothers Medical Publishers; 2019.

CHAPTER
2

Approach to a Child Having Fever with Coma

Vipin M Vashishtha

ACUTE ENCEPHALITIS SYNDROME AND CENTRAL NERVOUS SYSTEM INFECTIONS

INTRODUCTION

Presentation of a child with fever and unconsciousness presents a diagnostic dilemma. Many infectious and noninfectious entities may lead to this presentation. The World Health Organization (WHO) has now decided to club all these diverse conditions under a new entity referred to as acute encephalitis syndrome (AES). Amongst the infectious entities, acute viral encephalitis constitutes the largest chunk. The etiological agents for acute viral encephalitis are varied and often clinically indistinguishable. The lack of availability and high cost of testing for specific viral agent in resource-limited countries and further to the limitations faced by the treating physicians. Several mimics of acute encephalitis are clubbed under AES head. Amongst them, acute encephalopathy has got varied etiologies and often erroneously labeled as acute viral encephalitis. A differentiation between acute encephalitis and acute encephalopathy is of paramount significance since not only therapeutic but preventive measures are also quite distinct. Apart from these two broad groups, several other entities such as cerebral malaria, acute disseminated encephalomyelitis (ADEM), tuberculous meningitis (TBM), metabolic encephalopathy, and diabetic coma. Three different case scenarios are presented in this chapter to emphasize a proper approach to arrive at a correct diagnosis.

CASE 1

A 4-year-old previously healthy girl, daughter of a poor, daily-wage worker, hailing from a nearby village presented with fever for last 2 days, sudden onset of vomiting for last 12 hours, and altered sensorium which rapidly progressed to deep coma within few hours since morning in the early winter month. There was no history of any exanthematous illness such as measles, varicella, and dengue; no history of recent vaccination; no upper respiratory infection (URI) symptoms; and no history of intake of aspirin and antiemetics prior to the onset of the disease. No history of developmental delay, consanguinity, and seizures. The attendants informed about the appearance of similar illness followed by sudden deaths in few other kids in the neighboring village.

On examination, the child was febrile (rectal temperature 100.5°F), nonicteric, pale with weak radial pulses, no organomegaly, and meningeal signs were also absent. The child was having decerebrate rigidity along with frothing at mouth. The pupils were also dilated and poorly reacting to light, and doll's eye sign was also absent. Rest other systemic examination was essentially normal.

Q1. What is the probable diagnosis?

Ans. Probably, we are dealing with a case of AES. Since investigations are in process, we can think of few common causes of AES such as acute viral encephalitis, meningitis (both viral and bacterial meningitis), and cerebral malaria. Since the duration of illness is very short and rapidly progressing, we can rule out certain conditions such as enteric (typhoid) encephalopathy and TBM.

Q2. What do we mean by AES?

Ans. The AES is a very broad group that includes several infectious and noninfectious entities. However, the term AES is a misnomer. How can a very specific entity, i.e. "encephalitis," strictly a pathological diagnosis, be termed as a "syndrome," a constellation of different signs and symptoms having different pathophysiology and different sites of lesion?

Acute encephalitis syndrome is a term used by WHO for the surveillance of acute neurological disease with a focus on Japanese encephalitis (JE). The main aim is to widen the net and not to miss any case of acute viral encephalitis, particularly the JE. So the term AES includes not only viral encephalitis, but also all etiologies of fever and altered sensorium. A better term would have been "acute febrile encephalopathy" to describe these illnesses such as cerebral malaria, acute bacterial meningitis (ABM), ADEM, and TBM (Box 1).

Box 1: Different definitions used in describing a case of fever with altered sensorium.

Encephalopathy: A clinical syndrome of altered mental status, manifesting as reduced consciousness or altered behavior. The exact site of pathology may be outside the brain.

Febrile encephalopathy: When encephalopathy occurs in temporal association of fever.

Encephalitis: It means inflammation of the brain. Encephalitis is strictly a pathological diagnosis, but surrogate clinical/imaging markers may provide evidence of inflammation.

Acute encephalitis syndrome: Clinically, a case of AES is defined as a person of any age, at any time of year with the acute onset of fever and a change in mental status (including symptoms such as confusion, disorientation, coma, or inability to talk) and/or new onset of seizures (excluding simple febrile seizures).

Q3. How can one differentiate viral encephalitis from viral meningitis?

Ans. Unfortunately, the clinical syndromes and results of routine laboratory tests are typically nonspecific and often do not help distinguish encephalitis and viral meningitis. Patients may have symptoms of both parenchymal and meningeal processes, i.e. a patient with stiff neck and photophobia, classic signs of meningitis, could in fact also have encephalitis (called meningoencephalitis) (Tables 1 and 2). It is important to recognize other infectious and noninfectious causes, particularly those which are treatable.

Investigations: Coming back to the original case, her investigation reports are as follows: Serum glucose—16 mg%, peripheral smear (P/S) negative for malarial parasites (MP), complete blood count (CBC)—total leukocyte count (TLC) 3,400, differential leukocyte count (DLC)—P 64, L 32, M 4, platelet count—1.8 lac/cumm, electrolytes—normal range, urinalysis—normal, cerebrospinal fluid (CSF) examination—opening pressure normal, protein—18 mg%, sugar—6 mg%, total cells—4 (all mononuclear), liver function tests (LFTs)—serum bilirubin—1.2 mg% (direct 0.8 mg%), serum alanine transaminase (ALT)—3460 IU/L, serum aspartate transaminase (AST)—3220 IU/L, prothrombin time (PT)—56 (control: 16 sec), partial thromboplastin time (PTT)—98 (control: 46 sec), negative malaria serology, and blood and urine cultures were negative.

TABLE 1: Localization of a CNS lesion.

Clinical syndrome*	Part of CNS affected
Encephalitis	Brain parenchyma
Aseptic meningitis	Meninges
Myelitis	Spinal cord
Neuritis	Peripheral nerves

*A single infection can affect multiple locations of the CNS, making clinical diagnosis difficult (i.e. meningomyeloencephalitis)
(CNS: central nervous system)

TABLE 2: Differentiating features between encephalitis and viral (aseptic) meningitis.

Features	Encephalitis	Viral meningitis
Constitutional symptoms		
Fever	Yes	Yes
Headache, nausea, vomiting, and lethargy	Yes	Yes
Photophobia and neck stiffness	No	Yes
Neurologic dysfunction		
Seizures	Yes	Minimal
Cranial nerve palsies and paralysis	Yes	No
Altered mental status (i.e. confusion and coma)	Yes	Minimal

Q4. What is the diagnosis now?

Ans. Reye or Reye-like encephalopathy syndrome. Normal CSF and negative sepsis screen have rule out conditions such as ABM and sepsis-associated encephalopathy. Absence of malaria parasite in P/S and negative rapid-antigen detecting tests and markedly raised liver enzymes point a diagnosis away from cerebral malaria.

Q5. Why not acute viral encephalitis?

Ans. Clinical features pointing against the diagnosis of acute viral encephalitis which are as follows:
- Normal CSF examination (absence of pleocytosis)
- Markedly deranged liver enzymes
- Rapid progression to deep coma
- No focal neurological signs
- Presence of mild fever.

Q6. What are the other tests needed to rule out acute viral encephalitis?

Ans. Serological investigations and central nervous system (CNS) imaging are the other two broad groups of investigations needed to pinpoint the exact etiology. Serology, mainly enzyme-linked immunosorbent assay (ELISA) and polymerase chain reaction (PCR) [for JE, dengue, and other arboviruses, herpes simplex virus (HSV), Echo, and other enteroviruses, etc.], may be positive during acute phase. In magnetic resonance (MR) scan, brain may show typical changes associated with JE, HSV-encephalitis, etc.

In the above case, the results of further investigations are as follows:
- *Magnetic resonance scan*: Normal
- *Serology (ELISA and PCR)*: Negative
- *Plasma ammonia*: 88 μg/dL (borderline raised)
- *Arterial blood gas (ABG) and lactate levels*: Normal
- *Urinalysis*: Normal (including reducing sugars)
- *Serum salicylates level*: 1.52 mg/dL; (therapeutic range 20–120 mg/dL).
- *Viral isolation*: No organism detected.

Further investigations did not lead to a particular diagnosis, but we could now rule out certain conditions. Acute viral encephalitis is virtually ruled out since MR scan, serology, and virus isolation were negative. So, we are now left with the diagnosis of Reye-like syndrome which is characterized by acute encephalopathy and hypoglycemia associated with fatty degeneration of liver due to intracellular deposition of fats. Certain metabolic syndromes and inborn errors of metabolism (IEMs) such as organic acidemias (presence of hyperammonemia with marked acidosis), medium-chain Acyl CoA (coenzyme A) dehydrogenase deficiency, and other defects of fatty acid oxidation, can also present with the features of Reye syndrome. Classic idiopathic Reye syndrome, though a rarity, is usually follows administration of salicylates in individuals with viral prodromes such as varicella and influenza.

Course and prognosis
The child was treated in an intensive care unit (ICU) setup. Later she developed seizures, hyperpyrexia, hematemesis, and Cheyne–Stokes respiration during the course of treatment, and ultimately, she died after 72 hours of admission.

Q7. How to confirm the exact diagnosis?

Ans. To confirm the final diagnosis, the next step would be to do biopsy for histopathological examination of viscera, mainly liver and brain, or autopsy (after the child had died). In the above case, postmortem needle biopsies of liver and brain were performed. The hepatic histopathology revealed marked hydropic changes with centrilobular necrosis suggestive of massive liver necrosis following acute toxic injury (Figs. 1 and 2). There was macrovesicular fatty changes in the hepatocytes, quite different from the classical "microvesicular" fat deposition as seen in Reye syndrome (Fig. 3). Brain histo pathology revealed mild spongiosis with focal gliosis, but no inflammation and no viral inclusion bodies (Fig. 4). So, the histopathology findings disproved classical "Reye syndrome" and the characteristic hepatic changes pointed toward some toxin-mediated massive liver injury. In the background of rural origin, poor dwelling and a young age favor some environmental poisonings presumably congested orally. Hence, the final diagnosis in the above case was "acute toxin-mediated hepatic encephalopathy." Since the brain tissue did not show any evidence of inflammation and/or viral inclusion bodies, the brain involvement was secondary to liver pathology.

Q8. How to pinpoint the exact toxin?

Ans. This process would be quite tedious and may involve several other experts having experience in undertaking environmental and epidemiological studies. Since there was history of similar illness with deaths in few other children of surrounding village, a common source of the environmental toxin cannot be ruled out. Apart from epidemiological studies along with detailed inspection of the households of deceased children, some forms of toxicological studies such as high performance liquid chromatography (HPLC) and gas chromatography would also be needed to identify the putative toxin.

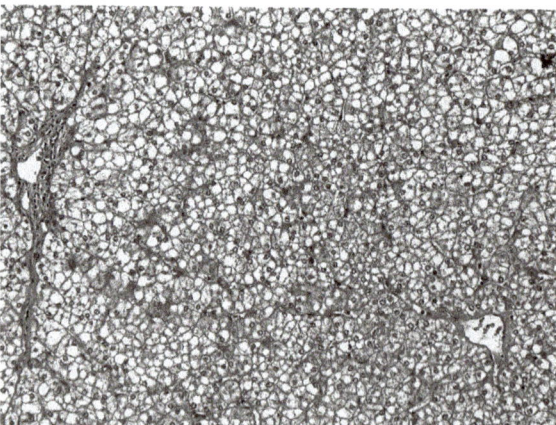

Fig. 1: *Liver histopathology*: Marked hydropic changes with centrilobular necrosis.

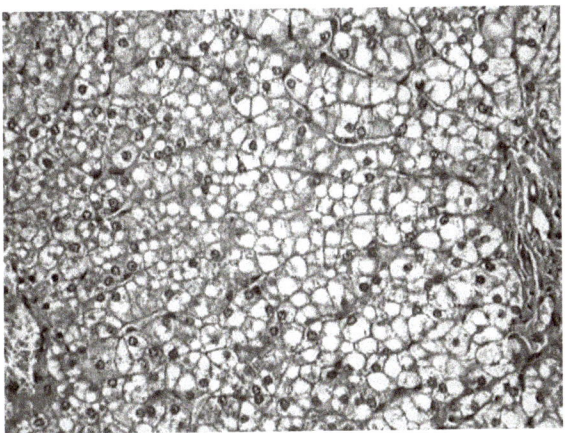
Fig. 2: *Liver histopathology*: Ballooning of hepatocytes (foamy cells).

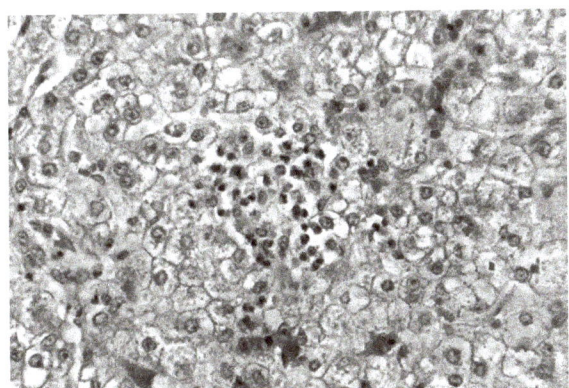
Fig. 3: *Liver histopathology*: Classical "microvesicular" fat deposition in Reye syndrome.

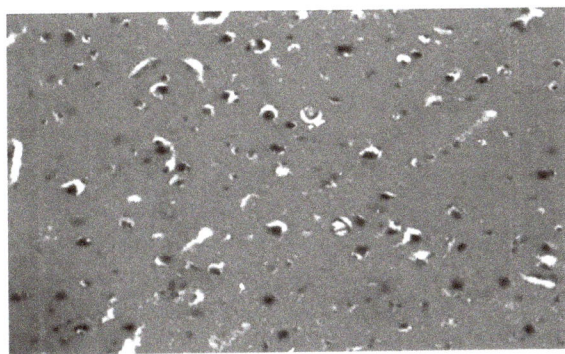
Fig. 4: *Brain histopathology*: Mild spongiosis with focal gliosis, no viral inclusion body and no inflammation of brain parenchyma.

Toxin-induced encephalopathy: Most of the toxin-induced encephalopathies have an abrupt onset with rapid progression to deep coma. Some of them present with features of acute Reye-like encephalopathy. Any clustering of cases should raise the possibility of a common environmental toxin. There can be many such agents that can cause this presentation such as drugs, herbal products, pesticides, insecticides, aflatoxins, amatoxins of Amanita phalloides, pyrrolizidine alkaloids and plants producing them, and weedy plants and their fruits.

CASE 2

A 7-year-old female child from rural West Bengal presented with moderate-to-high grade fever for 2 days, generalized seizures, and excessive somnolence leading to altered sensorium for last 1 day during the monsoon season.

There was nothing contributory in the history. No concurrent cases in neighborhood (that may have indicated JE), no history of exanthematous illness (may have indicated varicella, measles, dengue, and *Mycoplasma* as an etiology), no history of aspirin/drug intake (Reye syndrome), no history of animal bites (rabies), and there was no history of upper respiratory tract infection or recent vaccination (ADEM). An antecedent or concurrent respiratory illness may be present in *Mycoplasma* encephalitis. Unrecognized trauma or intracranial bleed due to coagulopathy may present similarly but with no history of fever.

Q1. What are we dealing with?

Ans. Acute febrile encephalopathy, probably an infectious type. Acute meningoencephalitis should be kept at the top of the diagnostic possibilities. Acute bacterial meningitis (ABM), cerebral malaria, acute disseminated encephalomyelitis (ADEM), and other rare acute febrile encephalopathies such as Reye syndrome, metabolic encephalopathy, and epileptic encephalopathy are other entities that should be kept in differential diagnosis.

Q2. Which particular acute meningoencephalitis should be considered first?

Ans. Japanese encephalitis is a strong possibility in view of the epidemiologic information (rural area, West Bengal, monsoon season). HSV is the most common cause of sporadic viral encephalitis in older children and adults. Studies show that it is fairly uncommon in children but is nevertheless important as it is the only treatable cause of viral encephalitis. Recent data suggests that *Mycoplasma* can cause up to 15% of childhood encephalitis and is often due to immune-mediated mechanism. For ADEM, acute neurologic abnormalities and imaging evidence of demyelination are required for the diagnosis. ADEM follows vaccination or infections including rubeola, rubella, varicella, mumps, herpes zoster, Epstein–Barr virus (EBV),

Mycoplasma, or other URI viruses. Seizures, altered sensorium, coma, bilateral optic neuritis, myelopathy, and other lateralizing focal signs such as hemiparesis should be there. Dengue is a recognized cause of childhood encephalitis/encephalopathy in endemic areas, especially during dengue epidemics. Systemic manifestations of dengue and severe dengue such as dengue hemorrhagic fever (DHF) or dengue shock syndrome (DSS) are often absent. Epileptic encephalopathy is due to nonconvulsive status epilepticus that may not be clinically apparent and hence may be missed unless an electroencephalogram (EEG) is done. Typhoid encephalopathy is unlikely in this case as it usually occurs in the second week of untreated typhoid fever. So is TBM. Unrecognized trauma or intracranial bleed due to coagulopathy may present, similarly, but there should not be a history of fever.

Physical Findings and Investigations
On physical examination, there was no pallor, no icterus, no skin rash, and no organomegaly. Respiratory system examination was also normal. There was left-sided hemiparesis, but both neck rigidity and Kernig's sign were absent. No frank seizures were present.

On investigations, the hemoglobin (Hb)—11.0, TLC—7,000, P 50, L 40, M5, E5, platelet count—2 lac/cumm; MP—negative, Malaria antigen—negative; serum glutamate-pyruvate transaminase (SGPT)—34 IU, and blood sugar—76 mg%. Chest X-ray (CXR) was normal. CSF examination showed 70 white blood cells with 90% lymphocytes and 10 red blood cells, sugar—64 mg%, protein—100 mg%, and no organism was seen on Gram staining.

Q3. What is the likely diagnosis now in this case?
Ans. After investigations, our initial impression of acute meningoencephalitis is almost confirmed. Since, there was no meningeal irritation sign, the correct entity would be acute encephalitis. Among this group, we need to consider both JE and HSV along with ADEM. It would not be possible to clinically distinguish between JE and HSV in this case. JE is more likely given the epidemiology. For ADEM, an MR scan would be needed. Since, CSF sugar level is normal, both ABM and TBM are excluded.

Cerebral malaria is unlikely as both peripheral smear and malaria antigen were negative. Further, there was no pallor nor any organomegaly, and asymmetrical neurologic signs were present which go against the diagnosis of malaria. Absence of any respiratory prodrome or signs is a pointer against *Mycoplasma*, but does not rule out *Mycoplasma*.

Q4. What are the common viral agents causing acute encephalitis in India?
Ans. There is a long list of viruses responsible for acute encephalitis in India. The list of common and not-so-common viruses is given in Box 2. This list includes both the viruses responsible for epidemics and sporadic cases of AES.

Box 2: Different viral agents responsible for acute viral encephalitis in India (epidemic and sporadic).

Common Causes	Uncommon Causes
• Japanese encephalitis	• Chandipura virus
• Herpes simplex virus 1 encephalitis (HSV-1)	• Chikungunya virus
• Enterovirus encephalitis (mainly EV 71)	• Epstein–Barr virus
• Mumps virus	• Human immunodeficiency virus (HIV)
• Measles virus	• Nipah (Handra)
• Varicella-zoster virus (VZV)	• Kyasanur Forest disease
• Dengue virus (encephalopathy)	• Human herpesvirus 6 (HHV-6)
• Rabies virus	• West Nile virus

Q5. How can one pinpoint the exact cause of viral encephalitis?

Ans. Most of the time, it is not possible to make an etiological diagnosis of acute viral encephalitis. But following tests would facilitate the process:

Neuroimaging: Though CT scan can provide some useful information such as presence of cerebral hemorrhage, brain edema, temporal lobe hypodensities (HSV encephalitis), thalamic abnormalities (JE), and basal exudates and hydrocephalus (TBM). Magnetic resonance imaging (MRI) is the investigation of choice as far as neuroimaging in encephalopathy cases is concerned, since it provides more useful information regarding the etiology and alternative diagnoses than CT. Suggestive MRI findings are present in some etiologies of viral encephalitis such as HSV encephalitis, JE, and enterovirus encephalitis (Table 3). MRI may show nonspecific features of viral encephalitis such as cortical hyperintensities and cerebral edema. MRI is also useful for diagnosing alternative etiologies such as ADEM and antibody-associated encephalopathies.

TABLE 3: MRI changes in some types of acute viral encephalitis.

Etiology of acute viral encephalitis	MRI findings
Japanese B encephalitis	Abnormal signal intensity in thalami, substantia nigra, and basal ganglia
HSV encephalitis	Abnormal signal intensity in medial temporal lobe, cingulate gyrus, and orbital surface of frontal lobes
Acute disseminated encephalomyelitis (ADEM)	Multifocal abnormalities in subcortical white matter; involvement of thalami, basal ganglia, and brainstem
Enterovirus 71 (EV 71)	Abnormal signal intensity in the dorsal pons, medulla, midbrain, and dentate nuclei of the cerebellum
Nipah virus	Focal subcortical and deep white matter and gray matter lesions; small hyperintense lesions in the white matter, cortex, pons, and cerebral peduncles
West Nile virus	Abnormalities in deep gray matter and brainstem; white matter lesions mimicking demyelination may also be seen
Varicella	Multifocal abnormalities in cortex, associated cerebellitis, vasculitis, and vasculopathy

(MRI: magnetic resonance imaging)

Polymerase chain reaction (PCR) and other serologic tests: Detection of specific virus by PCR or virus-specific immunoglobulin M (IgM) antibody in the CSF may be very helpful in arriving at a correct etiological diagnosis. CSF PCR is highly sensitive and specific for certain viruses such as HSV, enteroviral, mumps, varicella, and Chandipura virus encephalitis whereas specific IgM antibodies in CSF or/and serum detected by ELISA (IgM-captured ELISA) are useful for the diagnosis of JE, dengue, measles, Nipah virus, etc. specifically for JE virus. However, the duration of CSF positivity of virus should be checked for individual viruses. It may be very brief for some viruses such as enteroviruses. Earlier, the facility for these tests was available in only some premiere government institutions, but now there are some tests also commercially available in private sector, which test for a panel of viruses (HSV 1 and 2, VZV, HHV-6, measles, mumps, rubella, Chandipura, chikungunya, Nipah, rabies, enteroviruses, Japanese B, dengue, West Nile virus, etc.) in CSF samples, using DNA (deoxyribonucleic acid) hybridization technique.

Q6. Does EEG help in making etiological diagnosis in a case of acute viral encephalitis?

Ans. Electroencephalogram is not routinely needed as it usually shows nonspecific slowing in viral encephalitis. The presence of periodic lateralized epileptiform discharges may indicate underlying herpes simplex encephalitis, but their absence does not rule out the diagnosis.

Case Progression
A contrast MR scan was performed which showed hyperintense lesion in the right temporal lobe (Fig. 5). There was no involvement of thalami and basal ganglia, the characteristic features of JE. In view of the asymmetric signs and MRI findings, HSV seems the most likely diagnosis. However, in the absence of CSF HSV PCR, one cannot make a definitive diagnosis. Though JE was more likely given the epidemiologic setting, the MRI findings were not consistent with it. The MRI was also not suggestive of ADEM. With the CSF and MRI findings and absence of MP cerebral malaria also was virtually ruled out. However for confirmation, a CSF PCR would be needed which is highly sensitive and specific for HSV.

Magnetic resonance findings in HSV encephalitis: Magnetic resonance abnormalities are found in 90% of patients with HSV encephalitis. MRI may be normal early in the course of illness. Temporal lobe involvement, sometimes hemorrhagic, and early involvement of white matter are typical. The inferomedial portion of the temporal lobe is most commonly affected on MRI, sometimes in association with abnormalities of the cingulate gyrus.

Polymerase chain reaction for HSV encephalitis: Polymerase chain reaction for HSV is highly sensitive (94–98%) and specific (98–100%). Results become positive within 24 hours of the onset of symptoms and remain positive for at least 5–7 days after the start of antiviral therapy. False-negative findings may occur early in the course of the disease when viral DNA levels are low (within 72 hours of the onset of symptoms) or when blood is present in the CSF, because Hb may interfere with PCR.

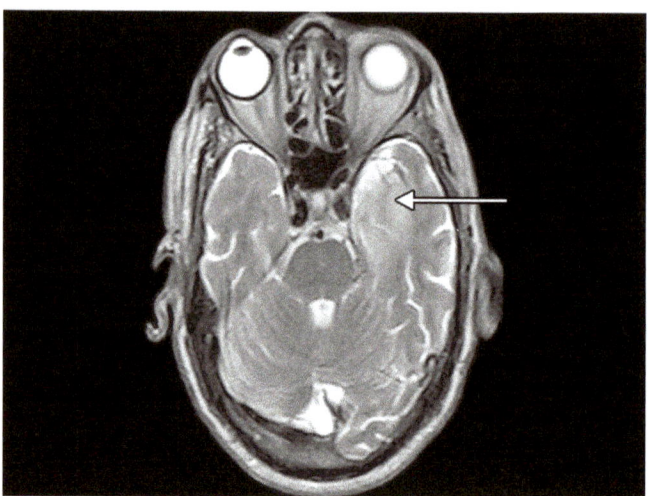

Fig. 5: A contrast magnetic resonance scan of Case 2 showing hyperintense lesion of right temporal lobe, a characteristic feature of herpes simplex virus encephalitis.

CASE 3

An 11-month-old male child born of nonconsanguinity presented with fever, cough and cold, vomiting, and few loose stools along with generalized uncontrolled seizures for last 24 hours. The child was also having fast breathing, and rapidly progressed to deep coma from irritability with few hours.

The child had almost similar incident at the age of 4 months in the past for which he was treated by his family physician. He has normal developmental milestones and there was nothing contributory in perinatal history. However, there was history of poor feeding and death of his elder sibling in early infancy.

Q1. What are the diagnostic possibilities?

Ans. Acute onset CNS infections such as ABM and acute viral encephalitis are the most probable diagnosis. Other conditions that merit consideration are "sepsis-associated encephalopathy," febrile convulsions with status, and few noninfectious acute febrile encephalopathies.

Physical findings and investigations: On examination, the child was febrile and comatose, and was having mild dehydration with tachypnea, enlarged liver, and generalized tonic-clonic seizures.

On investigations, serum glucose—22 mg%, peripheral smear showed TLC—2,400/cumm, DLC—P 24%, L 76%, platelet count—80,000/cumm, P/s for MP—negative, and serum electrolytes were Na = 141, K = 4.2, and Ca = 8.0 mg%. CSF examination had opening pressure high with protein—18 mg%, sugar—12 mg%, and total count—nil. His LFTs were serum bilirubin—1.6, serum ALT—450 IU/L, serum AST—396 IU/L, PT—24 seconds (control: 16 sec), and PTT—56 seconds (control: 46 sec). Other investigations were CRP—negative, CXR—normal, and bacterial cultures (for both blood and urine)—negative.

Q2. What are the possibilities now?

Ans. In the above case, we are having marked hypoglycemia, leukopenia/neutropenia with mild thrombocytopenia, normal CSF with low sugar, and mildly elevated liver enzymes. Bacterial sepsis and ABM are excluded since both cultures and CSF examination are normal. We can now think of some metabolic syndromes (IEMs), Reye-like syndrome, or febrile seizures-associated status. Though CSF examination was normal, still possibility of acute viral encephalitis should be kept in the differential diagnosis.

Q3. How to proceed further?

Ans. To differentiate further, we need some more investigations. An ABG was done which showed the following values: pH = 6.8, $PaCO_2$ = 14 mm Hg, PaO_2 = 159 mm Hg, Na = 141, K = 4.2, Cl = 111, and HCO_3 = 3.5 with an anion gap of 26.5. Plasma ammonia was 198 µg/dL, serum lactate level was high, and urinalysis showed ketonuria.

Q4. Likely diagnosis, now?

Ans. The above reports reflect marked metabolic acidosis with hyperammonemia. This presentation of a brief prodromal illness that rapidly leads to encephalopathy along with marked metabolic acidosis and hyperammonemia points toward a metabolic syndrome/IEM. This is to be noted that around 20% of infants presenting with a "sepsis"-like picture in the absence of risk factors (such as prematurity and chorioamnionitis) have an IEM.

Q5. Which type of IEM?

Ans. Since both hyperammonemia and marked acidosis with high "anion gap" are present, organic acidemias [also referred as organic acidurias (OAD)] is a strong possibility.

Q6. What are the organic acidemias (organic acidurias)?

Ans. Organic acidemia, also called organic aciduria, is a term used to describe a group of IEMs which disrupt normal amino acid metabolism that leads to a build-up of acids which are usually not present.

Organic acidurias are fairly common IEM in India and usually present with hypoglycemia, ketonuria, metabolic acidosis with high "anion gap," and raised ammonia level. These changes are associated with vomiting, seizures, lethargy, coma, hypotonia, hepatomegaly, respiratory distress, failure to thrive (FTT), developmental delay, and mental retardation. A subcategory of OAD termed as "cerebral OAD" presents with predominant CNS manifestations. There are several different types of OAD, few common and important, others rarer and less important.

Q7. How to proceed further to confirm the exact type of IEM?

Ans. Confirmatory diagnosis of OAD requires sophisticated investigations. They include the following tests:

Tandem mass spectrometry: Plasma amino acids and acyl carnitine profile by tandem mass spectrometry (TMS) for diagnosis of organic acidemias/acidurias, urea cycle defects, aminoacidopathies, and fatty acid oxidation defects.

Gas chromatography mass spectrometry: Gas chromatography mass spectrometry (GCMS) of urine for diagnosis of organic acidemias/acidurias.

High performance liquid chromatography: High performance liquid chromatography (HPLC) for quantitative analysis of amino acids in blood and urine; required for diagnosis of organic acidemias and aminoacidopathies.

Enzyme assays: Measuring of specific enzyme activity in leukocytes or cultured fibroblast will reveal the exact defect. This is required for definitive diagnosis, but not available for most IEMs.

Available enzyme assays include the following:
- Biotinidase assay—in cases with suspected biotinidase deficiency (intractable seizures, seborrheic rash, and alopecia)
- GALT (galactose 1-phosphate uridyl transferase) assay for cases with suspected galactosemia (hypoglycemia, cataracts, and reducing sugars in urine).

Analysis of organic acids in urine is of paramount importance for the diagnosis of OADs. It is important to conduct these investigations while the patient is ill, not after treatment. Many abnormalities will disappear when the child improves and may make the diagnosis difficult. It may take several days for results.

Final diagnosis: Tandem mass spectrometry was conducted which confirmed the diagnosis of methylmalonic aciduria.

Q8. When should one suspect metabolic syndrome/IEM in a case of acute encephalopathy?

Ans. Most of the IEMs are commonly present during the neonatal period and early infancy, but they may also present later during early childhood. Infections and stress may trigger an acute episode. These disorders may present with vomiting, seizures, acidosis, hypoglycemia, hyperammonemia, acute onset encephalopathy, and hepatic derangement. Box 3 provides a list of features that points toward the possibility of IEM in an encephalopathy case. Few IEMs are indistinguishable from "Reye syndrome" on clinical examination such as medium-chain Acyl CoA dehydrogenase deficiency and other defects of fatty acid oxidation (Box 4).

Box 3: Features pointing possibility of metabolic syndrome or inborn errors of metabolism (IEM).

Features Pointing Toward Metabolic Syndromes	
• Persistent vomiting	• Hypotonia
• Failure to thrive	• A peculiar odor of urine
• History of fasting before developing encephalopathy	• Hepatomegaly
	• Cardiac dysfunction
• Developmental delay	• Consanguinity
• Metabolic acidosis (lactic or organic)	• Past history of similar disease in other siblings
• Hyperammonemia	

Box 4: A list of common metabolic syndrome or inborn errors of metabolism.

Common IEMs Presenting with Acute Encephalopathy
• Organic acidemias and aminoacidurias
• Urea cycle defects
• Congenital lactic acidosis
• Fatty acid oxidation defects

Q9. How do you manage a case of IEM?

Ans. Since most of the commonly occurring OADs are treatable entities, correct diagnosis becomes important. Every effort should be taken to arrive at a correct diagnosis. Sometimes, it is not possible to salvage the child owing to extreme critical condition, but even in this scenario, identification of OAD is vital for offering genetic counseling to the parents and offering the prenatal diagnosis possible in a future gestation.

Dietary modification is effective in some of the OADs. Amino acid-based formulas provide energy, nitrogen, vitamins, and minerals which can promote anabolism and growth. Goal of nutritional therapy is to provide all essential nutrients to promote physical and mental development. Synthetic amino acid-based formulas should provide approximately 50% of daily protein requirement. At the same time, the offending dietary precursor amino acid has to be restricted. Fasting also has to be avoided.

Take Home Messages
- Acute febrile encephalopathy (AFE) is a vast diverse group of disorder.
- Viral encephalitis is not the only possible diagnosis in a young, febrile child with coma.
- Presence of fever not always indicate an infectious etiology.

- Many diverse, altogether different, disorders can mimic AVE.
- Non-infectious AFE can also present in epidemic form.
- A brief knowledge and high index of suspicion can help in arriving at proper diagnosis.
- Hypoglycemia, markedly raised liver enzymes, and acidosis point toward a diagnosis other than infectious AFE.
- Every attempt should be made to confirm the etiological diagnosis of acute viral encephalitis.
- Detection of specific virus by PCR or virus-specific IgM antibody in the CSF may be very helpful in arriving at a correct etiological diagnosis.
- Histopathological examination of viscera may at times mandatory to clinch a correct diagnosis.
- Acute presentation with a brief prodromal illness that rapidly leads to encephalopathy along with marked metabolic acidosis and hyperammonemia points toward a metabolic syndrome/Inborn error of metabolism (IEM).
- Dietary modification is effective in some of these IEMs.

SUGGESTED READING

1. Karmarkar SA, Aneja S, Khare S, et al. A study of acute febrile encephalopathy with special reference to viral etiology. Indian J Pediatr. 2008;75(5):801-5.
2. Sankhyan N, Vykunta Raju KN, et al. Management of raised intracranial pressure. Indian J Pediatr. 2010;77(12):1409-16.
3. Sharma S, Mishra D, Aneja S, et al. Expert Group on Encephalitis, Indian Academy of Pediatrics. Consensus guidelines on evaluation and management of suspected acute viral encephalitis in children in India. Indian Pediatr. 2012;49(11):897-910.
4. Vaidyanathan K, Narayanan MP, Vasudevan DM. Organic acidurias: an updated review. Indian J Clin Biochem. 2011;26(4):319-25.
5. Vashishtha VM, John TJ, Kumar A. Clinical and pathological features of acute toxicity due to Cassia occidentalis in vertebrates. Indian J Med Res. 2009;130(1):23-30.

GENERAL MANAGEMENT OF A CHILD WITH COMA

INTRODUCTION

A child with coma or with acute encephalitis syndrome (AES) is a medical and neurological emergency, requiring immediate efforts to stabilize, evaluate (clinically and diagnostic) and start empirical treatment proceed almost simultaneously. The mainstay of management of a child with coma is stabilization and maintenance of "ABC", i.e. airway, breathing, and circulation. The mainstay of the management of a comatose child is to maintain adequate intracranial pressure (ICP) which depends on adequate cerebral perfusion pressure (CPP) so that cerebral ischemia is avoided. Hence, judicious management of raised ICP is the cornerstone of the successful management of any comatose child, more so of a febrile encephalopathic case. Emergency management of raised ICP at the time of presentation is potentially life saving in all encephalopathies. Further, definitive treatment is as per the confirmed etiology. A stepwise approach to the management of a comatose child is presented here.

Q1. What are the key investigations needed in the management of an acute febrile encephalopathy (AFE) case?

Ans. We can divide the investigations into three different categories:

Step I: Basic investigations
- Serum glucose
- Complete blood count (CBC), p/s for malaria parasite (MP)
- Electrolytes—Serum Na, K, calcium, and chloride
- Cerebrospinal fluid (CSF) examination including culture and latex particle agglutination
- Urinalysis—routine
- Liver function tests
- Renal function tests
- Cultures of blood, urine, and CSF

Step II: Investigations
- Arterial blood gas (ABG) with anion gap
- Plasma ammonia and serum lactate
- Urine for reducing substances
- Serological studies [both enzyme-linked immunosorbent assay (ELISA) and polymerase chain reaction (PCR)]—serum, CSF, and other body fluids as per presentation
- *Neuroimaging*: CT/MR scan (contrast enhanced) (Figs. 6A to C)
- Electroencephalogram (EEG)

Step III: Investigations
- Metabolic screening tests and urinalysis—ketone bodies, aminoacidurias, and other specific tests to rule out inborn errors of metabolism (IEM) (depending on earlier results)

- Viral inoculation studies (available at higher institutes)
- Tissue biopsy and autopsy—liver, kidney, brain, and muscle.

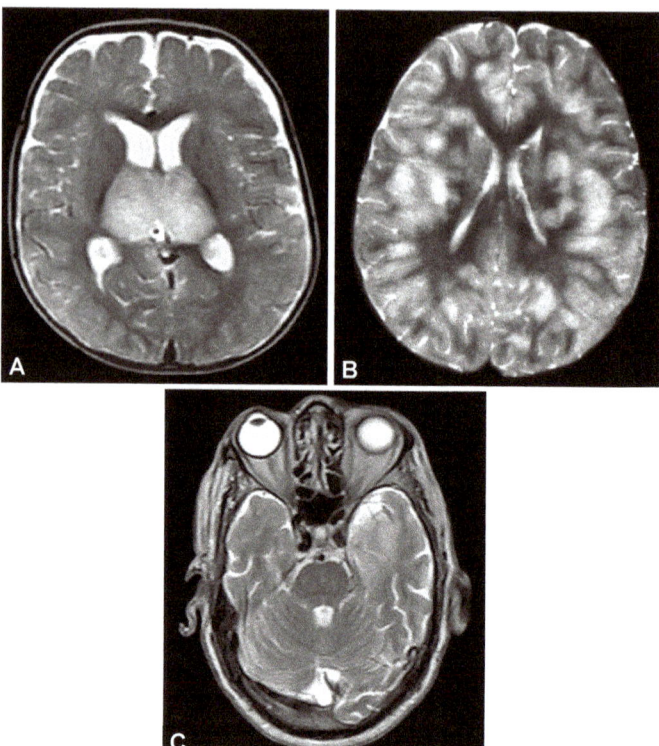

Figs. 6A to C: Classical MR findings in a case of (A) Japanese encephalitis (JE); (B) acute disseminated encephalomyelitis (ADEM); and (C) herpes simplex virus (HSV) encephalitis. (A) MRI (T2-weighted images) in JE shows high signal intensity lesions in thalamus, basal ganglia, cerebellum, pons (brainstem), midbrain, and occasionally spinal cord. (B) In ADEM, lesions are multifocal, bilateral, asymmetric demyelinating of the subcortical white matter, basal ganglia, and brainstem. Periventricular area is less affected (30–60% cases). (C) A contrast MR scan showing hyperintense lesion of right temporal lobe, a characteristic feature of HSV encephalitis.

Q2. How would you treat a child with acute febrile encephalopathy?

Ans. The mainstay of management of a child with AFE is stabilization and maintenance of "ABC".

General Management

- *Airway*: Clear airway and gentle suctioning.
- *Breathing*: Intubate and perform intermittent positive pressure ventilation (IPPV), if anyone of the following conditions is present:
  - Apnea or gasping respiration
  - Signs of herniation (i.e. bradycardia, hypertension, and irregular breathing, the Cushing's triad)

- Deep coma [Glasgow Coma Scale (GCS) <8]
   - SpO_2 < 92% despite high flow O_2
   - Refractory shock.
- *Circulation*: Measure mean arterial pressure (MAP) and maintain it as high as possible acutely!
   - Fluid bolus 20 mL/kg of normal saline (NS) and use inotropes, if needed.
- *Blood glucose*: Should be maintained at around 80–120 mg/dL [Hyperglycemia is associated with poor neurological outcome and increased mortality. Hypoglycemia causes disturbances of cerebral blood flow (CBF), increasing the regional CBF by as much as 300% in severe hypoglycemia].
- *Seizures control*: Intravenous (IV) midazolam = 0.2 mg/kg bolus (or IV lorazepam 0.1 mg/kg) followed by a loading dose of phenytoin 20 mg/kg slow IV. Supportive care is very important.
- Control of seizures is often difficult and serial administration of phenytoin, phenobarbitone, and midazolam infusion may be required; midazolam slow IV infusion at 1 μg/kg/min.
- *Temperature*: Treat fever and hypothermia.
- *Identify signs of cerebral herniation or raised ICP*: May need intubation and short-term hyperventilation [Partial pressure of carbon dioxide ($PaCO_2$) should be kept at 30–35 mm Hg].
- Correction of clotting factors deficiencies (with vitamin K, FFP, etc.).
- *Perform investigations*: CSF, blood/serum, urine, MRI (CT, if MRI not available/possible), avoid sedation, throat swab, nasopharyngeal swab, etc. If CSF is contraindicated (raised ICP, features of herniation, etc.), perform CT scan brain. Other investigations (as per presentation of the case)—serology and PCR.

Empirical Treatment

It must be started, if CSF cannot be done/report will take time and patient sick.
- Ceftriaxone
- Acyclovir (use in all suspected sporadic viral encephalitis)
- Artesunate [stop if peripheral smear and rapid diagnostic test (RDT) are negative].

Specific Treatment

- *Acute bacterial meningitis (ABM)*: IV antibiotics
- *Acute viral encephalitis*: IV acyclovir
- *Mycoplasma encephalitis*: IV azithromycin with steroids
- *Acute disseminated encephalomyelitis (ADEM)*: High dose IV methylprednisolone pulse therapy
- *Cerebral malaria*: IV artesunate
- *Sepsis-associated encephalopathy (SAE)*: Appropriate IV antibiotics

- *Enteric encephalopathy*: IV ceftriaxone and other antibiotics
- *Leptospirosis*: IV penicillin
- *Heat stroke*: Cooling and IV fluids
- *Diabetic ketoacidosis*: Fluids, insulin, and other measures
- *Metabolic syndrome*: Appropriate treatment (see below) and dietary modification
- Empirical use of steroids should be avoided.

Q3. What is the rationale behind empiric use of IV acyclovir in all cases of acute febrile encephalopathy?

Ans. Intravenous acyclovir should be used in all cases of encephalitis empirically until an alternative diagnosis is made or if the MRI is normal. In most cases of encephalitis, it is often difficult to make an exact etiologic diagnosis and IV acyclovir may need to be continued for full duration. It is vital to maintain good hydration during acyclovir infusion to avoid neurotoxicity and nephrotoxicity.

Q4. What doses and duration of the drugs should be used?

Ans.
- *HSV*: Acyclovir 10 mg/kg or 500 mg/m^2 8 hourly for 14 days
- *Mycoplasma*: IV azithromycin 10 mg/kg/day OD for 3-5 days or IV clarithromycin 15 mg/kg/day for 14 days ± pulse steroids
- *Cerebral malaria*: IV artesunate drug of choice, 2.4 mg/kg loading and 1.2 mg/kg OD. Once able to take orally switch to oral artesunate 4 mg/kg/day for another 3 days with either doxycycline 3.5 mg/kg/day for 7 days (not in children below 8 years) or clindamycin 10 mg/kg twice a day for 7 days. Avoid mefloquine in cerebral malaria as risk of neuropsychiatric reactions is increased.
- *ADEM*: Pulse methylprednisolone 30 mg/kg for 3 days and then oral prednisolone 1-2 mg/kg for 4-6 weeks.

Q5. Should IV azithromycin be added to empirical agents to use in a case of suspected acute viral encephalitis?

Ans. Since *Mycoplasma* is a treatable and common cause of childhood encephalitis, it is prudent to empirically treat it till an alternative diagnosis is made. Azithromycin is preferred as there are no drug interactions unlike clarithromycin.

Q6. What is the significance of ICP in the management of a febrile coma patient?

Ans. The ICP is the total pressure exerted by brain (around 80%), blood (around 10%), and CSF (around 10%) in the cranial vault. These values are constant and an increase in any one of these values should be counterbalance by an equal decrease in another otherwise the ICP increases.

Q7. What are the normal values of ICP in different age groups?

Ans. The ICP varies with age and normal figures for the children are not very well-known. Both intracranial hyper- and hypotension worsen the brain insult by producing cerebral ischemia. ICP values greater than 20–25 mm Hg require treatment in most circumstances. Ideally, the ICP should be kept <10–15 mm Hg in adults and older children for adequate cerebral perfusion. The target value for young children is <3–7 mm Hg and <1.5–6.0 mm Hg for term infants. Sustained ICP of >40 mm Hg indicates severe life-threatening intracranial hypertension.

Q8. What do you mean by "cerebral perfusion pressure (CPP)"?

Ans. Cerebral perfusion pressure is the major factor that affects CBF, hence maintains adequate oxygenation of brain. Cerebral perfusion depends on CPP.

Q9. How do you estimate CPP?

Ans. The CPP is the difference between systemic MAP and ICP. The equation is: CPP = MAP – ICP. The CPP can reduce as a result of reduced MAP or raised ICP or combination of these two.

Q10. What are the normal values of CPP in different age groups?

Ans. Measurement of CPP helps in determining the amount of blood volume present in the intracranial space. It is used as an important clinical indicator of CBF, and hence adequate oxygenation. Normal CPP values for children are not clearly established, but the following values are generally accepted as the minimal pressure necessary to prevent ischemia: adults CPP >70 mm Hg; children CPP >50–60 mm Hg; infants/toddlers CPP >40–50 mm Hg.

Q11. What is the most critical component of the management of an acute febrile encephalopathy case?

Ans. The main aim of a proper treatment of a comatose child is to maintain adequate CPP so that cerebral ischemia is avoided. As mentioned above, both intracranial hyper- and hypotension result in brain injury due to cerebral ischemia. Hence, judicious management of raised ICP is the cornerstone of the successful management of any comatose child, more so of a febrile encephalopathic case. Emergency management of raised ICP at the time of presentation is potentially lifesaving in all encephalopathies. Following key messages must be remembered while managing a case of AFE:
- Use only hypertonic or isotonic fluids
- No need for fluids restriction
- Papilledema is very rarely seen in AFEs
- Normal CT may not exclude raised ICP.

Q12. How does raised intracranial pressure cause brain damage?

Ans. Raised ICP or intracranial hypertension is thought to cause brain damage by at least two mechanisms:
- Firstly, reduced (CPP = MAP – ICP) causes cerebral ischemia, particularly in the border zones between the main arterial territories; this may be associated with seizures, for example in hypertensive encephalopathy, but is often clinically silent.
- Secondly, through herniation of different anatomical parts of the brain. If there are differences in pressure between the forebrain compartment and the posterior fossa, one (uncal herniation) or both (diencephalic and midbrain/upper pontine herniation syndromes) temporal lobes may herniate through the tentorium. Similarly, if there is a pressure differential between the posterior fossa and the spinal canal, the brain may herniate through the foramen magnum (lower pontine and medullary herniation syndromes).

Brain herniation: Brain herniation causes direct mechanical damage and also ischemia and hemorrhage secondary to vascular distortion (Figs. 7 to 9). Central or uncal herniation through the tentorium is compatible with intact survival; herniation through the foramen magnum is not. These syndromes, and the changes from one to the next which signify progressive herniation, can be recognized clinically.

Recovery is extremely unlikely if the patient has reached the lower pontine or medullary stage, so that if children are seen with some or all of the signs, either of uncal herniation or of the diencephalic or midbrain/upper pontine phases of central herniation, emergency management of presumed raised ICP is mandatory.

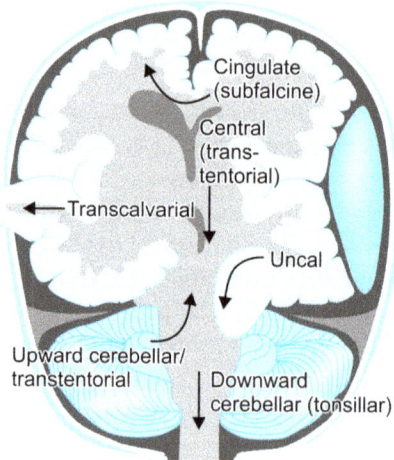

Fig. 7: Different types of brain herniation syndromes.

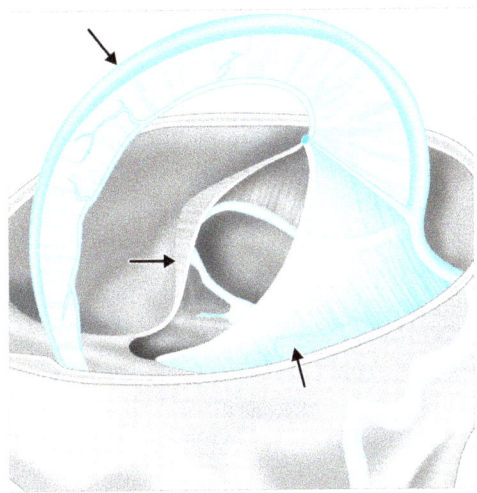

Fig. 8: Falx cerebri and tentorium cerebelli.

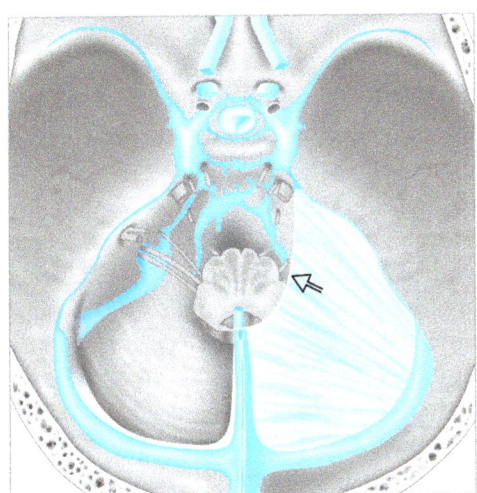

Fig. 9: Pressure exerted through tentorium cerebelli over intracerebral vessels and nerves.

Q13. What are the signs and symptoms of brain herniation syndromes?

Ans. Signs and symptoms may include:
- High blood pressure
- Irregular or slow pulse
- Headache
- Weakness
- Cardiac arrest (no pulse)
- Loss of consciousness
- Loss of all brainstem reflexes (blinking, gagging, and pupils reacting to light)
- Respiratory arrest (no breathing).

Q14. What are the key interventions in the proper management of raised intracranial pressure?

Ans. One should not delay the treatment of raised ICP when clinical features point to this entity. The efforts to identify underlying cause of the raised ICP can follow the interventions needed to reduce it urgently.

Following interventions are urgently needed:
- *Management of the ABC*: Airway, breathing, and circulation (see above)
- *Mild elevation of head* to 15–30°
- *Hyperventilation*: It acts by constricting the blood vessels that leads to lowering of CBF. However, one should only employ hyperventilation when emergent reduction is needed for sharp acute increase in ICP or when there is a danger of brain herniation. The aim is to maintain $PaCO_2$ = 30–35 mm Hg. Aggressive hyperventilation may dramatically decreases CBF that may cause or aggravate already existing cerebral ischemia.
- *Osmotherapy*: Following agents are used in reducing raised ICP.
  - *Mannitol*: Should be used when blood pressure is maintained and there is no hypovolemia, shock, and renal failure. The optimal dosing is not known. *Initial bolus*: 0.25–1.0 g/kg over 30 minutes, followed by 0.25–0.50 g/kg every 2–6 hourly for 48–72 hours only. One should use mannitol for minimum period of time with minimum doses as there is a risk of rebound rise of ICP.
  - *Hypertonic saline*: Should be preferred to mannitol in the presence of hypotension or hypovolemia. Other indications are renal failure or when serum osmolality >320 mOsmol/kg. Usually 3% saline is employed but its concentration has varied from 1.7% to 30% in various trials. It is administered as a continuous infusion at a rate of 0.1–1.0 mL/kg/hour and serum sodium level of 145–155 mEq/L is targeted. Hypertonic saline can be used up to 7 days under careful monitoring.
  - *Glycerol*: Glycerol can be used both orally and intravenously. The oral dose is 1.5 g/kg/day, q4–6 hourly. On IV administration, its effect on ICP lasts for about 70 minutes. There is a theoretical risk of rebound rise in ICP following its use.
- *Acetazolamide*: It acts by reducing the production of CSF. The usual doses are 20–100 mg/kg/day, three times per day. Commonly used in conditions such as hydrocephalous, benign intracranial hypertension, ICT associated with tumors, etc.
- *Furosemide*: This loop diuretic in used either alone or in combination with mannitol. Usual dose is 1.0 mg/kg/day three times per day.
- *Steroids*: These agents are highly effective against vasogenic brain edema usually associated with brain tumors, inflammatory conditions [ADEM and neurocysticercosis (NCC)], and some infectious conditions [tuberculous meningitis (TBM), adult bacterial meningitis (ABM)], etc. that

results in increased permeability of blood–brain barrier. Dexamethasone is preferred over other agents in a dose of 0.4–1.5 mg/kg/day in four divided doses. Their role in traumatic brain injury, intracranial hemorrhage, cerebral malaria, etc. has not yet established, hence, should be avoided.

Q15. What are the factors that aggravate ICP and should be avoided?

Ans. *Certain factors aggravate ICP, they include*: Hyperthermia (use antipyretics and hydrotherapy), irritability and pain arousal (use IV midazolam), seizures (use midazolam/lorazepam followed by IV Eptoin), hypovolemia and hyponatremia [use isotonic or hypertonic fluids Ringer's lactate (RL), NS, dextrose normal saline (DNS), etc.), and flexed head posture (keep head straight, slightly extended with mildly elevated).

Q16. How would you treat refractory rise in ICP?

Ans. Rarely needed in most of the instances of raised ICP which are adequately managed by the above-mentioned interventions. In the event of refractory ICP, a trial can be given of thiopentone. In extreme cases of refractory ICP, paralytic agents along with heavy sedation and surgical decompression-like craniectomy can be employed. Controlled hypothermia may be effective in infants and neonates with raised ICP secondary to hypoxic-ischemic insults.

Take Home Message

- After airway, breathing and circulation (ABC), look for the signs of raised intracranial pressure (ICP) and brain herniation.
- Emergency management of raised ICP at the time of presentation is potentially life saving in all encephalopathies.
- The main aim of a proper treatment of a comatose child is to maintain adequate cerebral perfusion pressure (CPP) so that cerebral ischemia is avoided.
- Cerebral perfusion pressure (CPP) is the major factor that affects cerebral blood flow, and hence adequate oxygenation (CPP = MAP − ICP) (MAP = mean arterial pressure).
- CPP can reduce as a result of reduced MAP or raised ICP or combination of these two.
- Should aim MAP = >75 mm of Hg (mild-moderate grade coma) and >85 mm Hg in severe grade.
- No need for fluids restriction.
- Use only hypertonic or isotonic fluids—aim should be to keep serum Na = 145–155 mEq/L.
- Papilloedema is very rarely seen in acute febrile encephalopathies (AFEs), even if the ICP is very high.
- Normal CT may not exclude raised ICP.

SUGGESTED READING

1. Chayovan T. Brain herniation syndrome: a pictorial review. [online] Available from https://www.slideshare.net/fernferretie/brain-herniation-imaging. [Last accessed on December, 2019].
2. Rangel-Castilla L, Gopinath S, Robertson CS. Management of intracranial hypertension [published correction appears in Neurol Clin. 2008;26(3):xvii. Rangel-Castillo, Leonardo [corrected to Rangel-Castilla, Leonardo]]. Neurol Clin. 2008;26(2):521-x. doi:10.1016/j.ncl.2008.02.003
3. Sankhyan N, Vykunta Raju KN, Sharma S, et al. Management of raised intracranial pressure. Indian J Pediatr. 2010;77(12):1409-16.
4. Sharma S, Mishra D, Aneja S, et al. Consensus guidelines on evaluation and management of suspected acute viral encephalitis in children in India. Indian Pediatr. 2012;49(11):897-910.
5. Singhi SC, Tiwari L. Management of intracranial hypertension. Indian J Pediatr. 2009;76(5):519-29. doi: 10.1007/s12098-009-0137-7.

Chapter 3

A Child with Recurrent Fever

Yashwant Rao

INTRODUCTION

Recurrent fever in a child is often a diagnostic challenge. Fever, defined as a rise of core body temperature more than that of normal body temperature, is a common manifestation of different pathologies. Viral infections are frequent causes of acute fever which subsides before 2 weeks. Uncomplicated bacterial infections can also be the reason for acute fevers. Conditions, where fever is prolonged or repeats after a variable interval fever-free period, can be a cause of great concern. Although in majority proportions of recurrent or prolonged fever the cause is unknown, detailed clinical history and examination can point toward the diagnosis. This chapter summarizes few case-based approaches toward infectious and noninfectious causes of *A child with a recurrent fever*.

CASE 1

The worried parents of a 3-year-old male admitted their child with complaints of recurrent fever for the last 3 months which was gradual onset, low grade, mostly during the afternoon and falls by night. The child also had developed lassitude, refusal to feed, and lost 2 kg. There were no other systemic symptoms. His father is a farmer and also owns cattle. He had no contact with tuberculosis (TB).

On physical examination, the child looked chronically sick. He had wasting, some pallor but no jaundice, no ascites, no lymphadenopathy, or any other abnormalities were found in general physical examination.

On systemic examination, he had hepatosplenomegaly. Nontender, firm, liver 3 cm below costal margin (Liver span of 10 cm) and mild splenomegaly. Rest of the systemic examination was normal.

Q1. What are the possible differentials?

Ans. The history is suggestive of (s/o) a chronic inflammatory process which can be infectious or noninfectious. Hepatosplenomegaly is the only positive finding in this child. The absence of jaundice rules out hepatocyte disease and absence of ascites rules out portal hypertension. So, hepatosplenomegaly in this child is likely due to reticuloendothelial cell involvement secondary to infection or noninfective disorder such as systemic inflammatory disease or malignancy.

Possible infections can be slowly progressive chronic infections such as TB, brucellosis, CMV (cytomegalovirus), malaria, and kala-azar besides fungal infections due to histoplasmosis, blastomycosis, or coccidioidomycosis. Alternatively, it can be due to noninfectious causes such as malignancy, especially hematological such as lymphomas and leukemia.

Now with malaria or kala-azar in chronic history, there would have been massive splenomegaly and severe pallor and CMV would have involved a specific organ such as liver and would have result in jaundice. However, all these features are missing in the child, so possibilities are less for the diseases mentioned earlier.

In malignancies of hematological origin, there might have been history of gum bleeding and petechiae and on examination, hepatosplenomegaly, severe pallor, lymphadenopathy, and bony tenderness were likely. These are lacking in this child, thus making the possibilities less likely.

Again, fungal infections are more common in immunocompromised children which is unlikely as of now in this child.

There can be possibilities of TB because it is more prevalent and brucellosis has high possibilities because of history of fever pattern (undulant), contact with cattle, and physical examination revealing hepatosplenomegaly.

Q2. What are the investigations to be done?

Ans. Complete blood count (CBC) with peripheral blood smear with thick and thin smear for malarial parasite, erythrocyte sedimentation rate (ESR), and chest X-ray (CXR). The result of these tests can differentiate among the above differentials. Laboratory result in this case showed moderate neutrophilic leukocytosis with elevated ESR. CXR was normal. An ultrasound abdomen suggested abscesses on liver and spleen which on CT abdomen was confirmed to be a granuloma. Pus culture from the abscesses drained under ultrasound guidance was negative for any other usual bacteria.

Q3. What further test should have been done here?

Ans. A test for *Brucella* antibody. The test may show false-negative as well as a false-positive result. No single titer is ever diagnostic, but most patients with acute infections have titer more than or equal to 1:160. PCR is most specific for diagnosis but not always available.

Q4. What is the final diagnosis and what treatment should be given?

Ans. The test result for *Brucella* antibody was positive and with the circumstantial evidence of prolonged fever with hepatosplenomegaly and history of contact with animals, brucellosis was made as a diagnosis.

Moreover, the child was treated with co-trimoxazole and with rifampin for 4 weeks.

Treatment for brucellosis requires an antibiotic which can cause intracellular killing of the organism. The choice of therapy is doxycycline (>8 years) with rifampin or aminoglycosides.

Take Home Message
Detailed history and thorough physical examination is the crux to reach up to correct clinical diagnosis.

CASE 2
A 9-year-old female child was brought by her parents to the hospital with complain of productive cough and fever for the last 10 days with fast and difficult breathing for the last 3 days. The fever was high grade with chills and was continuous. A cough was not associated with blood and was yellowish and foul smelling with no specific postural or diurnal variation.

On further asking her parents, they revealed that she had been suffering from similar episodes thrice in the last 1 year needing hospitalization with recurrent episodes of fever needing broad-spectrum antibiotics for prolonged periods and symptoms of upper respiratory tract infection (URTI) since she was 5 years of age. She also had a history of suffering from acute suppurative otitis media (ASOM) last year. Apart from that, she had a history of recurrent diarrhea, abdominal pain, and lack of appetite leading to failure to gain weight. Her immunization was complete. She had no other significant history. On physical examination, she was a chronically sick child with severe thinness. She had pallor and significant cervical lymphadenopathy, sinus tenderness—no other abnormalities in physical examination. On systemic examination, she had tachypnea with respiratory rate (RR) = 40/min, subcostal retraction, and bilateral crepitations all over the chest. She had hepatosplenomegaly and rest of the systems were normal.

Q1. What is the possible diagnosis?
Ans. The present history is suggesting that the child has pneumonia. Here the child has a recurrent fever which occurred in an irregular pattern as a result of different infections. She also has a history of recurrent pneumonia, recurrent episodes of URTI, an episode of ASOM, recurrent diarrhea, failure to thrive in the setting of severe wasting, lymphoreticular proliferation, and anemia.

From the history and examination, the child seems to suffer from an *immunodeficiency disorder*, either primary or secondary being susceptible to recurrent infections.

The condition should be suspected in patients presenting with *two of the following 10 warning signs*:
1. Four or more new infections in a year
2. Two or more serious sinus infections in a year
3. Two or more episodes of pneumonia in a year
4. Two or more months of antibiotics without effect
5. Failure of an infant to gain weight or grow normally
6. Recurrent deep skin infections or organ abscesses
7. Persistent oral thrush, or candidiasis elsewhere beyond infancy
8. Need for intravenous antibiotic
9. Family history of primary immunodeficiency
10. Two or more deep-seated infections including septicemia

The possible reasons for immunodeficiency could be the following:
- Primary immunodeficiency disorders
- *Secondary causes*:
  - Human immunodeficiency virus (HIV) infection
  - Severe malnutrition
  - Lymphoreticular malignancies
  - Immunosuppressive drugs (e.g. glucocorticoids, cyclophosphamide, and azathioprine)

Q2. What investigations should be considered and what finding did she have?

Ans. A careful inspection of past medical history is the first step in the diagnosis. Initially, we would ask for:

Complete blood count (CBC) and peripheral blood smear (PBS): Moderate anemia, dimorphic picture, moderate leukopenia, platelet count normal, and no abnormal malignant cell. Serum ferritin was high indicating coexisting nutritional and anemia of chronic disease.

Liver function test (LFT): Significant finding was low total protein level with normal enzymes and bilirubin level. HIV serology was negative.

Chest X-ray s/o right upper and middle lobe consolidations.
Mantoux
Sputum/gastric aspirate (GA) for cartridge-based nucleic acid amplification test (CBNAAT)
} **Negative**

Celiac serology and IgA level are negative but IgA levels were low.

The possible common causes for secondary immunodeficiency being ruled out, primary immunodeficiency becomes a possibility especially in the setting of low IgA level.

Q3. What primary immunodeficiency to be suspected in this case?

Ans. Recurrent fever, diarrhea, pneumonia, ASOM with hepatosplenomegaly and lymphadenopathy give a clue to common variable immunodeficiency (CVID) and chronic granulomatous disease. Chronic granulomatous disease is mostly present in early childhood and has recurrent staphylococcal infections of lungs, skin, or bone; persistent fungal *(Aspergillus)* pneumonia; and a liver abscess.

Q4. What are the specific investigations done for primary immunodeficiency disorder and what are the findings?

Ans. Serum immunoglobulins (IgG, IgA, and IgM) are low. Now, decrease of IgG (at least 2 SD below the mean for age) and a marked decrease in at least one of the isotypes IgM or IgA suggest CVID. In this setting, antidiphtheria and anti-tetanus antibodies (functional IgG) were also done to support the diagnosis which were found to be low.

By all these findings, a diagnosis of primary immunodeficiency disorder, probably CVID, was made. These children may develop various autoimmune disorders such as leukopenia, hemolytic anemia, arthritis, and also lymphoreticular malignancies. So, the patient was asked for close monitoring and follow-up.

Q5. What treatment is given in this condition?

Ans. The child was treated with IVIg (intravenous immunoglobulin) injections 3–4 weekly and she improved and showed weight gain. The limitation of this treatment is its high cost.

Q6. What are the special characteristics of different primary immunodeficiency disorder?

Ans. The prevalence of different primary immunodeficiency disorders is different depending on the age group and those have different clinical features as described in **Tables 1 to 3**.

TABLE 1: Immunodeficiency in an infant below 6 months.	
Features	*Diagnosis*
Hypocalcemia, unusual facies and ears, and heart disease	DiGeorge anomaly
Delayed umbilical cord detachment, leukocytosis, and recurrent infections	Leukocyte adhesion defect
Persistent thrush, failure to thrive, pneumonia, and diarrhea	Severe combined immunodeficiency
Blood stools, draining ears, and atopic eczema	Wiskott–Aldrich syndrome
Pneumocystis jiroveci pneumonia, neutropenia, and recurrent infections	X-linked hyper-IgM syndromes

TABLE 2: Immunodeficiency in children below 5 years.	
Features	*Diagnosis*
Severe progressive infectious mononucleosis	X-linked lymphoproliferative syndrome
Recurrent staphylococcal abscesses, staphylococcal pneumonia with pneumatocele formation, coarse facial features, and pruritic dermatitis	Hyper-IgE syndrome
Persistent thrush, nail dystrophy, and endocrinopathies	Chronic mucocutaneous candidiasis
Short stature, fine hair, and severe varicella	Cartilage-hair hypoplasia with short-limbed dwarfism
Oculocutaneous albinism and recurrent infection	Chédiak–Higashi syndrome
Abscesses, suppurative lymphadenopathy, antral outlet obstruction, pneumonia, and osteomyelitis	Chronic granulomatous disease

TABLE 3: Immunodeficiency in children older than 5 years.	
Features	Diagnosis
Progressive dermatomyositis with chronic enterovirus encephalitis	X-linked agammaglobulinemia
Sinopulmonary infections, neurologic deterioration, and telangiectasia	Ataxia-telangiectasia
Recurrent neisserial meningitis	C6, C7, or C8 deficiency
Sinopulmonary infections, splenomegaly, and autoimmunity, malabsorption	Common variable immunodeficiency

Take Home Message Used as Earlier

Always suspect immunodeficiency in a child with a recurrent fever with recurrent other infections and if the secondary cause is ruled out, a primary cause must be thought of.

CASE 3

A 10-year-old male child presented to the clinic with complaints of recurrent fever and swelling over the neck for the last 6 months. The fever was intermittent, associated with night sweats, high grade over a week, and then gradually decreased over another week with a fever-free interval of 1 or 2 weeks. The swelling over the neck had developed gradually and progressively increased in sign, no pain, redness, or increased temperature. The parents of the child were also concerned about his weight loss over the 6 months. On further asking, the parents conclude that he did not have any contact with TB. He did not have complaints of bleeding from any site, no history of bone pain, and no history of a chronic cough. Family history was uneventful. He was treated with oral amoxicillin and clavulanic acid but did not get any response. Rest of the history was not significant.

On physical examination, he looked chronically sick and severely thinned. He had some pallor, no icterus, and no edema but he had significant bilateral cervical lymphadenopathy, nontender, firm, and rubbery in consistency, nonmated, no discharging sinus, no signs of inflammation. Other groups of lymph nodes were not palpable. He had no hepatosplenomegaly. The rest of the systemic examination was within normal limits.

Q1. What are the possibilities?

Ans. The above history and examination are s/o chronic illness. The recurrent fever he has supports any infective or inflammatory cause. Significant cervical lymphadenopathy indicates lymphoreticular proliferation. The possible diagnosis can be TB, HIV, Hodgkin's lymphoma, or juvenile chronic myeloid leukemia. Recurrent fever with night sweats and weight loss can be present both in TB and in Hodgkin's lymphoma, but TB could have a history of contact which is missing in this child. Having said this, it should be remembered that contact of TB in children can be found in only one-third cases. An HIV infection can be presented with recurrent fever and cervical lymphadenopathy which can be generalized but the child here only had cervical lymph nodes and did not have an obvious risk factor in history. Chronic juvenile myeloid leukemia may present with recurrent fever, fatigue, weight loss, pallor, and nontender lymph node enlargement but the absence of hepatosplenomegaly is against it. Hodgkin's lymphoma can present similarly like this in initial stages.

Q2. What investigations were planned and what were the findings?

Ans. CBC, PBS, ESR, Hb (hemoglobin) 7 g/dL, normocytic normochromic, TLC (total leukocyte count)—5,200/cumm, and platelet—1.5 lakh/cumm. No abnormal cells.

ESR was raised. 45 mm at the end of 1 hour.
Mantoux: Negative
Chest X-ray within normal limits
HIV serology: Negative

Q3. What was a further investigation done?

Ans. *Lymph node biopsy*: As the child already had taken a course of antibiotic with no response, he was ordered a biopsy immediately. A biopsy was s/o Hodgkin's lymphoma mixed cellularity type. It is to be said that an entire node was excised for biopsy as a high index for lymphoma was there. Fine-needle aspiration cytology (FNAC) and frozen section material are not optimal for histology.

Q4. What specialized investigations were needed in this case?

Ans. The child underwent the positron emission tomography-computed tomography (PET-CT) scan which confirmed that only a single cervical lymph node region was involved and the disease was staged as stage 1B. Bone marrow biopsy showed no involvement. Liver function and renal function tests and alkaline phosphatase (ALP) were normal indicating no systemic spread. Immunophenotyping is also important in prognosticating the disease.

Q 5. How was the child treated?

Ans. The child was treated by the hemato-oncology team with chemotherapy. Although the child had a single lymph node region involving male sex, the presence of B symptoms (fever, night sweats and weight loss) and elevated ESR at presentation may affect the prognosis.

Take Home Message

Lymphoreticular malignancy in children is not so rare and should always be suspected in a child with recurrent fever as early diagnosis and treatment may result into the complete cure of the disease.

CASE 4

A 16-year-old girl attended the emergency with complaints of fever for 10–12 days high grade, intermittent, one or two spikes a day, with no chills or rigor, and no rash. She also complained of mild dry cough which had developed in the last 1 week. She did not have any neurological symptoms, no arthritis or arthralgia, no retro-orbital pain, no abdominal symptoms, and no c/o dysuria or pain. Her menstrual history was normal. On further asking, she told she was having recurrent episodes of similar fever for the last 4–6 months, initially low grade, more on the night, and lasting for few days. Then she would feel well for the next 2 or 3 weeks. She had developed a lack of appetite and lost few kilograms. She did not have contact with TB. Family history was not significant.

On examination, she had 103.4°F temperature with a proportionate increase in pulse. Respiratory rate and blood pressure were normal. She was thin and BMI (Body Mass Index) was between 3rd percentile and 10th percentile for her age and sex. On physical examination, she had some pallor, no icterus, no clubbing, no lymph node palpable, no edema, and no stigmata of TB. Rest of the physical examination was normal. On systemic examination, no significant finding was revealed.

Q1. What is the possible diagnosis?

Ans. The history and examination are not signifying toward any particular system although a picture of an infectious disease or inflammatory disease with recurrent fever is present. Clinically, this is fever without localization. Common infectious causes of fever such as enteric fever and malaria should be ruled out. The possibility of any deep-seated infection or abscess, tuberculosis, and systemic inflammatory disorder such as juvenile idiopathic arthritis (JIA) and other autoimmune diseases can be possible.

Q2. What investigations were done and their findings?

Ans. *CBC*: Hb—9.4 g/dL, TLC—7200/cumm, platelet—2.35 lakh/cumm, and RBC indices s/o normocytic normochromic
- ESR was mildly elevated, 32 mm at the end of 1 hour.
- C-reactive protein (CRP) was negative.
- *Blood culture*: Negative
- *Malarial parasite*: Negative
- *Widal titer*: Negative
- *Urine routine and culture*: Normal
- *Liver functions and renal functions*: Normal
- *Ultrasound of abdomen*: Normal. Subdiaphragmatic areas were normal. Now, from these initial investigations any usual cause or focus of fever was not identified. As CRP was negative, systemic inflammatory diseases became unlikely.

Q3. What was a further test done?

Ans. A chest X-ray was ordered which showed prominent bronchopulmonary markings and mild left-sided pleural effusion. Mantoux test was significantly positive. The maximum transverse diameter of the induration measured on the long axis of the forearm on the volar surface measured by rolling a ball pen was more than 10 mm. HIV test was negative. So, pulmonary tuberculosis was suspected.

Q4. What confirmatory diagnosis was done?

Ans. Induced sputum was sent for CBNAAT which came out to be positive with no drug resistance.

Q5. How was the girl treated?

Ans. She was treated as category one patient with antitubercular drugs. Other family members were also screened for pulmonary TB. She was declared completed cured after 6 months.

Take Home Message

Tuberculosis can present with recurrent fever or even fever without localizing sign and should always be kept in mind to rule out.

As we have discussed in the above cases, recurrent fever in children has infectious or noninfectious etiology. Although covering all of the causes is out of the scope of this discussion, special mention of the other infectious causes is warranted.

Viral diseases such as repeated independent respiratory viral infections, parvovirus B19 infection, Epstein–Barr virus infection, and recurrent herpes virus infection can cause recurrent fever.

Bacterial diseases such as relapsing fever (*Borrelia recurrentis* and other borreliae), brucellosis, trench fever (*Bartonella quintana*), syphilis (*Treponema pallidum*), rat-bite fever (*Spirillum minus*), melioidosis (*Burkholderia pseudomallei*); Whipple's disease, chronic meningococcemia, infective endocarditis, subacute cholangitis, abscesses, especially occult dental abscesses, and osteomyelitis are important causes of recurrent fever but not usual in India. Fungal diseases such as histoplasmosis and coccidioidomycosis are suspected in immunocompromised patients.

Parasitic diseases such as malaria and visceral leishmaniasis can present with recurrent fever in endemic areas.

The noninfectious causes which have a presentation with recurrent fever are immune mediated and granulomatous diseases such as Crohn's disease, Behçet's disease, systemic lupus erythematosus (SLE), juvenile dermatomyositis (JDM), sarcoidosis, and granulomatous hepatitis.

Rare causes such as periodic fever syndromes and autoinflammatory disorders which include cyclic neutropenia, periodic fever, aphthous stomatitis, pharyngitis, and adenopathy (PFAPA) syndrome, and familial Mediterranean fever (FMF) should be suspected when more common causes are ruled out.

To conclude the discussion, recurrent fevers have a self-resolving course in most children and occur mainly due to susceptibility to infections which are typical of their age group and usually have a good prognosis. In some cases, recurrent fever may be a manifestation of a much rare disease that requires special investigations and treatment.

When evaluating recurrent fever, it is important to consider the age at onset, family history, duration of febrile episodes, length of the interval between episodes, associated symptoms, and response to treatment. Additionally, knowledge of travel history and exposure to animals are helpful, especially about infections. It is important to rule out the possibility of an infectious process or a malignancy, especially if steroid therapy is being considered or in an immunocompromised child as we discussed earlier. After excluding an infectious or neoplastic etiology, immune-mediated and autoinflammatory diseases should be taken into consideration.

However, despite a thorough evaluation, recurrent fever may remain unexplained. A watchful follow-up is thus mandatory because new signs and symptoms may appear over time.

SUGGESTED READING

1. A Parthasarthy. IAP Textbook of Pediatric Infectious Diseases, 2nd Edition. New Delhi: Jaypee Brothers Medical Publishers; 2019.
2. Barron KS, Kastner DL. Periodic fever syndromes and other inherited autoinflammatory diseases. In: Petty RE, Laxer RM, Lindsely CB, Wedderburn LR (Eds). Textbook of Pediatric Rheumatology, 7th edition. Philadelphia, PA: Elsevier; 2016. pp. 609-26.
3. Cherry J, Demmler-Harrison GJ, Kaplan SL, et al. Textbook of Pediatric Infectious Diseases, 8th edition. Canada: Elsevier; 2019.
4. John CC, Gilsdorf JR. Recurrent fever in children. Pediatr Infect Dis J. 2002;21(11): 1071-7.
5. Long SS. Distinguishing among prolonged, recurrent, and periodic fever syndromes: approach of a pediatric infectious diseases subspecialist. Pediatr Clin North Am. 2005;52(3):811-35.
6. McCarthy PL. Fever: Pediatrics in Review (An official journal of the American Academy of Pediatrics). 1998;19(12):401-8.

CHAPTER 4

Fever with Positive Tuberculin Skin Test

Ajay Gaur, Prakash Petchimuthu

INTRODUCTION

The global tuberculosis (TB) report 2018 reports that in India, an estimated 2.2 lakh children become ill with TB each year (22% of global TB burden), with slightly higher burden among males. Pulmonary TB is the most common form in children. It is also known that 10% of cases reported to the NTCP (National Tuberculosis Control Program) are from children under 14 years of age. TB is a formidable problem keeping high suspicion of TB in children presented with persistent fever or cough for more than 2 weeks

Tuberculosis remains a leading cause of morbidity and mortality in the world, especially in developing countries. A combination of factors including high costs, limited resources, and the poor performance of various diagnostic tests make the diagnosis of TB difficult in developing countries. Short of demonstrating viable organisms in body tissues and fluids, the tuberculin skin test (TST) is the only method of detecting *Mycobacterium tuberculosis (MTB)* infection in an individual and is used to diagnose TB in individual patients, as well as in epidemiological settings, and to measure the prevalence of TB infection in populations. The TST is one of the few investigations dating from the 19th century that are still widely used as an important test for diagnosing tuberculosis. Though very commonly used by physicians worldwide, its interpretation always remains difficult and controversial. Various factors such as age, immunological status, and coexisting illness influence its outcome and interpretation.

CASE 1

An 18-month-old child presented with complaints of persistent pneumonia with mild fever and cough lasting for 15 days. The patient has been referred for these complaints. On detailed history, there were no similar episodes before but the patient had episodes of cough and cold for 3–5 days which usually will be relieved by oral medications. This episode started with history of fever for 4–5 days followed by cough and cold without expectoration. The patient was fully vaccinated. There was no history of contact with TB in the family and any foreign body aspiration. On admission, the patient was sick and on respiratory distress, so was started on oxygen and antibiotics. Respiratory rate was 48/min and heart rate was 116/min; subcostal retractions were present and bilateral air entry was present. No cyanosis, no anemia, no icterus, no lymphadenopathy, and no edema were present. Head-to-toe examination revealed no positive findings. Anthropometry showed weight for length <−3 SD, weight for age <−3 SD and length for age <−2 SD. Cardiovascular examination was normal. Per abdomen examination showed mild hepatomegaly with palpable liver 2 cm below right costal margin.

Q1. What differential diagnosis should we consider?

Ans. This could be due to bacterial or viral pneumonia but after giving 15 days of antibiotics there is no improvement, so we have to think of other causes also. Other causes could be due to human immunodeficiency virus (HIV), TB, congenital heart disease, chronic foreign body, congenital malformations of lung such as congenital cystic adenomatoid malformations, lung hypoplasia, fungal infections, gastroesophageal reflux disease (GERD), or immunodeficiency disorders.

Q2. What investigations to be done?

Ans. Complete blood count revealed normal values, except mild leukocytosis and normal eosinophil count with raised erythrocyte sedimentation rate (ESR); chest X-ray (CXR) revealed bilateral pneumonitic patches. Mantoux test was done and results after 72 hours showed 10 mm of induration. Blood culture and sensitivity was done before starting antibiotics which revealed no growth of bacterial and fungal organisms. Sputum and gastrointestinal (GI) aspirate for acid-fast bacillus (AFB) and cartridge-based nucleic acid amplification test (CBNAAT) was sent and reports were normal. HIV serology was normal. Diagnostic bronchoscopy was done and no foreign body was found. Serum IgE levels were normal. 2D-ECHO was done and showed no major abnormality. Contrast-enhanced computed tomography (CECT) thorax showed consolidation of the right middle lobe of lung.

Discussion

After all investigations, the patient was diagnosed with TB and ATT (antitubercular therapy) was started after which the child recovered within 15 days. So in this case of TB, only investigations positive were TST and consolidation. According to new guidelines, in case of suspicion of TB in children, CBNAAT sputum is the initial investigation of choice. As this was negative, next investigation to proceed in TB was CXR and TST. If CXR showed highly suggestive lesions, irrespective of Mantoux test, we should do GI aspirate/induced sputum/BAL (bronchoalveolar lavage) for AFB. If AFB is detected in any of the above investigations, then it would be diagnosed as morphologically diagnosed TB. But in this case, no AFB was detected and so we had to label it as clinically diagnosed TB. Now coming to TST, it demonstrates the existence of host hypersensitivity to the tuberculosis bacillus proteins, usually as a result of MTB infection although it can also be induced with

Bacillus Calmette-Guérin (BCG) vaccine or infection with environmental *Mycobacteria*. The TST only indicates that the person has been infected with TB previously or not, i.e. it gives idea about latent infection. It does not specify that the patient is having the disease. The sensitivity and specificity of TST were 80% and 85% respectively from a recent systematic review, which were similar to the newer serum immune-based diagnostic methods such as interferon gamma release assays (IGRAs). However, the sensitivity of the TST decreases in children of younger age and in HIV-infected children. False-positive results have been a concern with neonatal BCG vaccination and other environmental mycobacteria or incorrect method of administration. The correct method of administration of TST involves intradermal administration of 2 TU PPD-RT23 (properly stored and refrigerated) on the forearm and it is important to raise a wheal of at least 6 mm after the intradermal injection and the test is read 48-72 hours after an injection. Ballpoint or palpatory methods are used to read the induration. The width of reaction (induration) in the horizontal plane is noted for interpretation. Mantoux test or purified protein derivative (PPD) skin test is considered positive if the induration is 10 mm or more. Degree of reaction including necrosis and ulceration may not necessarily differentiate infected from diseased. If the patient returns for reading beyond 72 hours but by 7th day, a positive test can still be read. A repeat test may be needed, if there is an induration less than 10 mm and the suspect reports for reading beyond the stipulated time of 72 hours post injection. Repeat tuberculin test when required should preferably be done on the other arm. Another important cause of false positive tuberculin skin test includes previous BCG vaccine administration. In a meta-analysis of Mantoux test, it was found that patients who had received BCG vaccination were more likely to have a positive result. The relative risk was 2.12 [95% CI (confidence interval): 1.50-3.00] as compared to those without BCG vaccine. The effect of BCG on Mantoux test was less after 15 years of vaccination. The studies also show that 4 years after the neonatal BCG vaccination, there is no difference of TST reaction in the vaccinated and the unvaccinated children. Also it was stated that TST reaction due to BCG vaccination wanes of as age advances and the reaction usually does not exceed 10 mm. But in this case, it is very difficult to report that positive TST was due to BCG vaccination or prior infection. But current recommendation is for patients with a high risk for tuberculosis, the history of BCG vaccination should not be a consideration in the interpretation of the tuberculin test. Also this difference could be evidenced by the IGRA assays which assess the release of interferon-gamma (IFN-γ) to PPD in the peripheral blood. In case, the positive TST was due to BCG, IGRA will be negative, and in case of TB infection, IGRA will be positive. It recognizes *MTB* specifically and eliminates the cross-reactions in patient who have been exposed to atypical organisms as well as those who have received BCG immunizations. But according to our national guidelines, there is no role of immunological assays such as IGRAs. In this case, as it was clinically diagnosed TB, the patient was given ATT and he improved.

CASE 2

A boy of 3 years of age, for over the past 4 months had evening and nocturnal fever with night sweats, general asthenia, and progressive weight loss. This symptomatology had persisted despite several outpatient treatments with nonspecific antibiotics. He had normal perinatal medical history and a birth weight of 3,100 g. BCG vaccine was administered at birth. He is the youngest of four siblings, all of whom were alive and well. He did not have any family disorder and parental consanguinity. His family had a low socioeconomic status and history of contact with TB (grandfather). At admission, he exhibited alertness, clinical anemia, severe malnutrition with a body weight of 9.1 kg, a height of 85.5 cm with mid-upper arm circumference (MUAC) 11 cm. His anthropometry interpretation was that weight for age <-3 SD and weight for height <-3 SD. He exhibited firm, mobile, confluent, nontender, bilateral, and cervical lymphadenopathy with normal looking skin. General examination showed pallor, not icteric, no cyanosis, and no clubbing. The pulmonary examination was normal as were those of the other organs. Per abdomen examination showed no organomegaly.

Q1. What differential diagnosis would you consider?

Ans. This child has prolonged fever with loss of weight over 3 months. Fever of prolonged duration suggests chronic bacterial infection or systemic inflammatory disorder. But systemic inflammatory disorder would have manifested with skin rash, arthritis, mouth ulcers, or other organ involvement over few weeks and so is unlikely. Other possibility that should be kept in mind are malignancy and collagen vascular diseases, the most common malignancy among children being hematological malignancy. Absence of severe anemia, purpura or bleeding, no organomegaly rules out hematological malignancies such as leukemia and lymphoma. Absence of skin rashes or any cutaneous manifestation, joint pain, and mucosal involvement also rules out collagen vascular diseases. Lymphadenopathy in this case can be related to infectious mononucleosis, cytomegalovirus (CMV), and tuberculosis. Slowly progressive chronic infections include tuberculosis, CMV, malaria, and kala-azar besides fungal infection. Malaria and kala-azar would have severe pallor and large splenomegaly. Primary streptococcal infection may present with prolonged fever but fever may not last for 3 months, and hence unlikely in this child. So, differential diagnosis in this child would include infections such as tuberculosis, CMV, and infectious mononucleosis.

Q2. What laboratory investigations to do?

Ans. Complete blood count with ESR, blood culture, C-reactive protein (CRP), CXR, TST, ultrasound abdomen, fine-needle aspiration cytology (FNAC) of cervical lymph nodes, sputum for AFB, and HIV serology.

Results

The complete blood count revealed hyperleukocytosis of TLC (total leukocyte count)—12,000 (48% neutrophils, 35% lymphocytes, 15% monocytes, and 2%

eosinophils) and a hypochromic microcytic anemia of 7.3 g/dL. CRP was negative. ESR was raised. The HIV serology was negative. The blood cultures were negative. The intradermal reaction to tuberculin revealed an induration with a diameter of 15 mm. Testing for AFB in the expectorations was negative. The cervical lymph node biopsy with anatomical pathology examination indicated a caseating granuloma. The anteroposterior CXR was normal. The abdominal ultrasound revealed deep mesenteric lymphadenopathy of nonsignificant size. GI aspirate for AFB was negative for two consecutive samples.

Diagnosis of these cases described
A diagnosis of tuberculosis was made. The patient was treated with anti-tuberculosis agents according to RNTCP for 6 months and a nutritional support based on therapeutic milk and enriched local food items. After 6 months, there was a favorable change in his condition, with regression of the lymphadenopathies and a weight gain of 5 kg.

Take Home Message
- Tuberculosis is leading cause of morbidity and mortality in children.
- The presentation and symptomatology is vague, clinician should have high index of suspicion.
- Tuberculin skin test (TST) is one of the oldest method of diagnosis and still relevant, if method of inoculation and reading is correct.
- Various epidemiological factors should be considered in interpretaion of results.

SUGGESTED READING
1. Burl S, Adetifa UJ, Cox M, et al. The tuberculin skin test (TST) is affected by recent BCG vaccination but not by exposure to non-tuberculosis mycobacteria (NTM) during early life. PLoS One. 2010;5(8):e12287.
2. Central TB Division, Ministry of Health & Family Welfare, Government of India. Technical and operational guidelines for tuberculosis control in India 2016: Revised National TB control Programme. [online] Available from https://tbcindia.gov.in/index1.php?sublinkid=4573&level=2&lid=3177&lang=1.
3. Kiwanuka JP. Interpretation of tuberculin skin-test results in the diagnosis of tuberculosis in children. Afr Health Sci. 2005;5(2):152-6.
4. Kumar M, Biswal N, Bhuvaneswari V, et al. Persistent pneumonia: underlying cause and outcome. Indian J Pediatr. 2009;76(12):1223-6.
5. Nayak S, Acharjya B. Mantoux test and its interpretation. Indian Dermatol Online J. 2012;3(1):2-6.
6. Seddon JA, Paton J, Nademi Z, et al. The impact of BCG vaccination on tuberculin skin test responses in children is age dependent: evidence to be considered when screening children for tuberculosis infection. Thorax. 2016;71:932-9.
7. Wang L, Turner MO, Elwood RK, et al. A meta-analysis of the effect of Bacille Calmette-Guérin vaccination on tuberculin skin test measurements. Thorax. 2002;57(9):804-9.

CHAPTER 5

Fever Beyond One Week

Arun Shah

INTRODUCTION

Fever beyond one week is quite common presentation in office practice. This is most commonly caused by infections, less commonly by noninfectious causes. Complete history thorough physical examination with relevant investigation clinches the diagnosis in majority of cases. Occasionally, there is uncommon presentation of not so common disease.

Significant numbers of febrile children referred for evaluation have parenteral misinterpretation of normal temperature variation. Parents sometime add 1–2°F to axillaries temperature to approximate the core temperature while there is complete absence of fever at the time of evaluation. Fever is said to occur when rectal temperature is more than 100.4°F, axillaries more than 99°F and oral 99.7°F.

CASE 1

A 13-year-old girl Bittu was brought to me with complains of fever and loss of appetite since last 2 weeks. She was treated by local doctor with chloroquine and cefixime without any appropriate response. The child was from Sitamarhi, North Bihar. She had not visited in recent past any endemic zones with dengue fever, rickettsial infection, and leptospirosis.

On examination she was pale, ill looking, febrile oral temperature 101°F, vitals stable, liver +3 cm firm in consistency, nontender, and spleen 4 cm firm in consistency. Heart sounds normal and air entry bilateral symmetrical with no adventitious sound, no generalized lymphadenopathy. No rash, no icterus, no edema, no joint pain, and no signs of meningeal irritation were seen.

She was stopped all the previous medicines and planned for relevant investigation. Her temperature was recorded every 6 hourly. She was offered bland nutritious diet and paracetamol SOS for fever, if oral temperature is beyond 101°F associated with discomfort.

Day 16 of fever, she was investigated complete blood count (CBC): white blood cell (WBC)—7,200, hemoglobin (Hb)—6.5, normocytic hypochromic. Polymorphs—52%, platelet—1.5 × 10^3 cmm, erythrocyte sedimentation rate (ESR)—raised, peripheral blood smear examination did not show any malarial parasite and any abnormal cell, widal test was negative, rapid malaria test—negative, rK39—negative, serology for dengue—negative, X-ray chest posteroanterior (PA) view showed increased bronchovascular prominence, blood culture not sent as no facility for proper collection and transportation, urine microscopy—no significant pyuria, tuberculin test—negative, urine culture—sterile.

Q1. What could be the differential diagnosis?

Ans. (1) Chloroquine-resistant malaria, (2) Kala-azar, (3) Hidden abscess: subdiaphragmatic or perirenal, and (4) Collagen vascular disease or malignancy.

Q2. What more investigation shall you suggest at this stage when diagnosis is not yet confirmed?

Ans. She was advised ultrasonography of abdomen to look for any hidden abscess and significant mesenteric lymph nodes enlargement and bone marrow aspiration for any abnormal blast cells. All these tests turned out to be within normal limit. Finally serological tests for collagen vascular disease were sent. Child continued to have fever with spikes without rigor and chills. Her serological findings for cardiovascular disease (CVD) were: rheumatoid arthritis (RA) factor—negative, antinuclear antibody test—positive, anti-double stranded antibody—positive. Her final diagnosis was systemic lupus erythematosus (SLE).

She was referred to a pediatric rheumatologist; incidentally later she developed pain, burning sensation in palm, and erythematous rash in both hands and fingers. Later she also developed classical butterfly rash in face. Presently, she is on remission with low dose of prednisolone hydroxychloroquine 200 mg and regular follow-up with intermittent flare ups.

Take Home Message

Noninfectious causes such as collagen vascular diseases and malignancy should be considered in a child with persistent fever along with or without organomegaly after ruling out infective causes with relevant investigations.

CASE 2

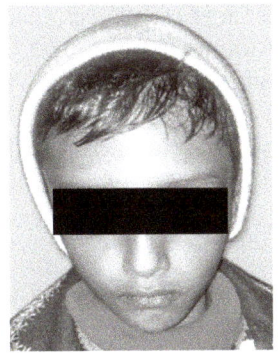

Anurag, 8-year-old child, was brought to me with complain of irregular fever since 14 days and loss of appetite. The child started having fever since 2 days and examined by a local pediatrician. He investigated the child; *CBC*: Normal, serum glutamic pyruvic transaminase (SGPT): 58. The child was advised cefixime 200 BD and paracetamol 125 mg SOS when temperature was more than 100°F along with multivitamin syrup.

The child continued to have persistent fever. The treating pediatrician added ofloxacillin 200 mg BD. The fever and loss of appetite persisted. He was brought to me on 14th day of fever. He had not visited in recent past any endemic zones with dengue fever, rickettsial fever or leptospirosis.

On clinical examination, he was febrile oral temperature 101°F well looking. His heart sounds normal and air-entry bilateral symmetrical, no organomegaly, no lymphadenopathy, no sign of any meningeal irritation, and no skin rash. He was fully protected with age appropriate vaccine.

He was advised to stop all the previous medicine especially antibiotics. He was prescribed paracetamol 250 mg SOS for fever with discomfort. He was advised to maintain a temperature chart. To continue family diet with plenty of fluid and to report after 3 days with temperature chart. Meanwhile he was thoroughly investigated to rule out infectious cause of persistent fever.

Again the child was brought to me for further evaluation on day 17. He was afebrile with return of appetite since the day child stopped antibiotics. His all tests were within normal limits:

CBC: WBC—12,100, P—38%, L—60%, E—1%, Hb—11 g, and platelets—350,000. Comment on PBS—negative for MP and no abnormal cells. Widal test O & H antigen—1/80. Serology for dengue—negative. X-ray chest PA view was normal. Urine—microscopy no pus cells and urine culture sterile tuberculin test—negative.

Q1. What could be the diagnosis of persistent fever in a well-looking child with no systemic findings?

Ans. The final diagnosis was drug-induced fever.

Discussion

A well-looking febrile child without any focus since last 2 days was started empirical cefixime by local pediatrician based on presumptive diagnosis of enteric fever was irrational. Child continued to have persistent fever despite use of cefixime. However, the pediatrician did not further investigate but added ofloxacin which was another irrational approach of combination therapy not recommended.

What was most likely viral fever which would have resolved on its own became drug induced fever.

Take Home Message

There is urgent need for judicious use of antibiotics/antimicrobials. Antibiotics are neither antipyretics nor panacea for all febrile episodes.

CASE 3

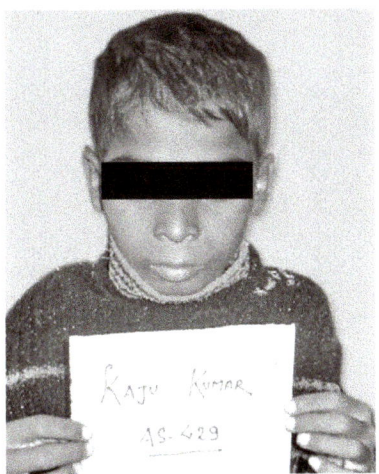

A 5-year-old boy, Kaju weighing 15 kg from village in North Bihar with complains of fever since 15 days. Fever was without rigor/chills. He was under the treatment by a local doctor since last 10 days but fever persisted. He had not visited in recent past any endemic zone with rickettsial infection, dengue fever or leptospirosis. He lived in endemic zone with malaria and kala-azar.

He was investigated by local doctor. His blood picture CBC Hb—9 g%, platelet count—60,000 cmm, WBC—5300, PBS as negative for MP and rapid malaria test was negative.

He was initially given cefixime 200 mg in divided doses by local doctor. After 3 days, doctor added chloroquine but fever was persistent. Then he was brought to me.

Clinical examination: He was pale, well looking, child temperature—102.5°F (oral), weight—15 kg, liver—2 cm, spleen—4 cm, no petechial spots or rash or any lymphadenopathy. He was partially immunized with no Bacillus Calmette-Guérin (BCG) scar. *Chest and CVS*: NAD. No other positive findings.

He was further investigated: CBC: WBC—3,200, polymorph—30%, lymphocyte—65%, monocyte—1%, eosinophil—4%, platelets—80,000, Hb—9 g/dL, PBS—negative for MP, Rapid malaria test was negative , Widal test—positive, O & H antigen—1/80, Tuberculin test—negative, rK39—positive, chest X-ray PA—increased BVP, urine—NAD, bone marrow—not done.

The final diagnosis is visceral leishmaniasis (Kala-azar).

Take Home Message

Visceral leishmaniasis should be suspected in a child with persistent fever, splenohepatomaly in an endemic zone, anemia, leukopenia and positive rk39 (an immunochromographic test) with very high sensitivity and specificity.

CASE 4

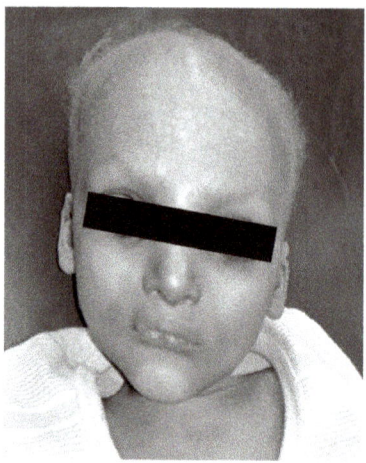

This child, 3-year-old, was brought to me in hot and humid month with complain of irregular fever since last several months. He had visited several doctors and had been prescribed oral and parenteral antibiotics, antimalarial drugs without any response. His fever used to be more pronounced during day time. His fever was not responding to antipyretics.

Clinical examination: He had dysmorphic facies. There was absence of teeth, sparse hair in scalp, dry skin, and hypopigmented hair. He was undernourished and pale.

Systemic examination: NAD. The parent confirmed the loss of sweating despite high-grade fever.

Though the diagnosis was obvious based on history and clinical examination, preliminary investigation was done to rule out any superadded/ secondary infection. His Hb was 10 g%. There was no clinical hematological and radiological evidence of any infection. The urine had no pus cells and was sterile on culture.

Discussion
Ectodermal dysplasia is heterogeneous disorders due to abnormalities of group of genetic ectodermal structures. Mode of inheritance is multiple. Treatment is supportive reassurance and genetic counseling.

Take Home Message

All fevers are not infections. Of the various causes, a genetic cause-like ectodermal dysplasia may also cause fever and should not be missed.

SUGGESTED READING

1. Brinks R, Fischer-Betz R, Sander O, et al. Age-specific prevalence of diagnosed systemic lupus erythematosus in Germany 2002 and projection to 2030. Lupus. 2014;23:1407-11.

2. Cervera R, Khamashta MA, Font J, et al. Systemic lupus erythematosus: clinical and immunologic patterns of disease expression in a cohort of 1,000 patients. The European Working Party on Systemic Lupus Erythematosus. Medicine (Baltimore). 1993;72:113-24.
3. Chehab G, Fischer-Betz R, Schneider M. Changes in mortality and morbidity in systemic lupus erythematosus. Z Rheumatol. 2011;70:480-5.
4. Cluff LE, Johnson J 3rd. Drug fever. Prog Allergy. 1964;8:149-94.
5. Fischer-Betz R, Herzer P, Schneider M. Systemic lupus erythematosus. Dtsch Med Wochenschr. 2005;130:2451-8.
6. Hanson MA. Drug fever: Remember to consider it in diagnosis. Postgrad Med. 1991;89:167-70.
7. Johnson DH, Cunha BA. Drug fever. Infect Dis Clin North Am. 1996;10:85-91.
8. Labony SS, Begum N, Rima UK, et al. Apply traditional and molecular protocols for the detection of carrier state of visceral leishmaniasis in black Bengal goat. J Agric Vet Sci. 2014;7:13-8.
9. MedlinePlus. (2015). Ectodermal dysplasia. [online] Available from https://www.nlm.nih.gov/medlineplus/ency/article/001469.htm. [Last accessed December, 2019].
10. National Foundation for Ectodermal Dysplasias. (2016). Genetics and inheritance. [online] Available from http://nfed.org/index.php/about_ed/genetics. [Last accessed December, 2019].
11. National Foundation for Ectodermal Dysplasias. (2019). About Ectodermal Dysplasias. [online] Available from http://nfed.org/index.php/about_ed/about-ectodermal-dysplasias. [Last accessed December, 2019].
12. Orphanet. (2013). Ectodermal dysplasia syndrome. [online] Available from https://www.orpha.net/consor/cgi-bin/OC_Exp.php?lng=EN&Expert=79373. [Last accessed December, 2019].
13. Reithinger R, Dujardin JC, Louzir H, et al. Cutaneous leishmaniasis. Lancet Infect Dis. 2007;7:581-96.
14. Roush MK, Nelson KM. Understanding drug-induced febrile reactions. Am Pharm. 1993;NS33:39-42.
15. Tabor PA. Drug-induced fever. Drug Intell Clin Pharm. 1986;20:413-20.
16. Talmi-Frank D, Kedem-Vaanunu N, King R, et al. Leishmania tropica infection in golden jackals and red foxes, Israel. Emerg Infect Dis. 2010;16:1973-5.

CHAPTER 6

Typhoid Fever with Jaundice

Kheya Ghosh Uttam, Prabhas Prasun Giri

INTRODUCTION

Enteric fever is a systemic infection caused by *Salmonella typhi*, which involves different organ systems including liver. Liver involvement in enteric fever usually manifests as a raised level of liver enzymes and hepatomegaly. Frank jaundice in typhoid fever is relatively rare. Typhoid-induced hepatic involvement is associated with high relapse rate. So, it is of utmost importance to diagnose and treat it early and also to differentiate it from other causes such as viral hepatitis and malaria.

CASE 1

A 9-year-old boy admitted with history of fever for last 8 days associated with anorexia and occasional loose stool with pain in abdomen. The fever was high grade, regular in nature, not associated with any chill, rigor or rash, and was responsive to antipyretics. On admission, he was looking sick, dehydrated, pale, and icteric.

There was hepatosplenomegaly and capillary refill time (CRT) was prolonged and abdomen was distended.

Heart rate was 148 beats/min, peripheral pulses were feeble, and BP (blood pressure) was 92/58 mm Hg.

Q1. What is differential diagnosis?

Ans. From the history, it is obvious that the boy had some inflammatory disorders characterized by fever for 8 days. Prolonged CRT, tachycardia, and feeble pulses were suggestive of hemodynamic compromise in the form of shock. Presence of icterus points toward some sort of hepatobiliary disorder. Presence of hepatosplenomegaly with jaundice and abdominal distension with fever is likely to be due to some infectious disease with liver involvement. Among the suspicious infectious agent, malaria comes first followed by dengue scrub typhus, enteric fever, and leptospirosis. On the other hand as there is hepatosplenomegaly with pallor and jaundice, it may be a case of hemolytic anemia.

Q2. What investigations would you consider?
Ans.
- Complete blood count (CBC)
- Liver function test (LFT)
- C-reactive protein (CRP)
- Peripheral smear for malarial parasite (MP) and MP dual antigen, dengue, Widal test, and scrub typhus immunoglobulin M (IgM)
- Blood culture and sensitivity (C/S).

Initial management
As the patient was dehydrated and in the state of shock, IV (intravenous) fluid boluses had been given. He was started on empirical IV ceftriaxone with other supportive measures. After fluid resuscitation, hemodynamic parameters improved.

Laboratory test results
- Initial blood reports revealed total leukocyte count (TLC)—3,800 (n 45 L 46), hemoglobin (Hb)—7.2 g/dL, and platelet count 1.5 lacs/cumm.
- C-reactive protein was 256 mg/L (normal less than 6).
- Alanine aminotransferase (ALT) 1,245 IU/L, aspartate aminotransferase (AST) 867 IU/L, and bilirubin 2.4 mg/dL (direct 1.6 mg/dL)
- Ultrasonography (USG) of whole abdomen was suggestive of hepatitis, hepatosplenomegaly, and acalculous cholecystitis.
- MP and dengue came out to be negative.
- Widal test was positive (TO and TH antigen titer more than 1:320).
- Blood C/S revealed growth of *S. typhi* sensitive to ceftriaxone, so it had been continued.

Q3. What further tests you ordered?
Ans. As this patient is having gross hepatic dysfunction, the other causes of hepatic dysfunction must be excluded. There may be some coinfection with some hepatotrophic viruses. So one must do serological tests for hepatitis A, B, C, and E. Serological tests for leptospirosis and scrub typhus should also be done. Prothrombin time/international normalized ratio (PT/INR) and activated partial thromboplastin time (APTT) should be done to assess the severity of liver dysfunction. One may proceed to do fibrinogen and D-dimer.

Laboratory test results
Serology for hepatitis A, B, C, and E came out to be negative. Scrub typhus IgM came out to be negative as well as *Leptospira* INR was 1.8.

Final diagnosis
Complicated enteric fever with hepatitis.

The boy improved gradually and became afebrile on Day 8 of hospital admission. He had been discharged on Day 11 of admission.

Liver function became normalized at the time of discharge and icterus subsided.

Discussion: Though the presence of transaminitis is common in enteric fever, the presence of frank jaundice and hyperbilirubinemia is uncommon. There are slight variations in the liver function profile in 21–60% of cases of patients with typhoid fever. However, acute hepatitis does not occur very frequently and has only been reported in 1–26% of patients. When present, it is a frequent cause of recurrence of the disease. Although clinical manifestations of hepatitis are indistinguishable from viral hepatitis due to hepatotropic viruses (A, B, C, D, and E), the diagnosis may be suspected when a patient has fever, jaundice, and hepatitis (increased transaminases) simultaneously. Hepatic compromise by *Salmonella* was first described in 1889 by William Osler when he reported 8 cases of hepatomegaly and jaundice in 1,500 patients with enteric fever. Ahmed et al. in their study stated that among 254 patients with confirmed diagnosis of typhoid fever, 31 (12.2%) presented with jaundice. In another study by Anjum et al., they wanted to see the frequency of typhoid fever among patients presenting with jaundice. They found that typhoid fever was found in 22 (19.1%) out of 115 patients with jaundice. This liver compromise secondary to *Salmonella* infection is known as hepatitis due to *Salmonella* or typhoid hepatitis. In the stage of *Salmonella* infection, hepatitis is an entity with good prognosis, if antibiotic therapy is initiated promptly. Otherwise, mortality can reach 20% when treatment in patients with severe manifestations such as intestinal perforation and hemorrhage is delayed. Liver compromise occurs more frequently in patients with previous immunosuppression, and it is 15–100 times more common in patients with HIV. Hence, early diagnosis of this extraintestinal manifestation is important in a patient with enteric fever.

CASE 2

A 9-year-old boy admitted with fever for 11 days associated with anorexia and constipation. He also complained of pain in abdomen and passing of dark-colored urine for last 3 days.

On admission, he was looking sick and icteric.

There was hepatosplenomegaly. Liver was soft and tender.

Vitals were stable at the time of admission.

Q1. What is differential diagnosis?

Ans. As the patient admitted with the chief complaint of fever for 11 days, an inflammatory disorder either infective or noninfective had been suspected. There was no history of rash, body ache, joint pain, etc., so possibility of noninfectious inflammatory disorders such as rheumatological disease is unlikely. So we are left with some infections that cause fever along with hepatosplenomegaly with icterus. So, infection with any hepatotrophic organism is suspected.

Q2. What are the investigations you want to do?
Ans.
- Complete blood count and CRP
- Renal function test (RFT) and LFT
- PT/INR and APTT
- Blood C/S
- MP dual antigen and dengue
- Hepatitis A, B, C, and E and IgM.

Laboratory tests results
Blood report revealed TLC 4,600 (N55L42), Hb 10.4 g%, and platelet count 1.56 lacs/cumm. CRP was 56 mg/L (normal less than 6).

Alanine aminotransferase 445 IU/L, AST 386 IU/L, bilirubin 9.4 mg/dL (direct 8.0 mg/dL), Widal-TH—1:320, and TO—1:160 positive.

Ultrasonography of whole abdomen was suggestive of hepatitis and hepatosplenomegaly.

Q3. What further tests you like to order?
Ans. As this patient is having gross hepatic dysfunction, the other causes of hepatic dysfunction must be excluded. There may be some coinfection with some hepatotrophic viruses. So, one must do serological tests for hepatitis A, B, C, and E. Serological tests for leptospirosis and scrub typhus should also be done. PT/INR and APTT should be done to assess the severity of liver dysfunction. One may proceed to do fibrinogen and D-dimer.

Assuming a diagnosis of complicated enteric fever, he was started on IV ceftriaxone and other supportive therapies.

Blood C/S came out to be positive for *S. typhi* sensitive to ceftriaxone.

Fever started subsiding after 4 days of IV antibiotics, but icterus increased. INR came out to be 3.2, injection vitamin K started. Other causes of hepatic dysfunction and icterus has been sought and hepatitis A IgM came out to be positive strongly. Gradually fever subsided and INR normalized. Icterus persisted for 3 weeks and liver function completely normalized after 1 month.

Final diagnosis
Enteric fever (*S. typhi*) with hepatitis A coinfection.

Discussion
Whenever a patient presents with acute febrile episodes with jaundice, the possibilities of viral hepatitis is very much high. Though there are other infections as discussed earlier may present with fever with jaundice. Typhoid fever can present with hepatitis as discussed earlier. Coinfection of hepatitis A with typhoid fever has also been reported, which is one of the most common causes of jaundice in typhoid fever. Jaundice is a rare clinical presentation in typhoid fever; therefore, hepatitis A should be considered in typhoid fever and jaundice because both are enterically transmitted disease and may thus occur simultaneously. Fever with jaundice can be seen in both typhoid hepatitis and viral hepatitis. Although the liver is commonly involved

in patients with typhoid fever, severe hepatic derangement simulating an acute viral hepatitis is rare. Other causes of jaundice in typhoid fever include cholangitis, cholecystitis, *Salmonella* liver abscess, and hemolysis. Presentation of an acute viral hepatitis is similar to typhoid hepatitis, but with a few differences. In viral hepatitis, the fever usually subsides with an appearance of jaundice, and the period between onset of fever and jaundice is usually 1–7 days. However, in typhoid fever, jaundice usually occurs at the peak of fever. Also, the fever persists after an appearance of jaundice. In children, serum aminotransferase levels are markedly elevated in viral hepatitis (8–10 times normal) as compared to typhoid hepatitis, and the ratio of AST : LDH (lactate dehydrogenase) is more than 9 in viral hepatitis.

Balasubramanian et al. found that on admission, children with typhoid hepatitis had ALT : LDH values below 9, and those with an acute viral hepatitis had the values above 9. The coagulation profile is usually normal in typhoid fever even in the presence of elevated hepatic enzymes. A study was done by Jagadish et al. on the hepatic manifestations of typhoid. They found that although the hepatic enzymes were elevated in more than 60% of cases, prolonged PT was observed in only 9.7% of cases. Hence, an abnormal coagulation profile in a patient with typhoid hepatitis should alert one to an underlying infection with a hepatotropic virus or disseminated intravascular coagulation associated with sepsis. The interaction of infections such as typhoid and viral hepatitis is unknown but may be synergistic, and thus leads to more severe liver damage than when the infections act separately.

Take Home Message

- Clinical jaundice is an extremely rare phenomenon in confirmed enteric fever.
- Transaminitis without hyperbilirubinemia is common.
- Co-infection with other heptatotrophic virus (like hepatitis A) can give rise to clinical jaundice with hepatitis.

SUGGESTED READING

1. Ahmed A, Ahmed B. Jaundice in typhoid patients: differentiation from other common causes of fever and jaundice in the tropics. Ann Afr Med. 2010;9(3):135-40.
2. Anjum MU, Khan H, Shah SH. Typhoid fever with jaundice; a clinical study in Abbottabad. Professional Med J. 2015;22(4):439-42.
3. Balasubramanian S, Kaarthigeyan K, Srinivas S, et al. Serum ALT: LDH ratio in typhoid fever and acute viral hepatitis. Indian Pediatr. 2010;47(4):339-41.
4. Deepak NA, Patel ND. Differential diagnosis of acute liver failure in India. Ann Hepatol. 2006;5(3):150-6.
5. Huang DB, DuPont HL. Problem pathogens: extraintestinal complications of *Salmonella enterica* serotype typhi infection. Lancet Infect Dis. 2005;5(6):341-8.

6. Jagadish K, Patwari AK, Sarin SK, et al. Hepatic manifestations in typhoid fever. Indian Pediatr. 1994;31:807-11.
7. Karoli R, Fatima J, Chandra A, et al. *Salmonella* hepatitis: An uncommon complication of a common disease. J Fam Med Prim Care. 2012;1(2):160-2.
8. Mishra D, Chaturvedi D, Mantan M. Typhoid fever and viral hepatitis. Indian J Pediatr. 2008;75(5):509-10.
9. Osler W. Hepatic complications of typhoid fever. Johns Hopkins Hosp Rep. 1899;8:373-87.
10. Parry CM, Hien TT, Dougan G, et al. Typhoid fever. N Engl J Med. 2002;347(22): 1770-82.
11. Pramoolsinsap C, Viranuvatti V. *Salmonella* hepatitis. J Gastroenterol Hepatol. 1998;13(7):745-50.
12. Shetty AK, Mital SR, Bahrainwala AH, et al. Typhoid hepatitis in children. J Trop Pediatr. 1999;45(5):287-90.

Chapter 7

Children with Pyrexia and Unilateral Pleural Effusion

Rohit Bannerji, Mallar Mukherjee, Monjori Mitra

INTRODUCTION

Pleural effusion in children is frequently associated with lung infection. Mostly, it is caused by spread of inflammation and infection to pleura. Due to inflammation, there is leakage of proteins, fluid and leukocytes and causes effusion. With time bacteria invade the effusion and cause empyema. The bacterial organism has changed over time with the advent of antibiotic therapy. The common organisms are *Streptococcus pneumoniae* and *Staphylococcus aureus*, *Haemophilus influenzae* and methicillin resistant *S. aureus* (MRSA). Viral and mycoplasma pneumonia though less frequently but do complicate to cause pleural effusion. The less common bacteria but at times virulent are caused by *Viridans streptococci species, Group A streptococcus species*, and *Actinomyces species*. The parapneumonic effusion (PPE) has normally three stages exudative, fibrinopurulent, and organizational in different time period. The treatments and outcome of the disease also depend at which stage the patient has been diagnosed.

Complications associated with effusion and empyema are infrequent in children. They include bronchopleural fistula, lung abscess, and empyema necessitates (perforation through chest wall).

CASE 1

An 11-year-old boy was admitted to our hospital with complaints of fever, cough, and gradually increasing heaviness and pain on the right side of his chest. There was no other significant history except that her appetite had reduced a lot since a week.

Past medical history: No history of contact with any case of tuberculosis (TB).

Family history: Only child of nonconsanguineous parents.

Physical examination: Child was of average build and nutritional status, febrile, with no signs of respiratory distress. Trachea was central and the apex beat was found on the left 5th ICS half inch lateral to the midclavicular line. Respiratory movements, breath sounds, vocal fremitus, and vocal resonance were all decreased on the right side with a stony dullness on percussion. Rest of the physical examination was unremarkable.

Q1. What is the most likely diagnosis in this case?

Ans. Right-sided pleural effusion, as the findings in the respiratory system examinations are consistent with the same.

Q2. What are the differential diagnoses, which need to be kept in mind?

Ans.
- Consolidation
- Empyema.

Q3. What are the next steps of investigations, which need to be done?

Ans. It is first needed to establish the nature of the pleural effusion as being transudative or exudative as the causes for each are different. Common causes of transudative pleural effusion in children (usually bilateral) are congestive heart failure and nephrotic syndrome. Exudative effusions are commonly due to bacterial infections most commonly pyogenic bacteria (e.g. S. pneumoniae and S. aureus) and TB. Malignancy may rarely be encountered in children.

Hence the following investigations are needed:
- Routine blood counts will give a clue to pyogenic infections as the cause
- X-ray chest posteroanterior (PA) and lateral decubitus view if needed, to ascertain the amount of fluid, signs of TB, underlying consolidation if any, and the necessity of a therapeutic tap, if the lateral decubitus X-ray shows more than 1 cm of fluid.
- *Routine workup for TB*: Mantoux test, GeneXpert from induced sputum, three consecutive sputum samples for acid-fast bacilli (AFB), and pleural fluid biochemistry including adenosine deaminase (ADA) levels and cytology.
- Pleural fluid biochemistry, cytology, and microbiology.
- Ultrasound chest, if the fluid levels are minimal or if ultrasonography (USG)-guided tap is done in cases of encysted pleural effusions.
- Computed tomography (CT) scan thorax, if thoracotomy for decortication or video-assisted thoracoscopic surgery (VATS) is planned, or diagnosis is in doubt.

Investigations result:
Routine blood counts revealed—hemoglobin (Hb) 12.5 g/dL, total lymphocyte count (TLC) 8100/cumm (N76, L18, E4, B0, and M2), erythrocyte sedimentation rate (ESR) 28, platelet 2.65 lakhs/cumm, C-reactive protein (CRP) 77.8.

Figure 1 shows chest X-ray (CXR) of right lower lobe.

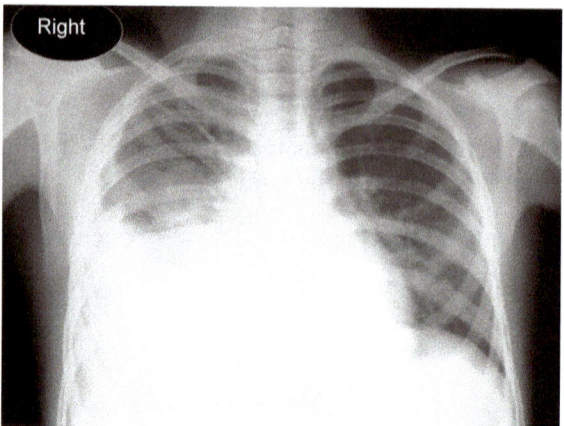

Fig. 1: Chest X-ray revealed collapse of right lower lobe with 450 mL of fluid in the right side.

Pleural fluid was straw colored with coagulum, with cell count 2,700/cumm; with 94% mononuclear cells, gram stain and Ziehl–Neelsen stain showed no organisms, glucose 90 mg/dL, 5.2 g/dL, lactate dehydrogenase (LDH) 361 units/L, ADA 62.3 units/L. Serum protein and LDH were 6.8 and 226, respectively.

GeneXpert assay was negative.

Q4. How relevant is GeneXpert test in children?

Ans. *GeneXpert Mycobacterium tuberculosis*/rifampicin (MTB/RIF) is an automated nucleic acid amplification test that can identify *M. tuberculosis* and rifampicin resistant. While the GeneXpert test appears to be highly specific, its sensitivity for sputum smear negative TB in children remains low. Overall, with induced sputum specimens, the sensitivity and specificity were 59% and 99%, respectively, for one GeneXpert test and 76% and 99% for two GeneXpert tests. It is a rapid test, and hence a better replacement for microscopy but cannot replace microbial culture. WHO now endorses this real-time polymerase chain reaction (PCR) test for diagnostic criteria for TB both pulmonary and extrapulmonary TB.

Q5. How do you differentiate between transudative and exudative pleural effusion?

Ans. The differentiation criteria were laid down by Light and his colleagues way back in 1972.

Fluid is exudate if one of the following Light's criteria is present:
- Effusion protein/serum protein ratio greater than 0.5
- Effusion LDH/serum LDH ratio greater than 0.6
- Effusion LDH level greater than two-thirds the upper limit of the laboratory's reference range of serum LDH

- *Common causes*:
  - *Exudate (local disease) (high protein)*: Local factors influence the accumulation or clearance of fluid.
    - Malignancy—lung, breast, and pleural
    - Infection—pneumonia, empyema, pleuritis, and viral disease
    - Autoimmune—rheumatoid and systemic lupus erythematosus
    - Vascular—pulmonary thromboembolism (PTE)
    - Cardiac—pericarditis
    - Respiratory—hemothorax and chylothorax
    - Abdominal—subphrenic abscess.
  - *Transudate (systemic illness) (low protein <30 g)*: Imbalance between oncotic and hydrostatic pressures.
    - Cardiac—congestive cardiac failure
    - Liver—ascites and cirrhosis
    - Renal—glomerulonephritis and nephrotic syndrome
    - Ovarian—Meigs syndrome
    - Autoimmune—Sarcoidosis
    - Thyroid—myxedema.
- *Note*: There is no ideal biochemical marker that allows complete discrimination between transudates and exudates. Light's criteria have high sensitivity but lower specificity and therefore do not have a high diagnostic efficiency. Rather it was found that the combination of fluid LDH measurements and fluid to serum total protein ratios is useful in differentiating exudates from transudates.
- Using this combination could help in patient management and avoid unnecessary testing.

Q6. What are the treatment options for pleural effusion?
Ans.
- *Thoracocentesis*: It is the most basic procedure used for both diagnostic and therapeutic purposes. The most common indication for diagnostic thoracocentesis is pleural fluid thickness of more than 1 cm in lateral decubitus X-rays of unknown etiology. It can be used to remove a large volume of pleural fluid, if present and then it becomes a therapeutic procedure as well.
- *Drainage catheter placement*: This is used for complicated pleural effusions which will not resolve unless the pleural fluid is drained. Examples include exudates, empyema, and hemothorax which are the most common indications for the placement of drains. Other indications include malignant/recurrent effusion, chylothorax, pneumothorax, hemopneumothorax, and leakage into the pleural space from esophageal or gastric rupture.
- *Intrapleural fibrinolytic therapy*: Used in conjunction with drainage catheters, fibrinolytic agents such as streptokinase, urokinase, and recombinant tissue plasminogen activator have been instilled in the

intrapleural space to enhance the drainage in patients with multiloculated PPEs or empyema. During the transitional fibropurulent stage of empyema, simple drainage placement is inadequate to allow removal of the entire fluid due to its multiloculated nature. Hence, the fibrinolytic agents need to be added to breakdown the fibrous septations and improve drainage in these cases.
- *Pleurodesis*: The procedure where the pleural space is artificially obliterated by adding sclerosing agents like talc, minocycline, tetracycline, etc. to prevent recurrence. This is done particularly in case of malignant pleural effusions.
- *Surgical decortication by open thoracotomy or VATS*: Decortication is a surgical procedure that removes a restrictive layer of fibrous tissue overlying the lung, chest wall, and diaphragm. The aim of decortication is to remove this layer and allow the lung to reexpand. When the peel is removed, compliance in the chest wall returns, the lung is able to expand and deflate, and patient symptoms improve rapidly. It is done in advanced cases of empyema.

Video-assisted thoracoscopic surgery is preferred due to minimal scar, lower morbidity and faster patient recovery but occasionally the VATS may be needed to convert to open thoracotomy during the operation, if the fibrous layer is too thick or the surgeon is unable to free the lung through the small incisions (ports) during the VATS.

Amongst the VATS, open surgery and conventional treatment for empyema, most authors now recommend VATS as the first line of management for empyema.

Q7. What is the most likely diagnosis and why?

Ans. The pleural fluid shows an exudative picture and with the straw color, 94% mononuclear cells and high ADA of 62.3; it is most likely to be *Mycobacterium tuberculosis* infection.

Note: Pleural biopsy report received subsequently showed granulomatous inflammation with epithelioid granuloma and Langhans giant cells which was compatible with our diagnosis.

CASE 2

A one-year 7 months old girl presented with fever and cough for 7 days, shortness of breath for 3 days. Fever was high grade and intermittent, and responding to paracetamol. She was lethargic and unable to take feed.

Past history: Apparently well before that episode. Thrived well till now. Known case of reactive airway disease

Family history: History of atopy of mother. No history of contact.

Physical examination: weight—10.5 kg; length—79.5 cm. lethargic; HR—132 beats/min; RR—65/min.

Respiratory system:
- Evidence of respiratory distress
- Decreased chest movement in left side
- Dull percussion note on left side
- Diminished breath sound in left side.

Q1. What is the provisional diagnosis?

Ans. Since the child has high-grade fever and cough, and respiratory distress community-acquired pneumonia is the probability and since the history dates back to 7 days and there was no resolution of symptoms with OPD basis treatment with the evidence of diminished left-sided breath sound, here is possibility of development of left-sided pleural effusion as a complication of left-sided consolidation.

Q2. What is the definition of empyema thoracis?

Ans. The presence of pus in the pleural space.

Q3. What is the prevalence?

Ans. Prevalence in children is estimated at 0.7–3.3 per 100,000 worldwide.

Q4. What are the stages of development of empyema?

Ans. Empyema evolves through the following stages:
- Sterile phase (termed "exudative")
- Pus is present within the pleural fluid (termed "fibrinopurulent")
- A final "organized" phase with thick exudate and heavy sediment (ultrasound or CT appearance or direct visualization).

Q5. What are the common organisms?

Ans. Most frequent causative organisms include *S. pneumoniae, S. pyogenes, S. aureus,* and MRSA.

Other organisms that should be considered include *H. influenzae, Pseudomonas aeruginosa,* and anaerobes.

Mycoplasma pneumonia is a rare cause of empyema, and recent data confirmed the low incidence of this organism in true empyema.

Q6. What is the approach and how to manage to a case of pleural effusion?

Ans. Flowchart 1 shows an algorithm taken from the British Thoracic Society (BTS) guidelines, which is followed in most of the developed countries and sporadically in some cases in our country.

Q7. What are the investigations to be done?

Ans.
- Complete blood count and CRP, procalcitonin—to find out the evidence of infection
- Blood culture

Flowchart 1: Algorithm for the management of pleural infection in children.

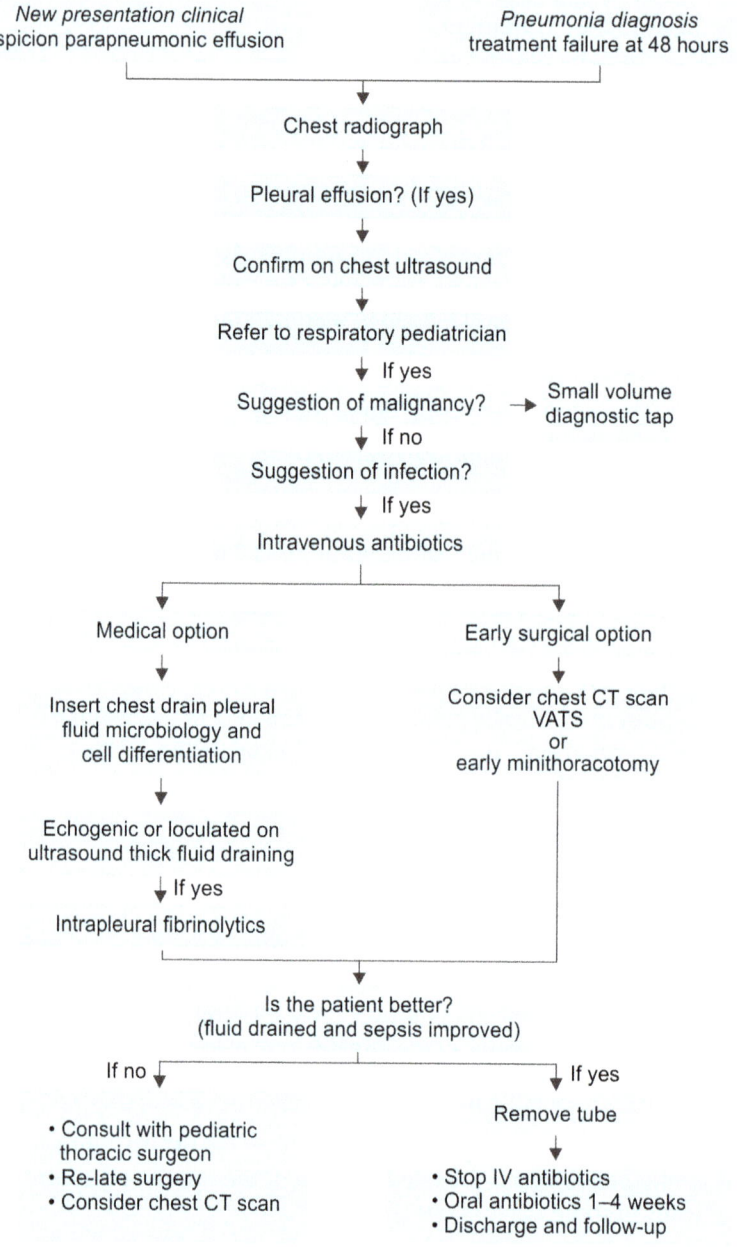

- Urea and creatinine and electrolytes—to assess syndrome of inappropriate antidiuretic hormone secretion (SIADH) and hemolytic-uremic syndrome (HUS) (rarely associated with *S. pneumoniae*)

- X-ray chest—PA view
- Mantoux test.

Q8. What did the initial investigations reveal?

Ans.
- Hemoglobin—9.7; TLC—14,500 (N74, L21, M5, E0, and B0); ESR—46; Platelet—2.4 lakh; CRP—275.3 (<6)
- Blood culture was sent
- Urea and creatinine and electrolytes were within normal limit (Fig. 2).

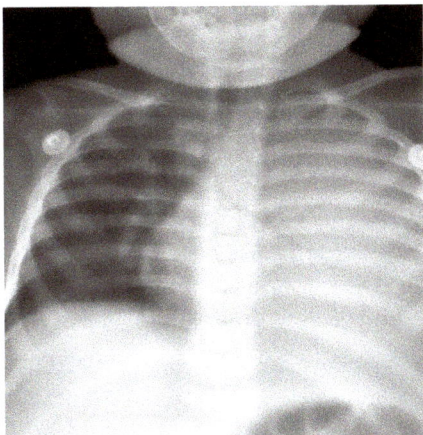

Fig. 2: X-ray shows left-sided homogeneous opacity and obliteration of costophrenic angle suggestive of consolidation with pleural effusion.

Q9. What is the role of chest X-ray in empyema?

Ans.
- Blunting of costophrenic angle initially
- "Meniscus sign" is a rim of fluid ascending the lateral chest wall
- Should be an erect film
- Scoliosis, mediastinal shift and raised hemidiaphragm away from side of effusion
- Complications, i.e. pyopneumothorax
- Lateral CXR is not routinely indicated.

Q10. What other investigation is to be done?

Ans. Since from chest X-ray (PA view), it seems to be a case of consolidation with pleural effusion, an USG chest is to be done.

Q11. How does it help?

Ans.
- Delineates size and location of effusion
- Identifies loculations
- Presence of complication (abscess, pneumatocele).

Q12. What is the role of CT chest and bronchoscopy?

Ans. No role for routine CT scanning in the management of empyema.
Indicated if:
- Surgical intervention required to guide surgical approach, after consultation with the surgical team
- Complicated pneumonia and failure to respond to further treatment to look for coexisting pathology such as abscess formation, underlying tumor, etc.

Diagnostic bronchoscopy is not indicated unless there is concern of an inhaled foreign body or unusual history.

Q13. USG chest shows collection of 300 mL of fluid in left pleural space.

Ans. By the time, Mantoux test has become nonreactive.

Q14. What are the parameters to be checked in pleural fluid?

Ans. Pleural fluid for:
- Sugar, protein, pH, and LDH
- Cell type and cell count
- Gram stain, C/S, and AFB.

Q15. What are the parameters of diagnostic pleural aspirate?

Ans.
- Pale yellow, hazy; clot present
- Cell count 22,000 [polymorphonuclear neutrophils (PMN)—48%; mononuclear—52%]
- Glucose—1 g/dL, protein—3.3 g/dL; ADA—117.8; LDH—7506; pH—7.15.

Q16. How are pleural fluid studies useful in diagnosing empyema?

Ans. The presence of pus, positive Gram stain or culture in the pleural fluid establishes the diagnosis of empyema which should be treated with tube thoracostomy followed by surgical intervention when appropriate.

A pleural pH <7.2 in a patient with suspected pleural space infection predicts a complicated clinical course, and tube thoracostomy should be performed followed by surgical intervention, when appropriate.

A pleural fluid LDH >1000 IU/L, glucose <40 mg/dL or a loculated pleural effusion suggests that the pleural effusion is unlikely to resolve with antibiotics alone and tube thoracostomy is recommended.

Q17. How should pleural fluid cultures be obtained?

Ans. Obtain pleural fluid cultures only from direct aspiration or drainage procedure, not from previously inserted tubes or drains.

Inoculate freshly drained pleural fluid into aerobic and anaerobic blood culture vials in addition to standard, sterile containers used for Gram stain and culture.

Q18. How will you manage a case of empyema?

Ans.
- Supportive therapy
- Antibiotic administration (see later)
- Surgical intervention (see later).

Supportive Therapy

- *Hospitalization*:
    - Oxygen to maintain saturations ≥95%
    - Antipyretics
    - *Adequate analgesia*:
        - Adequate pain relief will have beneficial effects on mobilization and chest expansion and will reduce the risk of hypoventilation-induced atelectasis complicating the speed of recovery.
        - Compensatory scoliosis and shallow breathing may indicate inadequate pain control.
        - Regular oral paracetamol and a nonsteroidal anti-inflammatory drug (NSAID), if hydration is well maintained and if there are no contraindications.
- *Ideal antibiotic management of empyema*:
    - *For community-acquired empyema*:
        - A parenteral second or third generation cephalosporin (e.g. ceftriaxone) with metronidazole or parenteral aminopenicillin with β-lactamase inhibitor (e.g. ampicillin/sulbactam) or third generation cephalosporin and lincomycin or clindamycin.
        - *Second line*: Consider vancomycin or linezolid, if poor treatment response, defined as:
            - Continuing clinical deterioration despite first-line antibiotics
            - Failure to defervesce as anticipated, taking into account the likely clinical course for the organism isolated.
    - *For hospital-acquired, or post-procedural empyema*:
        - Include antibiotics active against MRSA and *Pseudomonas aeruginosa* (e.g. vancomycin, cefepime, and metronidazole or vancomycin and piperacillin/tazobactam.
        - Avoid aminoglycosides in the management of empyema.
        - There is no role for intrapleural administration of antibiotics.
        - Consider continuing anaerobic coverage empirically when the anaerobic cultures are negative unless results reflect a low probability of anaerobic infection.
        - Recent data suggests a low incidence of *Mycoplasma pneumoniae* causing empyema. If suspected, however, a macrolide antibiotic (clarithromycin, roxithromycin, or erythromycin) may be given in addition.
        - The organism, adequacy of source control, and clinical response influence the duration of antibiotic therapy for acute bacterial empyema.

- Antibiotic therapy should be adjusted when identification of the infecting organism and its sensitivities are confirmed by the laboratory.
- Antibiotics should not be discontinued following a negative culture, as pleural fluid cultures are negative in 40% of cases. In these patients, prolonged empirical antibiotic therapy may be required.
- Antibiotic therapy should cover the most commonly encountered organisms.

Q19. What are the risk factors for MRSA infection?
Ans.
- Previous history of skin lesions (e.g. boils)
- Patients from area with known prevalence of MRSA
- Hospital-acquired infection.

Q20. What is the duration of antibiotic course?
Ans. The duration of antibiotic therapy should be individualized, depending on the adequacy of drainage and clinical response of the patient. Common practice is to continue antibiotics for at least 10 days after resolution of fever; antibiotics may be changed from the IV to oral route when the child has been afebrile and without a chest drain for two to five days, or possibly sooner if close clinical follow-up is assured. For community-acquired pneumonia associated with a parapneumonic effusion or empyema, oral antibiotics appear to be as effective as IV antibiotics after hospital discharge. Moreover, oral antibiotics avoid potential complications that can be associated with IV catheters. For most cases of parapneumonic effusion or empyema, a total antibiotic course of two to four weeks is adequate. Infections caused by certain pathogens, including CA-MRSA, may require a longer course of treatment.

Q21. When should chest tube drain be given in pleural effusion or empyema?
Ans. A chest drain should always be inserted in any child with suspected empyema on clinical, radiological, or fluid characteristics. Antibiotics alone can be considered in very small PPEs with pH >7.2.

Conservative treatment with antibiotics and chest tube drainage will be effective in 60–80% of cases, but is associated with an increased rate of treatment failure needing surgical intervention and longer hospitalization (14–24 days) compared with other interventions.

Q22. What is current practice with intrapleural fibrinolytics in management of empyema?
Ans. Fibrinolytic therapy has become standard practice in many developed countries and is recommended by the BTS as first-line therapy for any complicated PPE or empyema. Fibrinolytic agents lyse fibrinous strands and clear lymphatic pores, thus facilitating better drainage. In case of

loculated empyema, instilling fibrinolytic agent is also a choice of therapy adopted by some.

A recent review of the published evidence for fibrinolysis in prospectively designed randomized studies found only four small pediatric studies—three from developed countries and one from India. The studies compared fibrinolysis versus 0.9% saline or VATS. The authors concluded that fibrinolysis should be the initial treatment of choice for all PPE and empyema as its main benefit is a reduction of hospitalization time (6–13 days vs 14–24 days).

The study from India, however, showed no short-term benefit of intrapleural streptokinase versus 0.9% saline.

The role of routine intrapleural fibrinolysis in the setting of developing countries needs to be studied and cannot currently be recommended as routine therapy owing to its prohibitive cost and limited evidence of efficacy.

Q23. When should one consider surgical intervention?

Ans. Surgery is indicated when the children do not respond to the conservative treatment of antibiotic and chest tube drainage. The various surgical options are minithoracotomy and debridement; open decortication involving removal of the thickened pleural peel and pleural irrigation; and VATS (thoracoscopic decortication and irrigation). The indications and choice of surgical intervention are largely dependent on local surgical experience, preference, extent of the illness, and expertise.

A large meta-analysis comparing primary operative and nonoperative therapy demonstrated an overall benefit of primary operative therapy compared with conservative management, but this analysis is also limited as most of the studies included were either case series or retrospective reviews.

CONCLUSION

Childhood pneumonia and empyema continue to be an important problem in developing countries. Parapneumonic effusion and empyema are mostly associated with pneumonia, rarely infection from adjacent areas (retropharyngeal, vertebral, abdominal, and retroperitoneal spaces) may spread to the pleura resulting in development of effusion. The development of pleural effusion is determined by a balance between host resistance, bacterial virulence, and timing of presentation for medical treatments, hence, it is of clinical importance to reevaluate any child who remains febrile or unwell 48 hours after initiation of antibiotic therapy for pneumonia. Patients with PPE or empyema of bacterial etiology recover well, if appropriately treated. Less common but if viral and mycoplasmal origin of the effusions, it usually resolves spontaneously.

Empyema has a complicated course, if not treated and drained early, especially in children younger than 2 years. In a systemic review, studies have shown higher mortality and morbidity rate in children treated with antibiotics and chest tubes compared with those treated with fibrinolytic therapy,

VATS, or thoracotomy, and this also depends on the time of intervention. The mortality rate is higher in children younger than age 2 years. But death from empyema in previously healthy children is uncommon. Management of empyema in many resource-poor countries remains conservative, with antibiotics and chest tube drainage the primary therapy. The roles of fibrinolysis, VATS, or early open surgery need to be studied further.

Most TB effusions completely resolve with the use of proper antituberculous agents. Residual pleural thickening can occur in 50% of patients.

Take Home Messages

- Pleural effusion in children is frequently associated with lung infection, common causative organisms being *Streptococcus pneumoniae* and *Staphylococcus aureus, Haemophilus influenzae* and methicillin-resistant *S. aureus* (MRSA).
- Routine investigations in a case of pleural effusion/empyema include routine blood counts, chest X-ray and ultrasound, pleural fluid biochemistry, cytology and microbiology, TB workup, and CT scan (thorax) when surgery is being contemplated, no response to therapy or diagnosis is in doubt.
- Differentiating transudative and exudative effusions are imperative for treatment planning.
- Light's criteria have high sensitivity but lower specificity, and therefore do not have a high diagnostic efficiency. Rather, it was found that the combination of fluid LDH measurements and fluid-to-serum total protein ratios is useful in differentiating exudates from transudates.
- Treatment can be medical or surgical based on the algorithm laid down by the British Thoracic Society Guidelines.
- Management of empyema in many resource-poor countries remains conservative, with antibiotics and chest tube drainage the primary therapy. The roles of fibrinolysis, VATS, or early open surgery need to be studied further.

SUGGESTED READING

1. Ampofo K, Byrington C. Management of parapneumonic empyema. Pediatr infec Dis J. 2007;26:445-6.
2. Avansino JR, Goldman B, Sawin RS, et al. Primary operative versus nonoperative therapy for pediatric empyema: a meta-analysis. Pediatrics. 2005;115:1652-9.
3. Balfour-Lynn IM, Abrahamson E, Cohen G, et al. BTS guidelines for the management of pleural infection in children. Thorax. 2005;60(Suppl 1):i1-21.
4. Blackmore CC, Black WC, Dallas RV, et al. Pleural fluid volume estimation: a chest radiograph prediction rule. Acad Radiol. 1996;3(2):103-9.
5. Buckingham SC, King MD, Miller ML. Incidence and etiologies of complicated parapneumonic effusions in children, 1996 to 2001. Pediatr Infect Dis J. 2003;22(6):499-504.

6. Byington CL, Spencer LY, Johnson TA, et al. An epidemiological investigation of a sustained high rate of pediatric parapneumonic empyema: risk factors and microbiological associations. Clin Infect Dis. 2002;34(4):434-40.
7. Colice GL, Curtis A, Deslauriers J, et al. Medical and surgical treatment of parapneumonic effusions: an evidence-based guideline. Chest. 2000;118(4): 1158-71.
8. Cruz AT, Starke JR. Clinical manifestations of tuberculosis in children. Paediatr Respir Rev. 2007;8(2):107-17.
9. Desrumaux A, Francois P, Pascal C, et al. Epidemiology and clinical characteristics of childhood parapneumonic empyemas. Arch Pediatr. 2007;14(11):1298-303.
10. Jaffe A, Balfour-Lynn IM. Management of empyema in children. Pediatr Pulmonol. 2005;40(2):148-56.
11. Jaffe A, Calder AD, Owens CM, et al. Role of routine computed tomography in paediatric pleural empyema. Thorax. 2008;63:897-902.
12. Kim HJ, Lee HJ, Kwon SY, et al. The prevalence of pulmonary parenchymal tuberculosis in patients with tuberculous pleuritis. Chest. 2006;129(5):1253-8.
13. Le Monnier A, Carbonnelle E, Zahar JR, et al. Microbiological diagnosis of empyema in children: comparative evaluations by culture, polymerase chain reaction, and pneumococcal antigen detection in pleural fluids. Clin Infect Dis. 2006;42(8):1135-40.
14. Lee YC, Rogers JT, Rodriguez RM, et al. Adenosine deaminase levels in nontuberculous lymphocytic pleural effusions. Chest. 2001;120(2):356-61.
15. Light RW, Rodriguez RM. Management of parapneumonic effusions. Clin Chest Med. 1998;19(2):373-82.
16. Light RW. Clinical practice. Pleural effusion. N Engl J Med. 2002;346(25):1971-7.
17. Merino JM, Carpintero I, Alvarez T, et al. Tuberculous pleural effusion in children. Chest. 1999;115(1):26-30.
18. Metin M, Yeginsu A, Sayar A, et al. Treatment of multiloculated empyema thoracis using minimally invasive methods. Singapore Med J. 2010;51(3):242-6.
19. Mocelin HT, Fischer GB. Epidemiology, presentation and treatment of pleural effusion. Paediatr Respir Rev. 2002;3(4):292-7.
20. Obando I, Munoz-Almagro C, Arroyo LA, et al. Pediatric parapneumonic empyema, Spain. Emerg Infect Dis. 2008;14(9):1390-7.
21. Quintero DR, Fan LL. Approach to pleural effusions and empyemas. Paediatr Respir Rev. 2004;5(Suppl A):S151-2.
22. Qureshi NR, Gleeson FV. Imaging of pleural disease. Clin Chest Med. 2006;27(2):193-213.
23. Romero S, Martinez A, Hernandez L, et al. Light's criteria revisited: consistency and comparison with new proposed alternative criteria for separating pleural transudates from exudates. Respiration. 2000;67:18-23.
24. Schultz KD, Fan LL, Pinsky J, et al. The changing face of pleural empyemas in children: epidemiology and management. Pediatrics. 2004;113(6):1735-40.
25. Strachan RE, Cornelius A, Gilbert GL, et al. Bacterial causes of empyema in children, Australia, 2007-2009. Emerg Infect Dis. 2011;17:1839-45.
26. Strachan RE, Jaffe A. Recommendations for managing paediatric empyema thoracis. Med J Aust. 2011;195:95.
27. van Loo A, van Loo E, Selvadurai H, et al. Intrapleural urokinase versus surgical management of childhood empyema. J Paediatr Child Health. 2014;50(10):823-6.
28. Wurnig, SS,Wittmer V, Pridun N, et al. Video-assisted thoracic surgery for pleural empyema. Ann Thorac Surg. 2006;81:309-13.

CHAPTER 8

Prolonged and Confusing Fevers in Children

Rajesh Rai, Ankita Bhandari

INTRODUCTION

Fever is a controlled increase in body temperature over the normal values for an individual, fevers can be classified as:
- *Short duration fevers*: These are fevers lasting for less than 5–7 days most commonly seen in viral infections.
- *Fever of unknown origin:* These are defined as fever of >101°C lasting for 3 weeks or more for which no cause is apparent after 1 week of outpatient investigations.
- *Long duration fevers or prolonged fevers:* Although a terminology which is 0 now indicates fevers lasting for more than 2 weeks seen in chronic infections.

Most etiologies for different types of fevers are related to age specific infections with different organisms found to be involving different age groups. In the current scenario, the vaccine preventable infections do not pose a threat but a larger threat is faced due to uncommon infections which seem to be fast rising and which may exist in isolation or in combination with other infections. We tried to discuss few of the conditions in children which are not commonly thought of and therefore are responsible for prolonged childhood sufferings.

CASE 1

A 2-year-old male child presented to us with complaints of fever since the past 2 months associated with reduced appetite and history of easy fatigability (reduced physical activity). The child being a second order child born of third degree consanguineous marriage and there were no other associating complaints. On examination, he was mildly pale without any organomegaly. Systemic examination was non-contributory. Apparently normal looking child as seen (Fig. 1).

Prolonged and Confusing Fevers in Children

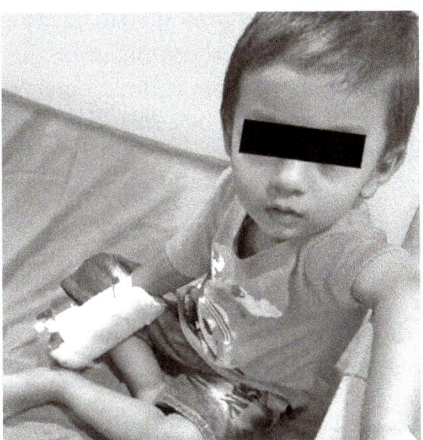

Fig. 1: Apparently normal looking child.

Q1. How will you approach this case?

Ans. The child had prolonged fever for the past 2 months with no other significant complaints. Any systemic inflammatory disorder would have manifested with skin rash, arthritis, mouth ulcers, or other organ involvement over a few weeks, which seems to be unlikely. Presence of pallor is suggestive of anemia wherein we can consider hemophagocytic lymphohistiocytosis (HLH) but again absence of hepatosplenomegaly makes it unlikely. Other chronic infections that could be thought of include tuberculosis, urinary tract infections (chronic), rickettsial diseases, cytomegalovirus (CMV), malaria, kala-azar, leptospirosis, or malignancy. Malaria and kala-azar would have shown severe pallor with splenomegaly while CMV would have been localized to a single organ leading to organ dysfunction none of which is seen in our case. Systemic fungal infections present in immunocompromised host again seem unlikely. Similarly, leptospirosis would show organ involvement with jaundice, lymphadenopathy which was not found in this case. One might think of collagen or rheumatoid disorders as well, but absence of rash and organomegaly disfavors the diagnosis. So the differential diagnosis in this child would include tuberculosis, rickettsial diseases, urinary tract infections, and malignancies.

Q2. Is there any other significant history that we missed out?

Ans. There was a positive history of travel to the village exactly 2 months back post which the fever spikes started, fever was low-grade intermittent relieved on antipyretics, 2–3 spikes per day the pattern of the fever hardly varied over the last 2 months (positive history of travel to the village leading to higher possibility of contact with farm animals, consumption of unpasteurized milk, etc. may indicate *Brucella*). The child underwent many investigations during this period which included serial complete blood count (CBC), blood culture, urine routine, tuberculosis workup, and all of which were inconclusive. The child presented to us for further evaluation and as there was no remission of the fever. On presentation, the child continued to have persistent fever spikes ranging from 100° to 101°, on physical examination, the child weighed 8 kg with a height of 83 cm, mid upper arm circumference was 13 cm, pallor was present with no other significant findings. All other systems were essentially normal as discussed earlier.

Q3. How to investigate?

Ans.
- Complete blood count, peripheral smear and erythrocyte sedimentation rate (ESR)—neutrophilic leukocytosis may favor brucellosis, anemia thrombocytopenia may suggest HLH, high ESR is seen in all three along with tuberculosis
- A screen for viral infections—human immunodeficiency virus (HIV), hepatitis B, and hepatitis C
- Liver function tests (LFTs)—to look for jaundice or derangement of liver enzymes
- Tuberculosis workup
- Urine routine and culture to rule out urinary tract infections
- Blood culture—look for bacterial infections
- Chest X-ray—to look for focus of tuberculosis or a fungal infection
- Abdominal ultrasound—to look for organomegaly or any other underlying abscess or pus collection (thinking of pus somewhere pus nowhere may be pus under diaphragm).

Interpretation of results:
- Complete blood count—anemia, hemoglobin (Hb) of 7.4 with lymphocytic predominance, microcytic hypochromic with normal platelets, and ESR of 35
- Liver function tests—showed a mild derangement of liver enzymes but not significant within range of hundreds
- Chest X-ray—normal
- Abdominal ultrasonography (USG)—normal
- Hepatitis B and C and HIV—Negative
- Mantoux test was negative
- Urine culture—growth of *Citrobacter* spp. sensitive to third generation cephalosporins
- Blood culture—no growth.

Q4. How will you manage?

Ans. As per the laboratory tests, a diagnosis of urinary tract infection was made and the child was started on injectable cefotaxime at 100 mg/kg/day in two divided doses based on the sensitivity. Five days after the starting of antibiotic therapy, the fever spikes still continued and the child had decreased oral acceptance.

Q5. What further tests can be considered?

Ans. Test for rickettsial diseases/*Brucella*—Slide agglutination test (SAT)

Result: The test came out to be positive for *Brucella abortus* which showed increased titers (1:160).

Final diagnosis: A diagnosis of brucellosis with urinary tract infection was made based on the antibody titers; child was treated with oral tetracycline (doxycycline) and rifampicin for a total of 45 days following which the child recovered well.

Take Home Message

Prolonged fevers could be due to infective and noninfective disorders. If due to infection, it could be chronic or any partially treated infections, but any partially treated infections such as typhoid or streptococci will not present with fever for 2 months. Noninfective causes may be ruled out like malignancies often hematological in origin. Since this child also has a history of travel to village area a diagnosis of brucellosis must be considered and we should not hesitate in taking the history again in difficult situations.

CASE 2

This child was 15 month-old female who presented to us with complaints of fever since 10 days, maculopapular rash, anasarca (Fig. 2A), and icterus (Fig. 2B), there was a positive history of travel to native place which was located in the forest region of remote Maharashtra. Fever was low grade initially followed by a afebrile period of 3-5 days post which she started having high-grade fever highest spike being of 106°F. Fever was then followed by maculopapular rash (Fig. 2C) which first appeared on the lower limb followed by trunks and then going on to involve the upper limbs (centripetal progression). After the development of rash, the child developed generalized edema presenting as abdominal distension first then progressing to face and then legs (not following the sequence seen either in renal involvement or cardiac involvement).

General physical examination showed presence of pallor and icterus which developed on the day when the child presented to us that is on the 10th day of fever. Also there was hepatomegaly, liver being 5 cm below the costal margin (span 9.5 cm) and soft in consistency, nontender. On day 2 of presentation the child also developed blackening of three fingers each of both upper and lower limbs (Figs. 2D and E) looking as if it is going to develop gangrene.

Anthropometrically, the child was normal; blood pressure was maintained in the 50th to the 90th percentile range, heart rate (HR) of 120 beats/min and respiratory rate (RR) of 32 breaths/min.

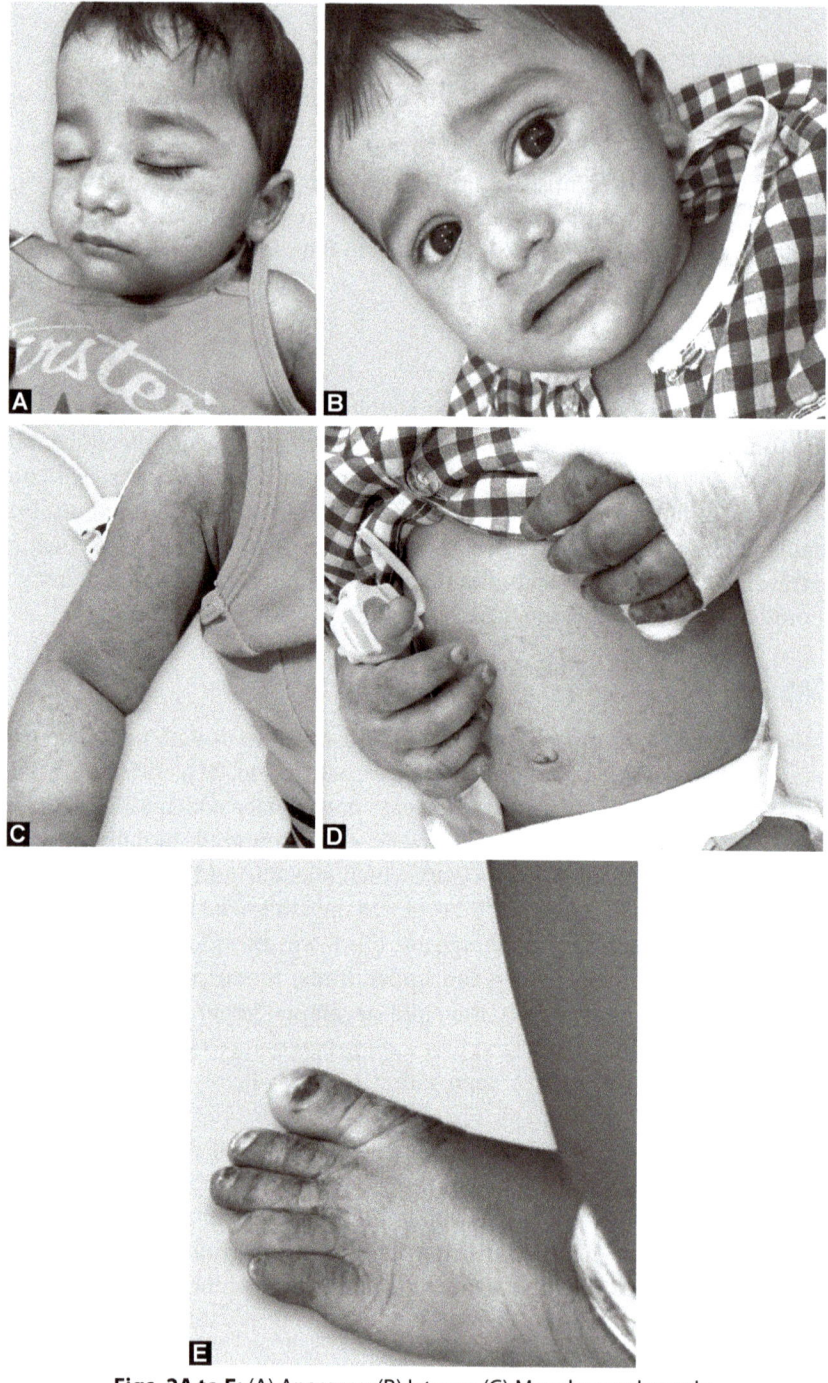

Figs. 2A to E: (A) Anasarca; (B) Icterus; (C) Maculopapular rash; (D) Gangrene of the fingers; (E) Gangrene of the lower limb.

Q1. How will you approach this case?

Ans. The child presented to us with prolonged fever with hepatomegaly, anasarca, rash with discoloration of digits in all four limbs, and icterus suggestive of a definitive liver involvement. This may indicate either a chronic hepatitis or infectious diseases such as leptospirosis or dengue fever since there was presence of rash with hepatomegaly, chikungunya or zika fever, secondary HLH can also be considered as one of the differentials. Since the rash has a centripetal progression first appearing on the extremities and then progressing toward the trunk, it could also be suggestive of rickettsial diseases presence of discoloration of digits could lead us to consider the possibility of microthrombi. Septicemia can also be considered as one of the differentials keeping in view high-grade fever and fast progression of symptoms in a sick looking child.

Q2. How to investigate?

Ans.
- Complete blood count—to look for anemia, thrombocytopenia, and white blood cell (WBC) counts
- C-reactive protein—for evidence of bacterial infections
- Liver function tests—to look for albumin, liver enzymes, and bilirubin
- Prothrombin time (PT) and activated partial thromboplastin time (aPTT)—to look for cause of bleeding
- Dengue NS1 with antibodies
- Color Doppler limbs—to find out blood flow in the vessels for evidence of thrombosis
- Ultrasonography abdomen—for the ECHO texture of the liver and to assess the spread of infection to other organs
- Chest X-ray—to look for underlying infections
- Blood culture—for etiological diagnosis
- Renal function tests—to look for renal status and involvement in view of anasarca.

Interpretation of results:
- Complete blood count—Hb 8 g/dL, platelets—40,000, WBC—19,800, with polymorphonuclear (PMN) leukocytosis
- C-reactive protein—88.3 mg/L
- Liver function tests—total bilirubin—12.5, direct bilirubin—8.8 indirect bilirubin 3.7, serum glutamic pyruvic transaminase (SGPT)—28.6, and serum glutamic oxaloacetic transaminase (SGOT)—57.9
- Dengue NS1 and antibodies—nonreactive
- Prothrombin time and APTT—16.5 (control 12 s), 75.2 (control 33 s)
- Renal function tests—serum creatinine 0.4, albumin—4, blood urea nitrogen (BUN)—20.4, total proteins 5.2
- Albumin creatinine ratio—normal
- Color Doppler limbs—normal blood flow in all four limbs
- Blood culture—no growth.

Q3. How will you manage?

Ans. In view of clinical presentation and the investigations with significant leukocytosis, with raised CRP levels, the child was started on intravenous (IV) antibiotics, meropenem, and vancomycin (as the child had already received many antibiotics including piperacillin tazobactam, ceftriaxone, and amikacin prior to referral to us). Low molecular weight heparin was also started thinking it to be impending gangrene in the digits. Even after receiving a wide range of antibiotics, there was no remission of symptoms.

Q4. What to do next?

Ans. *Tests for rickettsial diseases:* Weil-Felix reaction and antibody agglutination tests.

Results: OXK2 and OX19 came out to be positive which was suggestive of Rocky Mountain spotted fever.

Final diagnosis and management: A diagnosis of Rocky Mountain spotted fever with cholestasis was made and the child was then started on doxycycline with chloramphenicol, low molecular weight heparin was started in view of gangrenous changes, child showed gradual clinical improvement with resolution of edema and decrease in icterus and gangrenous changes.

Take Home Message

Prolonged fevers of unknown origin can present in any form, diagnosis in such children evolves over time as physical signs appear as disease progresses. Hepatic involvement with maculopapular rashes and petechiae are common features of rickettsial diseases, hence one should think of the uncommon when faced with such presentations. Noninfective causes should also be kept in mind such as malignancies or collagen disorders.

CASE 3

An 8-year-old female child came with complaints of fever since 8 days, which was high-grade intermittent type, 3-4 spikes per day not relieved on medication. There was occasional vomiting and abdominal pain since 3 days localized to the periumbilical region. There were two episodes of hematuria with passage of blood in stools as per history given by the mother which could not be confirmed on investigations. Also there was redness in both eyes.

General physical examination showed a sick looking child with hepatosplenomegaly liver being palpable 2 cm below the costal margin (span of 8 cm) and spleen 3 cm below the costal margin, cervical lymphadenopathy with maculopapular rash which appeared 2 days after presentation that is on day 10 of fever and conjunctival congestion was seen. The child weighed 19 kg with a height of 124 cm. No other significant findings were seen. Hematological tests revealed severe anemia with thrombocytopenia.

Q1. How to approach this case?

Ans. Sick looking child with high-grade fevers is suggestive of bacterial infection with toxemia, the child also had thrombocytopenia and anemia with hepatosplenomegaly and lymphadenopathy with bleeding manifestations such as hematuria, this could indicate toward infections such as dengue fever, malaria, enteric fever, and urinary tract infections. We may also consider diseases of hematological origin like hemophagocytic lymphohistiocytosis secondary to any of the above infections. Malignancies should be considered even though there was an acute presentation of the disease. Possibility of tuberculosis should always be kept in mind in case this fever persists beyond two weeks, again rickettsial diseases could also be one of the causes due to their varied nature of presentation and due to the different organisms involved in the spectrum each having their own target organ and a whole range of systemic involvement.

Q2. How to investigate?

Ans.
- Complete blood count with peripheral smear—to look for the blood picture, anemia, thrombocytopenia, abnormal cells, and blast cells
- Liver function tests—for deranged enzymes, indicative of the extent of involvement of the liver
- Erythrocyte sedimentation rate and Mantoux—to rule out the possibility of tuberculosis
- Prothrombin time and APTT—assess the degree of involvement of the coagulation pathway
- Tests for dengue, malaria—for confirmation of diagnosis
- Blood cultures—for bacteriological diagnosis
- Chest X-ray —to look for underlying infections
- Urine and stool routine—confirmation of hematuria and blood in stools.

Interpretation of results:
- Complete blood count—Hb 11.8 g/dL, platelets—85,000, and WBC counts—14,500
- Liver function tests—total bilirubin 0.5, SGPT—193, and SGOT—213
- Erythrocyte sedimentation rate —10, Mantoux—negative
- Dengue, malaria—negative
- Prothrombin time and APTT—15.8 (control of 12 s) and 78 s (control of 33 s)
- Blood culture—no growth
- Urine routine and stool routine—normal, with absent red blood cells (RBCs) in both
- Chest X-ray—normal.

Q3. How will you manage?

Ans. The child was started on IV antibiotics in view of clinical presentation and blood picture suggestive of leukocytosis. The fever continued to persist even after 72 hours of IV administration of ceftriaxone. Injection vitamin K was given along with fresh frozen plasma transfusion to prevent further bleeding manifestations.

Q4. What further tests can be considered?
Ans.
- Tests for rickettsial diseases—SAT and Weil–Felix reaction
- Workup for HLH—serum triglyceride levels, ferritin, and fibrinogen in view of hepatosplenomegaly with thrombocytopenia.

Test results:
- Titers of OXK came out to be positive which was s/o of scrub typhus
- Serum triglyceride levels elevated—486 mg/dL
- Serum ferritin elevated—2,360 ng/mL
- Fibrinogen—53 mg/dL which was low.

All of the above were consistent with the criteria required for diagnosis of hemophagocytic lymphohistiocytosis.

Final diagnosis: Hence a final diagnosis of scrub typhus with HLH was made the child was started on tablet doxycycline for 6 weeks the child improved drastically, fever spikes subsided and the child recovered well.

Take Home Message
As we have seen in the previous few cases, the rickettsial diseases have varied manifestations and they put us under a dilemma of different diagnosis. They present in different ways, therefore these groups of diseases must be considered and a diagnostic plan for the prompt identification of these diseases should be made as they prove to be fatal due to the faster rate of disease progression. Also they show quick recovery when started on the specific antibiotics of choice. Hence although the possibility of other noninfective and infective causes cannot be ruled out along with these, rickettsial group of diseases should be kept in mind and the child should be investigated accordingly.

CASE 4
An 8-year-old male child presented to us with complaints of fever since 10 days and altered sensorium since 4 days for which he was previously admitted outside and treated with IV antibiotics. A septic workup and cerebrospinal fluid (CSF) analysis were already done there which came out to be normal. The child was diagnosed as acute febrile meningoencephalitis. He was started on injection ceftriaxone, the child went into status epilepticus was intubated for 2 days and was on midazolam drip, which was tapered off over the next 2 days and the child was then extubated and referred to us in view of progressive clinical deterioration.

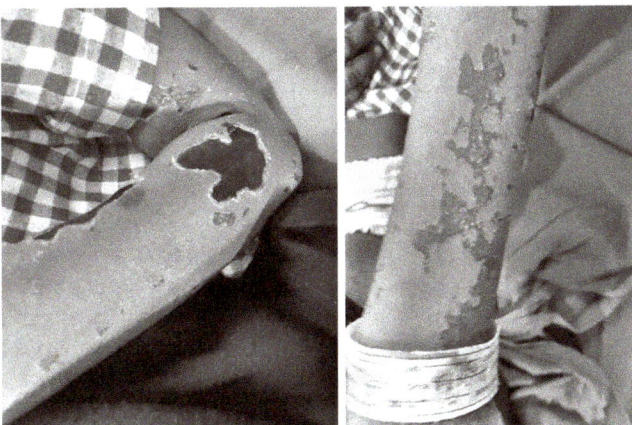

Fig. 3: Scaly lesions associated without pus discharge.

On admission at our hospital, the child had a Glasgow Coma Scale (GCS) of 9/15 rest all general physical examination was normal with no evidence of any organomegaly or lymphadenopathy. Two days after admission at our hospital, the child developed scaly lesions all over the body few of them without pus discharge (Fig. 3) and few with pus discharge (Fig. 4), injection ceftriaxone and injection acyclovir were continued along with antiepileptics in form of valproate and levetiracetam and investigations were repeated.

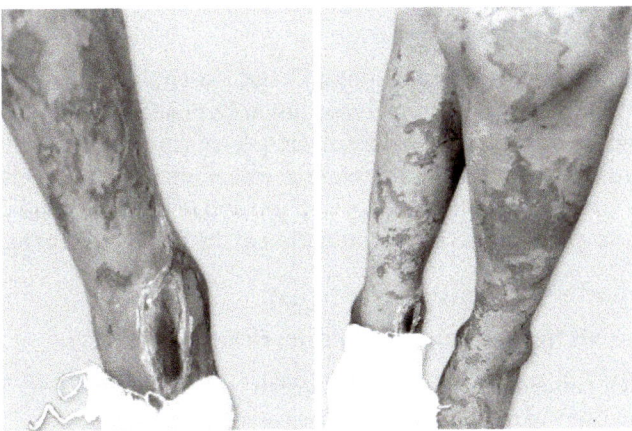

Fig. 4: Scaly lesions associated with pus discharge.

Q1. How will you approach this case?

Ans. The child had already been diagnosed as meningoencephalitis even though the CSF reports came out to be normal. The etiology kept in mind was probably viral with a possibility of partially treated septic meningitis. Meningoencephalitis can be seen as a complication of many bacterial, viral diseases, tuberculosis, malaria, dengue, measles, varicella, and rickettsial diseases. Since the child also developed scaly lesions filled with pus on the body, high suspicion of staphylococcal infections was kept in mind.

Q2. How to investigate?

Ans.
- Complete blood count—to look for raised cell counts and thrombocytopenia
- C-reactive protein—marker of infection
- Cerebrospinal fluid analysis—to look for residual infection or any appearance of new infection
- MRI brain—to look for involvement of meninges as seen in TBM, involvement of cortex because of repeated seizures as he was in status epilepticus, any vascular phenomenon that might have occurred. Possibility of space occupying lesions (though less likely in absence of focal neurological deficit keeping in mind the age of the child)
- Blood culture—for etiological diagnosis and confirmation of bacterial disease.

Interpretation of results:
- Complete blood count—Hb—9.2 g/dL, WBC—10,000, platelets—50,000
- C-reactive protein—202 mg/dL
- Cerebrospinal fluid—picture normal, no elevated proteins or high cell count
- MRI brain—suggestive of diffuse cerebritis
- Blood culture—came out to be positive for Methicillin-Resistant *Staphylococcus aureus* (MRSA) sensitive only to vancomycin.

Q3. How will you manage this case?

Ans. The child was already on antibiotics and antivirals (cephalosporins and acyclovir) after the blood culture came out to be positive for MRSA, the child was started on injection vancomycin as per sensitivity. The MRI showed diffuse cerebritis with edema therefore acetazolamide was also given to the patient, in addition to antiepileptics valparin and levipil. The child continued to have fever spikes after 3 days of initiation of the above treatment.

Q4. What further tests can be considered?

Ans. Weil–Felix test and antibody titers for rickettsial diseases.

Result: OXK came out to be positive which was indicative of scrub typhus (significant titers of more than 1:80 were seen).

Take Home Message

Meningoencephalitis is seen as a complication of many diseases 14% of which included scrub typhus, hence with such a presentation when the child after receiving many antibiotics and anti-MRSA treatment given after MRSA was positive in blood culture continued to deteriorate possibility of superimposed infection or two infection coexisting should be considered. Even though a screen for pathogenic bacterial infections has come out to be positive (MRSA in this case) a look out for uncommon infections with common complications should also be kept in mind.

Rickettsial diseases though ignored seem to be a cause for life-threatening complications hence a possibility of these should always be kept in mind

Q5. What this chapter adds?

Ans. In lieu of existence of common diseases and a narrow spectrum of thinking, we tend to forget the possibilities of existence of uncommon diseases. This chapter gives us an overview to increase our horizons of thinking. A single diagnosis, if explains the signs and symptoms of a disease mostly is the correct diagnosis. We should always consider coinfection with other organisms in cases, where it does not follow the natural course of the disease. Additional signs or symptoms or not responding patients make us think either to revise the diagnosis or look for other possible infections.

SUGGESTED READING

1. Centre of disease control and prevention (CDC). Rickettsial diseases. [online] Available from: http://www.cdc.gov/ncidod/diseases/sunmenus/sub_rickettsial.htm [Last accessed December, 2009].
2. Chahota R, Sharma M, Katoch RC, et al. Brucellosis outbreak in an organized dairy farm involving cows and in contact human beings in Himachal Pradesh, India. Vet Arh. 2003;73:95-102.
3. Kliegman, Stanton, St. Geme, Schor. Nelson's Textbook of Pediatrics. 20th Edition, Vol 2, First south Asia Edition, Elsevier: Pages 1419-1421 (chapter 207, table 207-1); 1500-1501 (Chapter 228.1); 1504-1505 (Chapter 229).
4. Kochar DK, Kumawat BL, Agarwal N, et al. Meningoencephalitis in brucellosis. Neurol India. 2000;55:271-5.
5. Kulkarni A. Childhood rickettsiosis. Indian J Pediatr. 2011;78(1):81-7.
6. Parthasarathy A. Textbook of Pediatric Infectious Diseases. New Delhi: Jaypee Brothers Medical Publishers; 2013.
7. Paul VK, Bagga A. Ghai Essential Pediatrics, 7th edition. New Delhi: CBS Publishers; 2009.
8. Rathore MH, Steele RW, Medscape. (2016). Rickettsial infection. [online] Available from: http;//emedicine.medscape.com/article/968385-overview [Last accessed on December, 2019].
9. Scola B, Raoult D. Laboratory diagnosis of rickettsiosis. J Clin Microbiol. 1997;33: 2715-27.
10. Walker DH. Rickettsiae and rickettsial infections current state of knowledge. Clin Infect Dis. 2007:45(suppl);S39-44.

CHAPTER 9

Fever with Splenomegaly

Dipti Agarwal

INTRODUCTION

Spleen is normally palpable in 10% children and 15–30% neonates. A normally sized spleen measures 11 cm in craniocaudal length. A length of 11–20 cm indicates splenomegaly and that >20 cm indicates massive splenomegaly. Spleen must be enlarged 2-3 times to be palpable. Splenomegaly on physical examination can be defined as palpable splenic edge >2 cm below left costal margin. Patients may at times complain of left upper quadrant pain with splenic enlargement. Radiological evidence of enlargement of splenic enlargement can be seen on ultrasonography (USG), CT scan, MRI and Technetium-99 scan. Infective causes of splenomegaly can be viral which includes cytomegalovirus, Epstein–Barr virus, and human herpes virus-6. Bacterial causes include enteric fever, disseminated tuberculosis (TB), brucellosis, and infective endocarditis. Among parasites, malaria, toxoplasmosis, and kala-azar are important causes for fever with splenomegaly. Noninfective causes may include inflammatory causes such as systemic lupus erythematosus, systemic vasculitis, and hemophagocytic syndromes. Hematologic malignancies such as lymphoma and leukemia may also result in fever with splenomegaly. The mechanism of splenomegaly will depend on the etiology; infection causes increase in reticulonodular cells; cardiac results enlargement due to congestion. Extramedullary hematopoiesis may be involved in hematological causes. Infiltration may result in splenomegaly in malignant causes. Detailed history and focused physical examination are the required rational approach to diagnosis which is then confirmed by relevant diagnostic tests.

CASE 1

A 10-year-old female child presented in the pediatric emergency department with high-grade fever for 5 days. She also complained of passing black-colored stools and extreme weakness. The child was well prior to onset of present illness when she developed high fever. There was no history of vomiting, pain in abdomen, or rashes. There was no history of similar episode in the past. There was no history of recent travel or contact with animals or any significant family history. Physical examination showed that the child was sick with severe pallor. The weight of the child was 32 kg and height was 132 cm. Per abdomen liver was about 10 cm in span, firm in consistency, nontender and spleen was 4 cm below the subcostal margin and firm. There was no evidence of jaundice, lymphadenopathy, or skin rash. Other systems were normal.

Q1. What is differential diagnosis?

Ans. This child has short duration of illness with high-grade fever, hepatosplenomegaly, severe pallor, and black stools as the key presenting features. Noninfective disorder such as systemic inflammatory disorder would have manifested with skin rash, arthritis, renal involvement over a period of few weeks, and seems unlikely in this patient. Absence of petechial rash, lymphadenopathy, and short history makes hematological malignancy unlikely. Chronic infections such as TB, brucellosis, and visceral leishmaniasis (VL) will have nonspecific features of reduced appetite, failure to thrive, and longer course of illness which are absent in this child. Fungal infection presents in an immunocompromised host and such features are not present in this patient. Viral hepatitis also seems unlikely due to absence of icterus and tender hepatomegaly. Absence of lymphadenopathy and pharyngitis does not favor the diagnosis of infectious mononucleosis. Anemia is unusual for enteric fever and the infection has predominantly gastrointestinal symptoms making the diagnosis less likely. So, differential diagnosis in this child would include infections such as malaria, dengue, and rickettsial diseases such as scrub typhus which can have short course of high-grade fever with hepatosplenomegaly. Rickettsial disease may often present as triad of fever, rash, and headache.

Q2. What investigations would you consider?

Ans. *Complete blood counts*: Total leukocyte count (TLC) may be normal or low; leukocytosis is seen in advanced rickettsial infections along with low platelets. Low platelets will be expected in dengue infection and can also be present in complicated malaria. TLC may be low in dengue infection which is usually normal in malaria. Hemoglobin levels will be low in malaria and rickettsial infections but is expected to be normal in dengue infection.

Peripheral smear: Both thick and thin smear should be examined for malaria. As concentration of RBCs is much more in thick smear, so chances of demonstration of malarial parasite are more. Thin smear helps in species identification. Thick smear have sensitivity of 5–10 parasites/µL and thin smears can detect 200 parasites/µL.

Liver function tests: Serum bilirubin may be raised in malaria due to hemolysis. There may be elevated transaminase levels in dengue and rickettsial infections.

Chest X-ray: There may be pleural effusion in dengue due to capillary leaks. Rickettsial infection may show infiltrations and sometimes reticulonodular shadows may be present. However, it is unremarkable in malaria.

USG abdomen: It will reveal hepatosplenomegaly in all these conditions. Ascites may be seen with dengue infection and in rickettsial disease.

Laboratory test results:
- *Complete blood count*: Hemoglobin was 4.6 g%, platelet count was 35,000/dL, and TLC was 6,000/dL.
- *Peripheral smear* did not demonstrate malaria parasite. It is perhaps important to obtain at least three smears 12–24 hours apart for successful demonstration of parasite. However, taking smears at the time of fever is not required for demonstration of the parasite.
- *Liver enzymes* were within normal range.
- *Chest X-ray* was normal.
- *USG abdomen* showed hepatosplenomegaly.

Q3. What further tests would you order?

Ans. *Rapid diagnostic test (RDT)*: Histidine-rich protein is used for diagnosis of *Plasmodium falciparum*. In India, RDTs use either LDH specific for *P. falciparum* or pan-specific for other species and is used to distinguish between *P. falciparum* and *P. vivax*. It can detect 100–200 parasites/µL.

Serological tests: Immunoperoxidase assay and immunofluorescence assay are considered gold standards for diagnosing rickettsial disease. NS1 antigen and IgM levels are specific for dengue infection.

Laboratory test result: Rapid diagnostic test was positive for *P. vivax*. Serological tests were negative for dengue infection and rickettsial diseases.

Final diagnosis: Diagnosis of complicated malaria was confirmed based on clinical presentation of high-grade fever, severe pallor, and splenomegaly. RDT also confirmed the diagnosis of *P. vivax*. The child responded when treated with artesunate.

Q4. What was the cause for anemia in this child?

Ans. Anemia can be caused due to hemolysis of red blood cells, impaired erythropoiesis, and peripheral destruction in spleen.

Q5. What are the clinical features and laboratory findings of complicated malaria?

Ans. Features of complicated malaria include impaired consciousness, prostration, multiple convulsions, circulatory collapse, acidotic breathing. Laboratory findings include hypoglycemia, severe anemia, hyperlactatemia, and thrombocytopenia renal impairment. In this case, severe anemia <5 g/dL and black stools with extreme weakness were the features of severe malaria.

Take Home Message

Fever with splenomegaly of short duration with pallor and thrombocytopenia may be due to malaria, dengue, and rickettsial disease. Absence of rash, eschar, lymphadenopathy, and negative serological tests for rickettsial disease show that the infection was unlikely. Low hemoglobin levels and negative IgM levels for dengue infection suggest that infection was unlikely. Positive RDT confirmed it to be *P. vivax* infection.

CASE 2

A 6-year-old child presented with fever for last 1 month and increasing paleness of body. He was well prior to onset of present illness. It started with low-grade fever that has varied in intensity over time. He had poor appetite and had lost some weight in 1 month. He seemed to get tired with accustomed exertion and was reluctant to go out to play. The patient had severe pallor and enlarged cervical lymph nodes. Cervical nodes involved both anterior and posterior triangles. The nodes were nontender and were not matted. The largest node was 2.5 cm in size. Physical examination showed moderate hepatomegaly firm in consistency, nontender with span of 12 cm as seen in Figure 1. Spleen was palpable below subcostal margin and was around 6 cm in size. Other systems were normal.

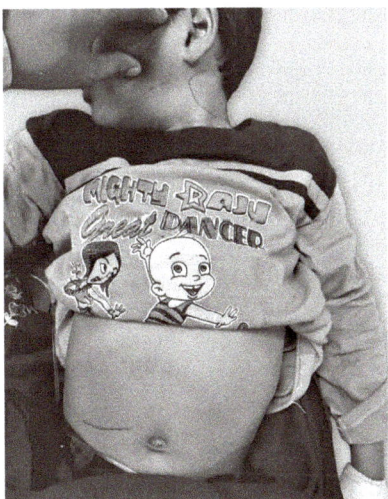

Fig. 1: Lymphadenopathy and hepatosplenomegaly (acute leukemia lymphoproliferative disorder).

Q1. What is differential diagnosis?

Ans. This child had presented with subacute onset of slowly progressive disease with severe pallor, hepatosplenomegaly, and lymphadenopathy. Chronic hepatitis could be a possibility but should have presented with jaundice, ascites, and gastrointestinal bleeding which were not seen in clinical presentation of the patient. Fever of long duration is in favor of chronic infection—most likely to be TB. Abdominal TB can present as nodal, visceral, or peritoneal form, Presence of anorexia, weight loss, lymphadenopathy, and organomegaly favor diagnosis of TB; however, there is absence of symptoms such as altered bowel habits and abdominal distension which are usually associated with abdominal TB. Hematological malignancies could be considered among differential diagnosis. Hepatosplenomegaly, lymphadenopathy, anorexia, progressive pallor favor its diagnosis. However, absence of petechiae, purpura, and bone tenderness does not favor diagnosis of leukemia but these features are present in advanced forms of disease. Infectious mononucleosis seems unlikely as the fever was not acute in onset and there was absence of pharyngitis. Visceral leishmaniasis (VL) also seems unlikely as it is not associated with massive splenomegaly, ascites, and cachexia which usually accompanies the disease. Absence of arthralgia and history of consumption of unpasteurized milk make diagnosis of brucellosis unlikely. Infective endocarditis may be a possibility although absence of features such as heart murmur and history of rheumatic heart disease/congenital heart disease make the diagnosis unlikely. Hemophagocytic syndrome should also be considered as a possibility in this patient. Rickettsial infections may be a possibility due to presence of hepatosplenomegaly and lymphadenopathy. Disseminated TB, hematological malignancies, and rickettsial disease are likely differential diagnoses considered for the case.

Q2. What investigations would you consider?

Ans. *Complete blood count*: Pancytopenia may be present in hematological malignancies and brucellosis. Anemia and low platelets may be seen with rickettsial diseases. TLC may be elevated in rickettsial diseases.

General blood picture (GBP): Immature cells or blast cells may be present in leukemia.

Chest X-ray: Mediastinal widening may be present in leukemia and lymphoma. Presence of hilar lymphadenopathy, and miliary and fibrocavitary lesions may be highly suggestive for TB. Infiltrates may be present in rickettsial infections.

USG abdomen: Lymphadenopathy >10 mm in short axis, omental thickening, bowel wall thickening will be suggestive for TB. Leukemia and lymphoma will show hepatosplenomegaly (Fig. 1).

Tuberculin test (2 TU/5 TU): Presence of induration >10 mm will be suggestive for TB.

Fine-needle aspiration cytology (FNAC) lymph node: Granulomatous formation with caseous necrosis will suggest TB. Lymphoma may show characteristic histopathology with lymphocyte depletion, lymphocyte cellularity, and nodular sclerosis or the characteristic Reed–Sternberg cells.

Laboratory test results:
- Complete blood count showed Hb 3.6 g%, TLC 13,000/dL with 60% polymorphs, and platelets 85,000/dL
- FNAC showed epithelial cells with no evidence of granuloma
- Chest X-ray showed mediastinal widening.
- Tuberculin skin test showed no induration.
- Serum ferritin was normal.
- Serum fibrinogen levels were normal.

Q3. What further investigations will be done?

Ans. *Bone marrow* was performed to confirm the diagnosis of hematological malignancy.

Biopsy of lymph node was performed and is preferred over FNAC for diagnosis of lymphoma and to differentiate it from TB.

Cartridge-based nucleic acid amplification test (CBNAAT): Results of FNAC of lymph node and tuberculin skin test were not suggestive for TB. Mediastinal widening could be presentation for TB, hence CBNAAT for *Mycobacterium tuberculosis* was performed on gastric aspirate samples.

Results: Bone marrow showed evidence of leukemic cells. Biopsy of lymph node was not consistent with lymphoma or TB. Results of CBNAAT were not suggestive for TB.

Diagnosis is acute lymphoblastic leukemia was made based on evidence of fever, weight loss, cervical lymph node enlargement and presence of hepatosplenomegaly. Chest X-ray showing mediastinal lymphadenopathy supported the diagnosis. The diagnosis was confirmed by bone marrow showing the presence of leukemic cells.

Take Home Message

Diagnosis in a child presenting with prolonged fever, lymphadenopathy, and hepatosplenomegaly with bicytopenia should be evaluated for hematological malignancies and chronic infections such as TB and infective endocarditis. Hemophagocytic syndromes can be ruled out in the patient due to lack of laboratory support such as normal levels of ferritin and fibrinogen. Tests such as biopsy/FNAC from lymph node, and bone marrow help to clinch the diagnosis.

CASE 3

A 14-year-old child presented with fever off and on for the last 6 months. He was well prior to present illness. It started as mild-to-moderate fever that increased over next few days to higher degree. Fever was high grade with few spikes during the 6 months' duration. There was gradual abdominal distension and enlargement of cervical lymph nodes. There was increasing paleness and swelling over feet was present. There was no association with arthralgia/arthritis and rashes. The patient was treated by local practitioners with antibiotics and antimalarial drugs but there was no response. Laboratory tests included repeated CBCs which showed anemia and other tests including serological tests for enteric fever and RDT for malaria were negative. Routine urine examination and blood culture were also normal; serology for various infections such as scrub typhus were also negative. This child was referred to our hospital for further evaluation. Physical examination revealed the following: Weight 35 kg (had lost 5 kg), height 144 cm, temperature 100°F, pulse 98/min, respiration 25/min, blood pressure 100/66 mm Hg. Moderate pallor and pedal edema with painless lymphadenopathy were positive findings on general examination. Massive splenomegaly and hepatomegaly with ascites were the major abdominal findings as seen in Figure 2.

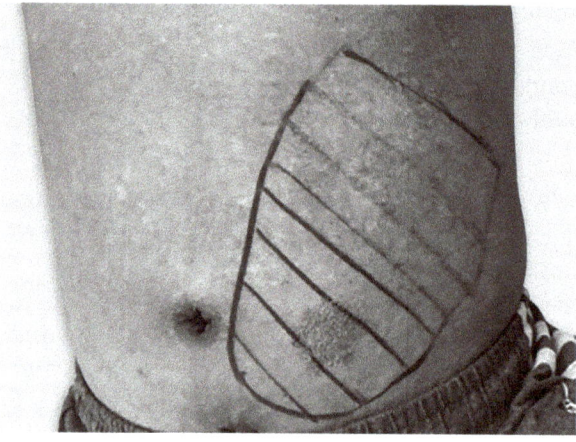

Fig. 2: Massive splenomegaly of patient diagnosed as Kala-azar.

Q1. What is differential diagnosis?

Ans. This child is progressively deteriorating as evident by loss of 5 kg over the last 6 months in a previously healthy child suggesting it to be a chronic process. Fever, splenomegaly, pallor, ascites, and lymphadenopathy could be seen in chronic infections such as TB or brucellosis. Lymph nodes in TB are matted in appearance and may be associated with fistula or sinus formation which was not seen in this patient. Massive splenomegaly is also not a feature of abdominal TB. Brucellosis as already mentioned in the previous case is unlikely due to absence of arthralgia and history of consumption of unpasteurized milk. Chronic myeloid leukemia (CML) may be possibility due to presence of fever of long duration with splenomegaly and increasing paleness. Non-Hodgkin lymphoma can also be considered as a differential diagnosis due to presence of enlarged lymph nodes, ascites, and abdominal mass. Presence of fever of long duration, massive splenomegaly, cachexia, edema, ascites, and lymphadenopathy favor diagnosis of VL. Infections with acute onset such as infectious mononucleosis, enteric fever, and rickettsial disease seems unlikely. Fever of long duration may also be systemic onset of inflammatory disorder but would have developed joint involvement and skin rash. Infective endocarditis may be considered as differential diagnosis in this case due to long-standing fever and splenomegaly. However, absence of murmur and difficulty in breathing make the diagnosis unlikely. There is no history of acquired disease or congenital heart disease making possibility of subacute bacterial endocarditis remote. Hematological malignancies and VL will be most likely diagnosis in this case.

Q2. What investigations would you consider?

Ans. *Complete blood count*: Hemoglobin will be low in VL and CML. In VL, total count will be low and also the platelets can be low as seen with hematological malignancies. However, TLC will be increased CML. Platelets may also be increased in CML.

Peripheral smear: Leishman–Donovan (LD) bodies may be seen.

Chest X-ray: It may show mediastinal widening in lymphoma.

Abdominal USG: To see organomegaly and lymph node involvement suggestive for TB or lymphoma

Fine-needle aspiration cytology: Lymph node to rule TB/lymphoma.

Laboratory test results:
- *Complete blood count*: Hb 5.6 g%, TLC 2,660/dL, and platelets 60,000/dL
- *Chest X-ray* was within normal limits.
- *Abdominal USG*: Hepatomegaly and massive splenomegaly were seen with subcentimetric lymph nodes (Fig. 2).
- *Liver enzymes*: SGPT (Serum glutamic pyruvic transaminase) was raised and found to be 78 mg/dL.

Q3. What further investigations needs to be done?

Ans. Laboratory investigations suggest presence of pancytopenia with raised liver enzymes suggesting a likely infective process such as VL. In order to rule out hematological malignancies and to confirm the diagnosis of VL, further investigations will be required which will include bone marrow biopsy/lymph node/splenic biopsy and demonstration of LD bodies to confirm diagnosis of VL. Serological tests such as rk39 will be performed for confirmation of diagnosis of VL. It is dipstick based on cloned antigen of 39 amino acids developed from the gene of *L* chopsi. The test has a sensitivity of 93% and specificity of 95%.

Test results obtained:
- *Bone marrow biopsy*: They were not suggestive for leukemia. It showed the characteristic LD bodies suggestive for VL.
- *Lymph node/spleen biopsy*: Lymph nodes did not show characteristic histopathology suggestive of lymphoma. Splenic biopsy showed characteristic LD bodies on Leishman stain.
- *rk39 dipstick*: It was found to be positive.

Final diagnosis: Visceral leishmaniasis was diagnosed based on clinical features of massive splenomegaly, long-duration fever, and presence of LD bodies on splenic biopsy and bone marrow biopsy.

Take Home Message

A child with massive splenomegaly and cachexia should be evaluated for VL and hematological malignancy. The diagnosis will require biopsy from various sites such as bone marrow, spleen, and lymph nodes.

SUGGESTED READING

1. Kliegman MR, St Geme J. Nelson's Textbook of Pediatrics, 21st edition. Netherlands: Elsevier; 2019.
2. Parthasarthy A. Textbook of Pediatric Infectious Diseases. New Delhi: Jaypee Brothers Medical Publishers; 2019.

CHAPTER 10

An Infant with Deep Jaundice and Acholic Stools

Alka Agrawal, Nimisha Arora

INTRODUCTION

Prolonged jaundice in newborn is always pathological and is an important cause of chronic liver disease in infants and young children. Neonatal cholestasis is defined as conjugated hyperbilirubinemia occurring in newborn due to diminished flow of bile. There are a number of underlying etiologies for neonatal cholestasis and early detection and intervention is necessary to halt the progression of liver damage. A detailed history and a thorough physical examination often give clues to the underlying etiology. Early diagnosis and timely referral are important for successful treatment and a favorable prognosis.

CASE 1

A 2-month-old female child was brought by her parents with complaints of jaundice since day 4 of life, along with the passage of clay-colored stools and high colored urine. There was no history of delayed passage of stools, constipation, lethargy or poor activity. No history of rash or convulsions could be elicited. The baby was born at full term, with an uneventful antenatal and postnatal period and birth weight of 3.2 kg. On examination, the baby was hemodynamically stable and icterus was present till soles and palms. Weight and height were between –1 standard deviation (SD) and –2 SD and head circumference was between mean and –1 SD. Systemic examination revealed a distended abdomen with firm hepatomegaly, 4 cm below the coastal margin with a span of 8 cm. Rest of the examination was normal.

Q1. What is the working diagnosis?

Ans. Since our case has presented with icterus, acholic stools, and hepatomegaly, the diagnosis of neonatal cholestasis seems most likely. A conjugated bilirubin of >1 mg/dL if total serum bilirubin (TSB) is <5 mg/dL or a conjugated hyperbilirubinemia of >20% of TSB if TSB is >5 mg/dL is used to define conjugated hyperbilirubinemia.

The causes can be either obstructive or hepatocellular, with biliary atresia being the most common cause in our country. The differential diagnoses in this case are biliary atresia, idiopathic neonatal hepatitis, and choledochal cyst.

Q2. What investigations would you consider to ascertain the cause of neonatal cholestasis?

Ans. Any patient with neonatal cholestasis should undergo a battery of investigations as described in Box 1.

Box 1: First-line investigation in a case of neonatal cholestasis.

- *Complete liver function tests*: Total bilirubin with direct fraction
- *Liver enzymes*: Aspartate aminotransferase (AST), alanine aminotransferase (ALT), alkaline phosphatase (ALP), gamma-glutamyl transpeptidase (GGT), prothrombin time (PT), international normalized ratio (INR), and serum albumin
- *Thyroid function tests*: Thyroid-stimulating hormone (TSH), T3, and T4
- Screening for metabolic causes urine for reducing substance and succinylacetone to look for galactosemia and tyrosinemia as the cause of neonatal cholestasis
- *Fasting ultrasound*: Look for the liver size and echotexture, associated portal hypertension, characteristics of the biliary tree, and gallbladder contractions postfeeding
- *Sepsis screen*: Done in a sick child

Q3. Initial investigations in our patient: Total bilirubin—28 mg/dL, direct bilirubin—20 mg/dL, aspartate aminotransferase (AST)—400 IU/L, alanine aminotransferase (ALT)—382 IU/L, alkaline phosphatase (ALP)—560 IU/L, gamma-glutamyl transpeptidase (GGT)—216 IU/L, international normalized ratio (INR)—1.9, and albumin—2.8 g/dL. Ultrasound was suggestive of hepatomegaly with normal echotexture, gallbladder size was 1 cm in fasting ultrasound with no contraction postfeeding and a nonvisualized common bile duct. What should be done next?

Ans. The initial investigations are suggestive of neonatal cholestasis with liver damage (as evidenced by transaminitis and deranged INR) and the ultrasound is suggestive of biliary atresia. However, to arrive at a definitive diagnosis, following investigations will need to be done.

- *Hepatobiliary iminodiacetic acid (HIDA) scan*: HIDA scan can be used to check the patency of biliary tree. However, use is limited nowadays due to low specificity. It is a good modality to exclude biliary atresia, because nonexcreting scans may be obtained in other conditions as well.
- *Liver biopsy*: Both North American Society for Pediatric Gastroenterology, Hepatology, and Nutrition (NASPGHAN) and Indian Academy of Pediatrics (IAP) recommend liver biopsy as an indispensable part of investigation profile for patient with neonatal cholestasis. Establishment of underlying cause and the extent of liver damage can be assessed by the histopathological examination.
- *Intraoperative cholangiogram*: Gold standard for the diagnosis of biliary atresia.

Q4. The liver biopsy was done in this case which showed bile duct proliferation, plugging of bile ducts, lymphocytic proliferation of biliary ducts and portal fibrosis, and suggestive of biliary atresia. How shall we proceed?

Ans. For patients with biliary atresia, definitive treatment is surgical. Kasai portoenterostomy is the procedure of choice. The atretic extrahepatic tissue is removed and a Roux-en-Y anastomosis to hepatic tissues is made. The best results with re-establishment of bile flow are obtained, if the Kasai portoenterostomy is done before 45–60 days of life. However, even after Kasai procedure, the progressive liver damage continues and only 20% of all the patients undergoing Kasai procedure will be able to survive into adulthood with their native liver and the rest will require liver transplantation.

Nutritional management includes adequate calories [125% of recommended dietary allowance (RDA)] and supplementation with fat soluble vitamins (A, D, E, and K). Ursodeoxycholic acid (20 mg/kg/day) may be required for pruritus.

Q5. This patient deferred the surgical procedure and has now come for follow-up at the age of 5 months. On examination, baby was deeply icteric with massive ascites with dilated veins over the abdomen with prolonged bleeding from the venipuncture site. Repeat investigations showed serum bilirubin—34 mg/dL with a direct fraction of 26 mg/dL, AST—500 IU/L, ALT—650 IU/L, ALP—1,020 IU/L, INR—2.8, and serum albumin—1.6 g/dL. How shall the case be approached now?

Ans. The physical examination and the investigations in our patient point toward decompensated cirrhosis (massive ascites, prolonged INR, and low albumin). The standard therapy for any patient with decompensated cirrhosis is liver transplantation. The patient needs to be referred to tertiary care center with the facility for liver transplantation.

Take Home Message

Biliary atresia is the most common cause of neonatal cholestasis in India. Early recognition of the condition is very important as the restoration of bile flow by Kasai procedure has a favorable outcome if done early in life. The most favorable outcomes are obtained, if the surgery for bile restoration is performed within first 90 days of life.

CASE 2

A two-and-a-half months old male child presented with progressive jaundice since day 4 of life associated with clay-colored stools and dark-colored urine. There was associated history of nonbilious vomiting on and off since day 15 of life. There were no associated complaints of constipation, lethargy, rash or convulsions. Mother was unbooked and no antenatal records were available. The perinatal period was uneventful and birth weight was 2.8 kg. On examination, baby was icteric without rash, pallor or superficial bleeds. Baby weighed 4 kg (between −2 SD and −3 SD), length—51 cm (–2 SD), and head circumference—37.5 cm (between –1 SD and –2 SD). Per abdominal examination showed liver palpable 3 cm below the costal margin and a span of 8.5 cm, without ascites or splenomegaly. Rest of the systemic examination was unremarkable.

Q1. What is the most likely diagnosis?

Ans. This is a case of neonatal cholestasis without any other system involvement or any dysmorphism. The important differential diagnosis includes biliary atresia, idiopathic neonatal hepatitis, and choledochal cyst.

Q2. What investigations would you consider to ascertain the cause of neonatal cholestasis?

Ans. The first-line investigations in a case of neonatal cholestasis remain essentially the same (as described in Box 1). Occasionally second-line investigations directed to a particular diagnosis may be required.

Q3. Initial investigations in our patient: Total bilirubin—18.4 mg/dL, direct bilirubin—15 mg/dL, AST—540 IU/L, ALT—674 IU/L, ALP—884 IU/L, GGT—310 IU/L, INR—1.3, and albumin—2.7 g/dL. Urine was negative for reducing substance and sepsis screen was also negative. Thyroid-stimulating hormone (TSH) and toxoplasmosis, rubella cytomegalovirus, herpes simplex, and human immunodeficiency virus (TORCH) profile were normal. Ultrasound showed hepatomegaly with a normal echotexture and a presence of cystic mass in the region of common bile duct, communicating with the biliary tree but distinct from the gallbladder suggestive of choledochal cyst. How will you manage this patient?

Ans. The treatment for choledochal cyst is surgical. The cyst is removed and there is reconstruction of biliary system by hepatic duodenostomy or Roux-en-Y hepaticojejunostomy. Prompt surgical treatment is important to prevent further damage. Also, it may sometimes be difficult on ultrasound to differentiate choledochal cyst from cystic biliary atresia, which may cause early onset of liver cirrhosis.

Q4. What is the prognosis of choledochal cyst?

Ans. Choledochal cyst, even in asymptomatic patients, if left untreated, can cause progressive hepatic fibrosis. The other complications include recurrent cholangitis and ductal inflammation leading to stricture formation and obstruction, development of cholangiocarcinoma and pancreatitis. This warrants early surgical intervention with the excision of cyst and a Roux-en-Y hepaticojejunostomy. Timely intervention with establishment of bile flow has a very good prognosis.

Take Home Message

Choledochal cysts are an important surgical cause of neonatal cholestasis. An ultrasound is a mandatory investigation in all cases of neonatal cholestasis since it can very easily detect surgical aberrations. A quick surgical referral is the key to successful management.

CASE 3

A 2-month-old female baby presented with history of jaundice and passage of acholic stools and dark-colored urine since day 4 of life. There was associated history of vomiting and poor weight gain. No history of constipation, fever or bleeding from any site could be elicited. The child was second in birth order, born out of nonconsanguineous marriage, with an uneventful antenatal and perinatal period. The birth weight was 3.2 kg. On examination, the weight of the child was 3.4 kg (at −3 SD), length—54 cm (between −3 SD and −2 SD), and head circumference—36 cm (between −2 SD and −1 SD). The baby was hypotonic and icteric, with bilateral pedal edema and bilateral cataract. Abdomen examination showed hepatomegaly, 5 cm below costal margin with an enlarged left lobe and a span of 9 cm, along with ascites and splenomegaly. Rest of the examination was unremarkable. On day 2 of admission, the child developed weak cry and poor activity. The blood sugar was 40 mg/dL, which was managed appropriately. Empiric antibiotics were added in view of suspected sepsis.

Q1. What is the most likely diagnosis in this case?

Ans. This is a case of neonatal cholestasis with hepatosplenomegaly and ascites. The associated history of vomiting, hypoglycemia, cataract, and poor weight gain point towards inborn error of metabolism as the most likely underlying cause. Galactosemia and tyrosinemia are the important metabolic causes of neonatal cholestasis. The associated bilateral cataracts and sepsis favor galactosemia as the most likely cause in our case.

Q2. Initial investigations in our patient: Total bilirubin—20 mg/dL, direct bilirubin—16 mg/dL, AST—328 IU/L, ALT—450 IU/L, ALP—786 IU/L, GGT—306 IU/L, INR—1.7, and albumin—2.5 g/dL. Urine was positive for reducing substance but negative for glucose. Ultrasound was suggestive of hepatomegaly with mildly altered echotexture, splenomegaly, and presence of free fluid, with normal biliary tract. What further investigations would you consider to confirm the diagnosis?

Ans. The clinical pointers and the presence of reducing substance in urine without glycosuria point toward galactosemia. Galactose-1-phosphate uridylyltransferase (GALT) assay is done to confirm the diagnosis of galactosemia. The assay will detect the GALT deficiency, which is the most common biochemical defect in galactosemia patients. The other enzyme deficiencies which may cause galactosemia include galactokinase and uridine diphosphate galactose-4-epimerase deficiency.

Q3. How will you treat this patient and what are the expected complications?

Ans. The dietary management is the mainstay of treatment in patients with galactosemia. The elimination of galactose containing food from the diet and usage of various nonlactose-containing milk substitutes along with adequate calcium supplementation may reverse the growth failure and cataracts may regress too. However, on long-term follow-up, the expected complications are developmental delay, learning disabilities, and hypergonadotropic hypogonadism. These complications can occur despite adequate treatment.

Take Home Message

Galactosemia is a relatively rare cause of neonatal cholestasis, accounting for 1–2% of cases. The key to better outcome is early diagnosis. Initiation of galactose free diet may reverse the growth failure, hepatic, and renal dysfunction and cataracts. A high index of suspicion and a thorough clinical examination to look for signs of galactosemia or other metabolic disorders should be done in all cases of neonatal cholestasis.

CASE 4

A 2-month-old male baby presented with jaundice and clay-colored stools since day 6 of life. There was no associated history of lethargy, rash or convulsions. The baby was preterm (born at 34 weeks of gestation) with a birth weight of 1.6 kg. There was no history of consanguinity in parents. Postnatally, he required admission in nursery for management of low birth weight, but did not develop any complications and was discharged on Day 4 of life. On examination, the baby had icterus and pallor, with gross abdominal distension. The weight was 2.5 kg (<–3 SD), length was 54 cm (<–3 SD), and head circumference was 32 cm (<–3 SD). The child had hepatosplenomegaly and ascites on abdominal examination. Rest of the systemic examination was normal.

Q1. What is your provisional diagnosis in this child?

Ans. This is a case of preterm, intrauterine growth restriction (IUGR) child with neonatal cholestasis, hepatosplenomegaly, and microcephaly. These features are suggestive of intrauterine infection. Among the cases of neonatal cholestasis in our country, infectious etiology is found in 17% of all the cases. Among the congenital infections, cytomegalovirus (CMV) is the most common cause. Apart from CMV and other TORCH infections, other hepatotropic viruses such as Epstein–Barr virus (EBV), herpes virus, and hepatitis A–E may cause neonatal hepatitis.

Q2. How would you investigate the baby?

Ans. Besides complete liver function test (LFT), TORCH titers should be done in this case. Titers for immunoglobulin M (IgM) and immunoglobulin G (IgG) antibodies should be done in both mother and baby.

Thyroid function, urine examination for reducing substance, and a fasting ultrasound may also help to exclude other causes of neonatal cholestasis.

Q3. Initial investigations in our patient: Total bilirubin—22.8 mg/dL, direct bilirubin—17 mg/dL, AST—780 IU/L, ALT—850 IU/L, ALP—1,020 IU/L, GGT—400 IU/L, INR—1.3, and albumin—2.5 g/dL. Urine was negative for reducing substance and sepsis screen was also negative. TORCH examination revealed raised CMV IgM titers of 7 UA/mL (>2 UA/mL). Urine sent for polymerase chain reaction (PCR) showed >10^5 copies/mL. Ultrasound was suggestive of hepatomegaly with mildly altered echotexture, splenomegaly, and minimal free fluid, with normal biliary tract. What further investigations would you consider to confirm the diagnosis?

Ans. In case of suspected neonatal CMV disease, diagnosis can be established by examination of the body fluids using PCR or culture to detect the presence of virus. Due to high shedding of virus in saliva and urine, these are the preferred samples in neonate. However, using these diagnostic methods, it is difficult to diagnose after 3 weeks of life whether the infection was congenital or was acquired postnatally.

Ultrasound skull: May support the diagnosis by demonstration of periventricular calcification.

Liver biopsy: Will establish CMV as a definitive cause with demonstration of multinucleated giant cells, periportal inflammation, parenchymal cell infiltrates, and the presence of inclusion bodies.

In our case, high CMV titers, positive CMV PCR in urine along with the supportive evidence of IUGR, low birth weight, hepatosplenomegaly, and periventricular calcifications in brain strongly point toward diagnosis of congenital CMV infection.

Q4. How will you treat and monitor this patient?

Ans. Supportive management should be started by supplementing with fat soluble vitamins A, D, E, and K in recommended doses. For definitive management, intravenous ganciclovir is indicated for 6 weeks in patients with symptomatic congenital CMV infection with severe end-organ involvement, indicated by neonatal hepatitis in our case. The dose is 10 mg/kg given intravenously for 6 weeks. The CMV as a cause of neonatal cholestasis can cause both intra- and extrahepatic cholestasis. The outcome is usually favorable with treatment.

After the treatment is initiated, complete blood count and LFTs should be done weekly for 6 weeks, then at 8 weeks, then monthly.

The CMV blood viral load should be done weekly for first 2 weeks and then at end of treatment. Regular ophthalmological examination should be done in patients with symptomatic CMV disease till 5 years of age.

Audiological testing should be done at 6-month intervals for the first 3 years of life, and annually thereafter to age 5 years. Regular developmental assessment for the first 3 years of life.

Take Home Message

The congenital infections are the causative factor in 17–18% of all the cases of neonatal hepatitis. CMV is the most common virus causing neonatal cholestasis. The clinical examination to look for the signs and symptoms of intrauterine infections should be an indispensable part of the evaluation of a patient with cholestasis. Timely intervention and treatment may ensure a favorable prognosis for these patients.

CASE 5

A 2-month-old female baby presented with complaints of progressive jaundice and acholic stools since day 2 of life. The baby was a product of consanguineous marriage (third degree) with insignificant antenatal history, born with a birth weight of 3.1 kg. During postnatal examination, a hematoma was noticed at the site of injection. Also, a murmur was detected for which echocardiography was done which was suggestive of pulmonic stenosis. On examination, the weight of the baby was 3.6 kg (–1 SD), length was 52 cm (between –2 SD and –3 SD), and head circumference 37 cm (–1 SD). The child had peculiar facial features with a triangular face, deep set eyes, frontal bossing, and a broad forehead. Cardiovascular system (CVS) examination revealed presence of 2/6 ejection systolic murmur in left suprascapular area. Hepatomegaly with a liver span of 8.5 cm was present. Respiratory and central nervous system (CNS) examinations were unremarkable.

Q1. What is the working diagnosis?

Ans. This is a case of neonatal cholestasis with facial dysmorphism and pulmonic stenosis. The triad is most likely suggestive of Alagille syndrome.

Q2. What further studies should be done to ascertain the cause of neonatal cholestasis?

Ans. As discussed in the above clinical scenarios, complete LFTs, TSH, urine examination, TORCH profile, and a fasting ultrasound should be done as first-line investigation in case of neonatal cholestasis.

Liver biopsy: To look for the classical bile duct paucity found in Alagille syndrome. However liver biopsy is not needed routinely.

Further work-up which is required in a suspected case of Alagille syndrome include:
- *X-ray spine*: To look for vertebral defects. Butterfly vertebra may be seen on anteroposterior radiograph. Other anomalies which may be found include hemivertebra, fusion of adjacent vertebra or spina bifida occulta.

- *Ophthalmological examination*: Posterior embryotoxon is most commonly found ophthalmological finding in patients with Alagille syndrome.
- *Echocardiography*: Most frequently peripheral pulmonic stenosis is found. Other cardiac defects associated are atrial septal defect, ventricular septal defect, and Tetralogy of Fallot.
- *Ultrasound kidney, ureter, and bladder (KUB)*: Renal system structural problems such as small, echogenic kidneys, cysts, and pelviureteric obstruction may be present.

Q3. Initial investigations in our patient: Total bilirubin—17.8 mg/dL, direct bilirubin—14 mg/dL, AST—508 IU/L, ALT—850 IU/L, ALP—990 IU/L, GGT—260 IU/L, INR—1.8, and albumin—2.2 g/dL. X-ray of the spine showed T4 and T6 butterfly vertebra. Posterior embryotoxon was present and echocardiogram was done at Day 3 of life which showed pulmonary stenosis. How will you confirm the diagnosis?

Ans. Presence of three out of five criteria makes the possibility of Alagille syndrome very high:
1. Congenital heart disease
2. Posterior embryotoxon
3. Dysmorphic facies
4. Cholestasis
5. Vertebral anomalies.

Peripheral pulmonic stenosis and neonatal cholestasis are the most prevalent features of Alagille syndrome.

For confirmation of diagnosis, mutational analysis for *JAG1* and *NOTCH2* gene mutations should be done.

Q4. How will you manage this patient?

Ans. A multidisciplinary approach is required in such patients.

Supplementation with fat-soluble vitamins (A, D, E, and K) and choleretic agents should be started immediately. The definitive treatment is liver transplantation. However, the success of transplantation depends on the presence of other comorbidities, especially cardiac and renal functions.

Growth and development monitoring, diet and nutrition status, and pancreatic function should be monitored regularly.

Take Home Message

Alagille syndrome is a rare cause of neonatal cholestasis, but the diagnosis is often missed, especially if the classical criteria are not met. A high index of clinical suspicion and early genetic testing are keys to establishment of diagnosis. The prognosis is guarded and depends on the extent of involvement of other systems.

A stepwise approach to a case of neonatal cholestasis is described in Flowchart 1.

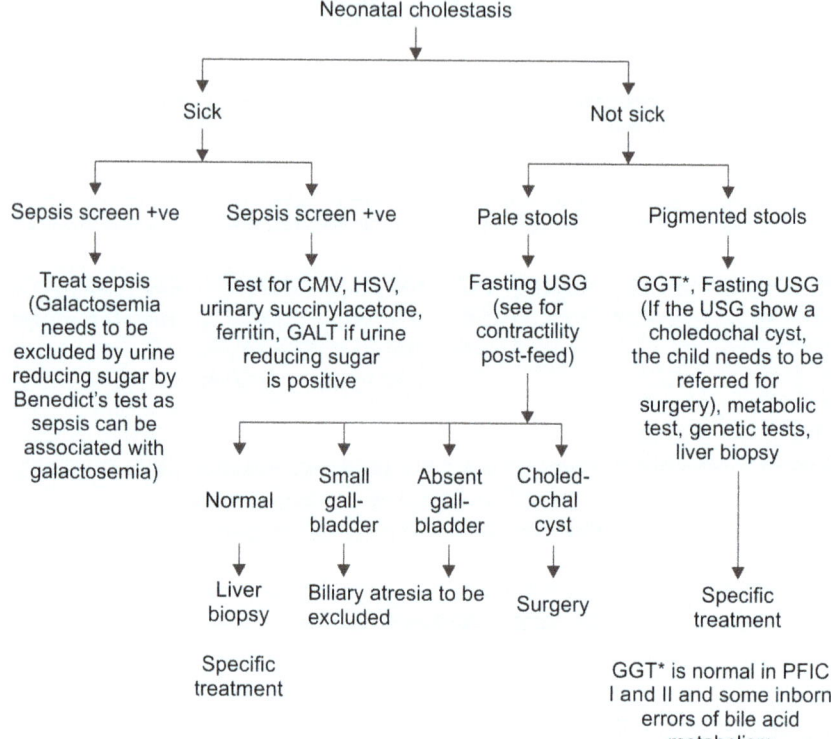

Flowchart 1: Approach to a case of neonatal cholestasis.

(CMV: cytomegalovirus; GALT: galactose-1-phosphate uridylyltransferase; GCT: glutaraldehyde coagulation test; GGT: gamma-glutamyl transpeptidase; HSV: herpes simplex virus; NC: neonatal cholestasis; PFIC: progressive familial intrahepatic cholestasis; USG: ultrasonography)

Source: Pediatric Gastroenterology Chapter of Indian Academy of Pediatrics, Bhatia V, Bavdekar A, et al. Management of acute liver failure in infants and children: Consensus Statement of the Pediatric Gastroenterology Chapter of Indian Academy of Pediatrics. Indian Pediatr. 2013;50(5):477-82.

SUGGESTED READING

1. Beltrán MA, Álvarez M, Palazón SC, et al. Galactosemia as a cause of neonatal ascites and cholestasis. Pediatria Catalana. 2007;67:235-40.
2. Bhatia V, Bavdekar A, Matthai J, et al. Management of Neonatal Cholestasis: Consensus Statement of the Pediatric Gastroenterology Chapter of Indian Academy of Pediatrics. Indian Pediatr. 2014;51(3):203-10.
3. Herman TE, Siegel MJ. Neonatal type 1 choledochal cyst. J Perinatol. 2007;27(7):453-4.
4. Kim J, Yang B, Paik N, et al. A case of Alagille syndrome presenting with chronic cholestasis in an adult. Clin Mol Hepatol. 2017;23(3):260-4.
5. Kumar M, Yachha SK, Gupta RK. Neonatal cholestasis syndrome due to galactosemia. Indian J Gastroenetrolo. 1996;15(1):26-7.

6. Moyer V, Freese DK, Whitington PF, et al. Guidelines for the evaluation of cholestatic jaundice in infants: recommendations of North American Society for Pediatric Gastroenterology Hepatology and Nutrition. J Pediatr Gastroenterol Nutr. 2004;39(2):115-28.
7. Ozkan TB, Mistik R, Dikici B, et al. Antiviral therapy in neonatal cholestatic cytomegalovirus hepatitis. BMC Gastroenterol. 2007;7:9.
8. Swanson EC, Schleiss MR. Congenital cytomegalovirus infection: new prospects for prevention and therapy. Pediatr Clin North Am. 2013;60(2):335-49.
9. Turnpenny PD, Ellard S. Alagille syndrome: pathogenesis, diagnosis and management. European J Human Genetics. 2012;20:251-7.
10. Welling L, Bernstein LE, Berry GT. International clinical guideline for the management of classical galactosemia: diagnosis, treatment, and follow-up. J Inherit Metab Dis. 2016;40(2):171-6.

CHAPTER 11

Child with Unusual Infections

Vinod Gunasekaran, Anupam Sachdeva

INTRODUCTION

Reports of infections caused by unusual organisms are becoming more common. Nevertheless, they are often missed or repeatedly misdiagnosed.

CASE 1

A 5-month-old male child presented with off and on fever, fast breathing, and poor weight gain for the last 2 months. Child was second in birth order, born to nonconsanguineous parents, asymptomatic during initial 3 months of life. Later, he developed the above complaints along with intermittent episodes of oral thrush and loose stools. No significant antenatal and natal history. No feeding difficulties. No previous sibling deaths or tuberculosis in the family. Child was immunized till 2½ months of life. Examination revealed an emaciated baby with tachypnea, nasal flaring, chest retractions, bilateral lung crepitations, and hypoxia. Child has been admitted in hospital twice so far and received prolonged intravenous antibacterials and antifungals. Serial chest X-rays showed progressively worsening bilateral diffuse interstitial infiltrates.

Q1. What is differential diagnosis?

Ans. This child has persistent pneumonia as suggested by prolonged fever and fast breathing over 2 months along with chest X-ray features. Child also has features of malnutrition and candidiasis. The differential diagnosis of persistent pneumonia in an infant can be broadly categorized as infections (congenital or acquired), aspiration syndromes, congenital lung malformations, immunodeficiency (primary or secondary), and cystic fibrosis.

Firstly, infections include acquired infections mainly tuberculosis and congenital infections mainly cytomegalovirus (CMV). Other common viral infections [respiratory syncytial virus (RSV), adenovirus, influenza, parainfluenza viruses, etc.) and bacterial infections such as *Pneumococcus*, *Staphylococcus*, and *Haemophilus influenzae* are unlikely in view of the long-standing history. Perinatally acquired human immunodeficiency virus

(HIV) can lead to opportunistic infections such as CMV, *Pneumocystis carinii* leading to persistent pneumonia.

Aspiration syndromes include gastroesophageal reflux disease (GERD) and H-type tracheoesophageal fistula. They are less likely as there are no feeding difficulties and other features such as arching, cough, and vomiting.

Congenital lung malformations such as cystic adenomatoid malformation and pulmonary sequestration can present with persistent pneumonia. However, chest X-ray in these conditions shows focal abnormalities unlike in our patient where there are diffuse interstitial infiltrates.

Acquired immunodeficiency (mainly HIV) has to be ruled out before considering primary immunodeficiencies. At the age of 3 months, T-cell defects [severe combined immunodeficiency (SCID) and DiGeorge syndrome] and phagocyte defects [chronic granulomatous disease (CGD), leukocyte adhesion defect (LAD), and severe congenital neutropenia (SCN)] are the primary immune deficiencies known to occur. Conditions involving B-cell defects [X-linked agammaglobulinemia (XLA), etc.] are unlikely to present before 4-6 months age in view of passive protection by maternal immunoglobulins (Igs).

Cystic fibrosis can present with persistent pneumonia, malnutrition, and greasy stools (due to fat malabsorption), and hence remains to be a strong possibility in the index case.

Q2. What investigations would you consider?

Ans.
- Complete blood counts (CBCs) with differential counts and peripheral smear examination—lymphocytosis in viral infections, monocytosis in tuberculosis, neutrophilic leukocytosis in LAD, neutropenia in SCN, and isolated lymphopenia in SCID
- Gastric lavage for *Mycobacterium tuberculosis* (most common cause of persistent pneumonia in our setting)
- Sweat chloride level—to rule out cystic fibrosis
- HIV enzyme-linked immunosorbent assay (ELISA)—to rule out HIV infection
- Contrast-enhanced computed tomography (CECT) chest—to rule out lung malformations
- If initial investigations are not contributory, bronchoalveolar lavage (BAL) should be performed for detailed microbiological evaluation.

Laboratory Test Results
- *CBC*: Hemoglobin (Hb)—10.7 g%, total lymphocyte count (TLC)—4,200/mm^3, platelet count—3.55 lakhs/mm^3, differential leucocyte count (DLC)—(neutrophils: 86%; lymphocytes: 10%; eosinophils: 2%, and basophils: 2%), and peripheral smear—no abnormal cells seen
- Blood C/S, gastric lavage for acid-fast bacillus (AFB), HIV ELISA, and sweat chloride levels—within normal limits. CECT chest—bilateral interstitial pneumonia. No lung malformations.

Q3. What further tests would you order?

Ans. Grossly, these investigations seem to be noncontributory. On careful interpretation of the differential blood counts, it shows absolute lymphopenia [absolute lymphocyte count (ALC): 420/mm^3]. Any ALC less than 4,500/mm^3 in an infant merits further evaluation. On reviewing the previous records, it was found that all the previous blood counts showed ALC between 300/mm^3 and 600/mm^3 with a normal neutrophil count. Even though this could be seen transiently in a viral infection, underlying SCID has to be ruled out. The clinical presentation is also compatible with this diagnosis. Evaluation of lymphocyte subsets with flow cytometry and measuring Ig levels will clinch the diagnosis.

Laboratory Test Result
Lymphocyte subset analysis showed CD3+ T cells—53/mm^3 (decreased), CD19+ B cells—3/mm^3 (decreased) and CD56+ natural killer (NK) cells—172/mm^3 (normal). Ig profile showed significantly decreased levels of all types (IgG, IgA, IgM, and IgE).

Final Diagnosis
Diagnosis of SCID (T–B–NK+) was made.

Q4. What are the opportunistic infections in the child leading to pneumonia?

Ans. Any virus, bacteria or fungi can cause life-threatening infections in SCID babies. Isolating the organisms and treating them is key to proceed with the definitive treatment.

Bronchoalveolar lavage was performed and was evaluated for bacterial (Gram stain and culture), fungal [potassium hydroxide (KOH) smear and fungal culture], mycobacterial [AFB staining, culture, and polymerase chain reaction (PCR)], virus (CMV by PCR) and *Pneumocystis carinii* (by immunofluorescence method).

Pneumocystis carinii was detected in BAL evaluation. Rest of the workup was negative.

Further Management
Child was started on therapeutic dosage of cotrimoxazole for *Pneumocystis* (20 mg/kg/day) along with prophylaxis for other infections (*Mycobacterium*, fungi, and viruses). Blood components, if needed, has to be irradiated prior to transfusion in such patients. Once infection settled, child underwent hematopoietic stem cell transplantation and is currently well 2 years after transplantation with complete immune recovery.

Take Home Message

Complete blood count with differential count and smear examination gives immense information while evaluating any child with fever with or without localizing signs. Calculating the absolute counts in a seemingly normal differential count should be incorporated into routine clinical practice, which helps in diagnosing such rare conditions which are otherwise missed. SCID is a medical emergency, which has to diagnose in early infancy before any life-threatening infection occur, to improve the chances of cure.

CASE 2

A 4-year-old boy presented with prolonged fever and right ear discharge for 3 months. Child also had three previous similar episodes since the age of 1½ years. He was admitted at the age of 7 months with pneumonia (grown *Pneumococcus* in blood culture). At the age of 2½ years, he was admitted with prolonged diarrhea, with stool evaluation showing *Giardia* cysts. Family showed two maternal uncles died at the age of 1 year and 1½ years of age due to pneumonia. On examination, child was moderately built (weight at −1 to −2 SD and height at 0 to −1 SD) and right ear showed purulent discharge. He was pale. No lymph nodes were palpable all over the body. Tonsillar fossa is empty. Systemic examination is unremarkable.

Q1. What is differential diagnosis?

Ans. This child has presented with recurrent history of infections since the age of 7 months with history of early deaths in maternal uncles. Multiple systems are involved [ear, lungs, and gastrointestinal tract (GIT)]. Bacteria and parasite are isolated. This clearly points to an underlying immunodeficiency. HIV has to be ruled out first. As the child was apparently well till the age of 7 months, T cell or combined defects are unlikely. Other conditions including B-cell defects (XLA), phagocytic defects (CGD, and cyclical neutropenia), hyper-IgE syndrome, etc. are likely conditions.

Q2. What investigations would you consider?

Ans.
- *Complete blood counts with differential counts and peripheral smear examination*: Neutropenia (in SCN and cyclical neutropenia), thrombocytopenia with small platelets [Wiskott-Aldrich syndrome (WAS)], lymphopenia [can be seen in SCID (mild variants presenting at this age), DiGeorge syndrome, XLA, idiopathic CD4 lymphopenia], eosinophilia (hyper IgE syndrome, WAS), and Howell–Jolly bodies in asplenia
- HIV ELISA—to rule out HIV
- Immunoglobulin profile—decreased levels (in B-cell immunodeficiencies), increased levels (in CGD), increased IgE with normal IgG, IgA, IgM (in hyper-IgE syndrome), increased IgA and E with low IgM (in WAS), increased or normal IgM level with low or absent IgG, IgA and IgE (hyper-IgM syndrome)
- Nitroblue tetrazolium test and dihydrorhodamine test—for diagnosing CGD.

Laboratory Test Results
- *CBC/DLC with peripheral smear*: Within normal limits
- *HIV ELISA*: Negative.
- *Immunoglobulin profile*: IgG 10 mg/dL, IgA <2 mg/dL, IgM <2 mg/dL and IgE <5 kU/L. All were significantly decreased as compared to age

appropriate ranges. Flow cytometry of peripheral blood for lymphocyte subset analysis showed absent of circulatory B cells (<2% of all lymphocytes).

Final Diagnosis

The final diagnosis is X-linked agammaglobulinemia. Diagnosis is based on a boy presenting with recurrent infections since late infancy and evaluation showing decreased level of all Igs along with absent circulatory B lymphocytes. Confirmation of diagnosis is made by demonstrating mutation in *Btk* (Bruton tyrosine kinase) gene.

Management

Treatment of XLA is lifelong regular intravenous Ig replacement. Infusions are given every 3-4 weeks at an initial dose of 400-600 mg/kg titrating the dose and interval to achieve a trough level greater than 400-500 mg/dL in XLA patients. These children do reasonably well on intravenous immunoglobulin (IVIG) replacement therapy. A higher trough level is maintained in patients with pre-existing permanent damages such as bronchiectasis, chronic gut diseases, etc.

Take Home Message

Any child with any one of the following 10 warning signs (given by Jeffrey Modell Foundation) should raise the suspicion of underlying primary immunodeficiency.
1. Four or more new ear infections in a year
2. Two or more serious sinus infections within 1 year
3. Two or more months on antibiotics with little effect
4. Two or more pneumonia within a year
5. Failure of an infant to gain weight or grow normally
6. Recurrent deep skin or organ abscesses
7. Persistent oral thrush or fungal infections in skin
8. Need for intravenous antibiotics to clear infections
9. Two or more deep-seated infections including septicemia
10. A family history of primary immunodeficiency.

Apart from these, any child with unusual infections or infections of unusual severity should raise the suspicion of underlying primary immunodeficiency. The age of onset, spectrum of infections noted and initial investigations (CBC/DLC and Ig profile) will give vital clues regarding the diagnosis.

CASE 3

A 2-year-old male child presented with fever and cough for last 3 months. He was well prior to present illness, except for episodes of upper respiratory tract infection (URTI). Fever was mild to moderate, occurring daily. Cough was wet, intermittent, and episodic with no diurnal or postural variation.

Child also had poor appetite and significant loss of weight. Child started having fast breathing for the past 15 days. He did not have a contact with tuberculosis. On examination, child had sparse depigmented hair, pedal edema, angular cheilitis, weight and height less than –2 SD and rashes over the groin. Auscultation showed coarse crepts over left lower lung fields. No cardiac murmurs heard. Hepatomegaly present. No splenomegaly. Initial chest X-ray was normal. Serial chest X-rays showed worsening consolidation over the left lower lobe along with cystic changes.

Q1. What is differential diagnosis?

Ans. Like *Case 1*, this child has persistent pneumonia with features of malnutrition. Again, the differential diagnosis can be broadly categorized as infections, aspiration syndromes, congenital lung malformations, immunodeficiency (primary or secondary), and cystic fibrosis.

Infection mainly would be tuberculosis or fungal infections, in view of chronic history. Aspiration syndrome is unlikely in view of absence of feeding difficulties or chronic cough prior to illness. Lung malformations are unlikely as the chest X-ray was normal to begin with. Immunodeficiency and cystic fibrosis must be ruled out by investigations.

Q2. What investigations would you consider?

Ans.
- Complete blood counts with differential counts and peripheral smear examination
- Gastric lavage for *Mycobacterium tuberculosis*, Mantoux test
- Sweat chloride level—to rule out cystic fibrosis
- HIV ELISA—to rule out HIV infection
- Contrast-enhanced computed tomography (CECT) chest
- Bronchoalveolar lavage should be performed for detailed microbiological evaluation.

Laboratory Test Results
- CBC, DLC, peripheral smear, gastric lavage for AFB, sweat chloride level, and HIV-ELISA were within normal limits
- CT chest showed left lower lobe consolidation with cystic changes
- BAL showed septate hyphae and culture grew *Aspergillus fumigatus*.

Thus, child was diagnosed as having *Aspergillus* pneumonia and child was started on injection amphotericin. Child started to respond (fever, edema and distress settled and child started gaining weight).

Q3. What further evaluation do you plan for?

Ans.
- An otherwise immunocompetent child developing *Aspergillus* pneumonia with a prolonged course is very unlikely

- Fasting blood sugar and hemoglobin A1c (HbA1c) were done, which were normal
- As HIV was also negative, an underlying primary immunodeficiency was considered
- Absolute neutrophil count and lymphocyte count calculated from differential counts were normal
- Immunoglobulin profile was performed, which showed increased levels of IgG, IgA, and IgM
- Defects in phagocytic function can present with fungal infection in early life, the most common being CGD. Nitroblue tetrazolium test and dihydrorhodamine test were done which were abnormal and suggestive of CGD.

Final Diagnosis
The final diagnosis is CGD with *Aspergillus* pneumonia.

Management of Chronic Granulomatous Disease
Use of life-long antibiotic (cotrimoxazole) and antifungal (itraconazole/voriconazole) prophylaxis have significantly improved the short-term survival rate of these patients. Hematopoietic stem cell transplantation is curative in CGD.

Take Home Message

Chronic granulomatous disease is a heterogeneous disease occurring due to defect in one of the subunits of nicotinamide adenine dinucleotide phosphate (NADPH) oxidase enzyme complex in phagocytic cells. Such defects lead to impaired production of superoxides and reactive oxygen intermediates thereby leading to impaired killing of intracellular microbes. Common infections include *Aspergillus, Staphylococcus aureus, Burkholderia cepacia, Serratia marcescens,* and *Nocardia*. Both X-linked and autosomal recessive inheritance are noted. Nitroblue tetrazolium dye test and dihydrorhodamine test are used in diagnosis.

CASE 4

An 11-month-old female child presented with fever and loose stools for the past 15 days. Child also had three episodes of loose stools previously since day 15 of life requiring hospitalization, intravenous fluids, and antibiotics. *Escherichia coli* was isolated once from blood culture. Child also had two episodes of skin infections in the form of nodules and ulcer formation with no pus discharge, requiring prolonged antibiotics. *Staphylococcus aureus* was isolated once from blood culture. Her umbilical cord was told to be separated at 4 weeks of life. On examination, she was malnourished, having oral thrush, skin nodules with no warmth or redness and moderate dehydration. No organomegaly or lymphadenopathy. Cardiac sounds and breath sounds were normal.

Q1. What is differential diagnosis?

Ans. We have an 11-month-old girl baby with recurrent skin and gastrointestinal infections since day 15 of life. This points to an underlying immunodeficiency. Apart from secondary causes (HIV), primary immunodeficiencies manifesting from neonatal period include SCID, LAD, DiGeorge syndrome, SCN and reticular dysgenesis.

Q2. What investigations would you consider?

Ans.
- Complete blood counts with differential counts and peripheral smear examination—neutrophilic leukocytosis in LAD, neutropenia in SCN, and isolated lymphopenia in SCID
- HIV ELISA—to rule out HIV infection
- Stool workup for identifying organisms—ova/cysts of *Entamoeba, Giardia, Cryptosporidium*, culture for *E. coli*, and stool for reducing substances
- Immunoglobulin profile.
  Further investigations should be based on clues from these investigations.

Laboratory Test Results
- *CBC*: Hb—9.2 g%, TLC—64,200/mm^3, platelet count—3.55 lakhs/mm^3, DLC—(neutrophils: 80%; lymphocytes: 16%; eosinophils: 2%, and basophils: 2%), and peripheral smear—no abnormal cells seen
- HIV—negative
- Stool workup—culture grew *E. coli*
- Immunoglobulin levels were appropriate for age.

Q3. What is the interpretation of clinical details and initial investigations?

Ans. A child with recurrent mucocutaneous and gastrointestinal infections (bacterial and fungal) without pus formation, history of delayed separation of cord, significant neutrophilic leukocytosis, and normal Ig levels are highly suggestive of leukocyte adhesion deficiency.

Q4. How will you confirm the diagnosis?

Ans. Flow cytometry of neutrophils for the expression of CD11b and CD18 shows the absence of CD11b/CD18 expression in neutrophils.

Q5. How will you manage this child?

Ans. Treatment of LAD includes:
- Management of active infections (GIT, skin, and oral thrush in this child)
- *Antibiotic prophylaxis*: Cotrimoxazole and antifungal (voriconazole or itraconazole)
- Close surveillance for early identification of infections and treatment
- Hematopoietic stem cell transplantation in severe cases.

Take Home Message

Leukocyte adhesion deficiency-1 is characterized by delayed separation of umbilical cord, omphalitis, leukocytosis, and recurrent mucocutaneous infections since infancy with no pus formation. It occurs due to mutation in gene coding CD18 (β2 integrin) leading to defective adhesion of leukocytes to endothelium. Absence of CD18 expression in leukocytes by flow cytometry is diagnostic.

SUGGESTED READING

1. Dvorak CC, Cowan MJ, Logan BR, et al. The natural history of children with severe combined immunodeficiency: baseline features of the first fifty patients of the primary immune deficiency treatment consortium prospective study 6901. J Clin Immunol. 2013;33(7):1156-64.
2. Sullivan K, Stiehm ER. Stiehm's Immune Deficiencies, 1st edition. Waltham, Massachusetts: Academic Press; 2014.

Chapter 12

An Infant with Cataract and Positive IgM Rubella

Bharat Mehra, AJ Chitkara

INTRODUCTION

Congenital cataracts are one of the most common treatable causes of visual impairment in infancy. The causes may vary from genetic etiology to metabolic disorders to intrauterine infections.

CASE 1

A 3½-month-old infant presented during his well-baby clinic visit, with mother complaining of poor eye contact and poor weight gain. On examination, weight 2.8 kg, OFC (occipitofrontal head circumference) 35 cm, active alert baby, soft murmur, with no hepatosplenomegaly, eye—bilateral hazy whitish opacity, s/o (suggestive of) cataract with normal pupillary reaction and no eye fixation.

Q1. An infant with cataract, what are the possibilities?

Ans. Majority of cataracts seen in infants are of unknown etiology. However, the known etiology for cataracts seen in the first year of life can be grouped as follows:

- *Intrauterine infections:* They cause central or nuclear cataract.
  - Rubella ⎫
  - Herpes simplex virus (HSV) 2 ⎭ Most common among intrauterine infections.
  - Toxoplasma ⎫
  - Cytomegalovirus ⎬ Very rare causes
  - Syphilis ⎭
- *Metabolic disorders*:
  - Galactosemia
  - Phenylketonuria
  - Homocystinuria
  - Peroxisomal disorders
  - Refsum disease
- *Endocrine disorders*:
  - Congenital hypothyroidism
  - Hypoparathyroidism

- *Chromosomal disorders*:
  - Down syndrome
  - Trisomy 13, 18
  - Turner syndrome
- Miscellaneous

Q2. What clinical clues in history and clinical examination can help us to reach a probable diagnosis?

Ans. Considering the known etiologies, the following information should be sought:

Antenatal: History of rubella immunization, consanguinity, fever with rash during first and second trimesters, poor weight gain during pregnancy, intrauterine growth restriction (IUGR), previous history of child with cataract or genetic problems.

Intranatal: History of instrumentation during delivery.

Postnatal: Birth weight, neonatal intensive care unit (NICU) stay, neonatal convulsions, and neonatal jaundice.

On examination, look for dysmorphic features, microcephaly, macrocephaly, bulging anterior fontanelle (AF), hepatosplenomegaly, murmur, petechial rash, and hypo-/hypertonia.

Progression of Case

The baby was born to a 25-year-old woman, primigravida, non-consanguinity, and spontaneous conception. No history of fever/rash in first and second trimesters, no GDM/PIH (gestational diabetes mellitus/pregnancy-induced hypertension), only one antenatal scan at 18 weeks was done which was normal.

Born at 38 weeks of gestation by vaginal route, immediate cry, with birth weight of 2.1 kg breastfed, with no history of neonatal jaundice/NICU stay.

Present weight: 2.8 kg, OFC: 35 cm (OFC at birth 33 cm), length: 50 cm (length at birth: 48 cm), no dysmorphic feature, apparently normal eyes and ear with open AF (1.5 ×1.5 cm) at level. However, eyes had a bilateral hazy whitish opacity symptom of cataract. Soft systolic murmur grade 2/6, liver palpable 3 cm below right costal margin (RCM), soft, spleen not palpable. Pupils equal size and reacting to light, normal tone, reflexes, and partial head control present.

Q3. How to proceed with investigations in the current case scenario?

Ans. Get CBC (complete blood count) (to look for anemia/thrombocytopenia), blood sugar, thyroid function tests, liver enzymes [SGOT/SGPT (serum glutamic oxaloacetic transaminase/serum glutamic pyruvic transaminase)], rubella and herpes serology of infant and mother. Also get an ophthalmology review to confirm the cataract and look for other ocular clues. IEM (inborn errors of metabolism) panel and karyotype if metabolic or chromosomal disorder suspected unlikely in this patient.

Progression of Case

Investigations: Hb (hemoglobin): 10.2, TLC (total leukocyte count): 8.2, P-56, L-34, platelet: 1.8 L; RBS (random blood sugar): 86, TSH (thyroid-stimulating hormone): 4.8 uIU/mL, SGOT/SGPT: 65/56, serology: rubella IgM positive, rubella IgG positive, HSV IgM negative, HSV IgG positive.

Ophthalmologist report: Nuclear cataract in both eyes, no evidence of retinopathy in peripheral retinal.

Hearing screening: OAE (otoacoustic emissions) failed.

Maternal tests: TORCH (Toxoplasmosis, Other Agents, Rubella Cytomegalovirus, and Herpes simplex) profile: Rubella IgM negative, IgG positive, HSV IgG positive, rest all tests negative.

Q4. Is cataract with rubella IgM +ve a sufficient evidence for labeling congenital rubella syndrome (CRS)?

Ans. As per the CDC (Centers for Disease Control and Prevention) guidelines, an infant with at least one of the symptoms clinically consistent with CRS; and laboratory evidence of congenital rubella infection demonstrated by either of following:
- Isolation of rubella virus from an appropriate clinical specimen [e.g. urine, nasopharyngeal swab, throat swab, CSF (cerebrospinal fluid)].
- Detection of rubella-specific immunoglobulin M (IgM) antibody.
- Rubella-IgG persisting for longer than 6 months [maternally derived immunoglobulin G (IgG)] in the absence of a recent immunization.
- A specimen that is PCR (polymerase chain reaction)-positive for rubella virus.

Q5. How to interpret rubella serology (IgG and IgM) in the infant and the mother?

Ans. While many antibody assays are available, enzyme immunoassays (EIAs) are the most acceptable, highly sensitive, and specific for rubella IgG and IgM antibodies. Capture EIA is the preferred test for rubella IgM. Presence of IgM and IgG in the cord blood is highly s/o CRS. While IgM is produced in the infected baby and persists for 6–12 months, maternally transmitted IgG invariably lasts for approximately 6 months. Persistence of elevated IgG beyond 6 months is highly symptom of CRS. False-positive rubella IgM can occur in other viral infections such as Epstein–Barr virus, cytomegalovirus, and parvovirus B19 while some infants with CRS may have undetectable IgM and very high IgG. Rheumatoid factor and SLE (systemic lupus erythematosus) are other causes of false-positive IgM.

Maternal rubella serology has wide implications as regards diagnosis of CRS and the rubella susceptibility of the mother. In a recently infected pregnant mother, the IgM shall be detected and shall also have a rising IgG (four-fold rise) on follow-up. While the IgM persists for only 2 months, IgG is detectable for very prolonged periods. IgM negative but IgG positivity in mother indicates rubella infection which can be past or recent. The IgG avidity test can resolve this issue of timing of infection. High-avidity rubella IgG indicates a past infection while low-avidity IgG signifies a very recent infection in the mother. A recently infected mother should have her baby tested for congenital infection by fetal cord sample or CV/AF analysis by culture/RT PCR (reverse transcriptase PCR) at the earliest to test for CRS and may be a reasonable ground for suggesting abortion. However, a mildly detected IgM in a pregnant mother should caution further follow-up and repeat testing before labeling as CRS to avoid unneeded abortions (Flowchart 1).

Therefore, the case presented here qualifies to be labeled as CRS in view of cataract, deafness, and positive rubella serology.

Flowchart 1: Approach to suspected rubella infection in pregnancy.

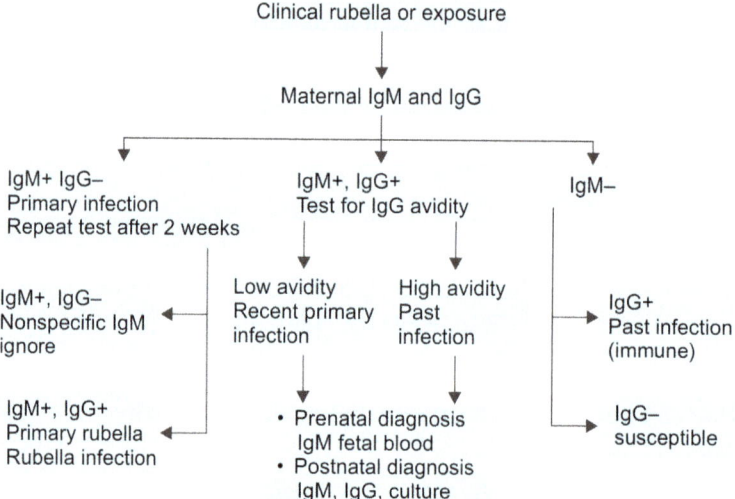

Source: Adapted from Mendelson E, Aboudy Y, Smetana Z, et al. Laboratory assessment and diagnosis of congenital viral infections: rubella, cytomegalovirus (CMV), varicella-zoster virus (VZV), herpes simplex virus (HSV), parvovirus B19 and human immunodeficiency virus (HIV). Reproductive Toxicology. 2006;21:350-82.

Q6. How are the babies with CRS managed?

Ans. Babies with proven CRS should be isolated as they can keep excreting rubella virus for a prolonged period and are infective for unimmunized contacts, especially pregnant ladies. The rest of the management is supportive and involves a multidisciplinary team to address the different needs of the baby.

Take Home Message

Besides several causes of congenital cataract, intrauterine rubella infection remains the foremost. It is important to diagnose these cases early as such babies can cause infection to the unimmunized contacts for prolonged periods.

SUGGESTED READING

1. Sinha R, Bali SJ, Sharma N, et al. Management of congenital cataract: a review. Indian J Ophthal. 2010;58(6):563-8.
2. Tesini BL. (2018). Congenital Rubella. [online] Available from https://www.msdmanuals.com/en-in/professional/pediatrics/infections-in-neonates/congenital-rubella. [Last accessed December, 2019].

CHAPTER 13

A Child with Prolonged Diarrhea

AK Patwari

INTRODUCTION

Acute diarrhea is generally self-limiting and resolves itself by 7–10 days but in some cases continued mucosal injury by enteric pathogens and/or impaired mucosal healing and diminished digestive and absorptive capacity may lead to continuation of diarrheal episode. It may also result from repeated enteric infections/mucosal injury without sufficient time to recover between episodes. Prolonged diarrhea in young children is a common clinical problem which remains one of the most common reasons for unnecessary use of antibiotics, antimotility agents, antiparasitic drugs, probiotics, and so on. A direct onslaught on the nutritional status of children is the most alarming consequence of prolonged diarrhea. Understanding the pathogenesis and following appropriate case management, protocol is critical to management of these cases.

CASE 1

A 7-month-old boy presented with history of passing loose stools for over 2 weeks. The child was apparently well when he suddenly started passing loose stools, which soon became watery, large in volume and without any visible blood. The child was treated with intravenous fluids, a combination of ofloxacin and metronidazole for 7 days along with oral rehydration solution (ORS) and probiotics, but he continued to pass 4–6 loose watery stools. The child was irritable, had poor appetite, and lost weight. There was history of passing less urine but no history of dysuria or excessive crying during micturition. He was on animal milk given with a feeding bottle. Complementary feeding was not started as yet. On physical examination, the child was not dehydrated, had mild abdominal distension with normal bowel sounds, and mild redness around anus. He weighed 7.0 kg and his length was 68 cm. Otoscopic examination of both the ears was normal. Systemic examination was normal.

Q1. What is differential diagnosis?

Ans. This child had acute onset watery diarrhea which could be viral in origin or due to self-limiting bacterial infection. Acute watery diarrhea as a result of parasitic infection is less likely in this age group. Secondary lactose intolerance can be considered in the differential diagnosis as it is a known consequence of acute diarrhea and presence of perianal rash supports this possibility. History does not suggest any food allergy because complementary feeding had not been started as yet. The child was underweight but did not suffer from severe acute malnutrition (SAM) and had no background to suspect human immunodeficiency virus (HIV). Persistent diarrhea (PD), defined as an episode of diarrhea of presumed to be of infectious etiology, which starts acutely but lasts for more than 14 days, is also a likely possibility.

Q2. What investigations would you consider?
Ans.
- Complete blood counts and peripheral blood smear examination—neutrophilic leukocytosis would suggest persistent enteric infection or extraintestinal infection. Blood culture can rule out systemic infection.
- X-ray chest and urine examination (routine and culture will rule out respiratory and urinary tract infections commonly associated with PD).
- Stool examination for reducing substances and pH would help in making a diagnosis of lactose intolerance. Stool culture can help in identifying organisms causing persistent gut infection.
- Stool examination for presence of blood, red blood cells (RBCs)/pus cells, ova, cyst, and fat globules can help to rule out parasitic infections and malabsorption.

Laboratory Test Results for Case 1

Complete blood count suggested leukocytosis with 75% neutrophils. X-ray chest was normal. Urine routine examination revealed 8–10 pus cells but urine culture grew *Escherichia coli* colony count >10^5 sensitive to most of the commonly used antibiotics.

Stool examination did not reveal any ova or cyst, had acidic pH with presence of reducing substances. Stool culture did not grow any organism.

Final Diagnosis

The final diagnosis is persistent diarrhea with underweight and urinary tract infection.

Q3. Why did this child have prolonged diarrhea?
This is a classic case of PD which began like a typical episode of infective diarrhea with acute onset, probably got worsened with antibiotics and episode continued beyond 2 weeks. The child had poor appetite which resulted in weight loss. Persistent diarrhea is believed to be multifactorial—a consequence of persistent mucosal injury due to specific pathogens (*E. coli, Shigella, Salmonella, and Campylobacter*), sequential infections with multiple pathogens, and host factors (micronutrient deficiency and compromised immune system). Use of antibiotics in acute diarrhea suppresses normal

gut flora which can result in overgrowth with pathogenic bacteria. The predominant problem in PD is the worsening nutritional status that, in turn, impairs the reparative process in the gut. This worsens nutrient absorption and initiates a vicious cycle that can only be broken by proper nutrition. One of the major obstacles to nutritional recovery is secondary lactose intolerance, and in some cases, impaired digestion of other complex carbohydrates due to decrease in brush border disaccharidases. This child did have features of secondary lactose intolerance (acidic pH and reducing substances in the stools and perianal excoriation) but did not have typical manifestations of lactose intolerance to account for overall clinical presentation of the child. Coexisting urinary tract infection contributed to poor appetite and weight loss.

Take Home Message

Acute diarrhea is a self-limiting disorder in children and should be managed with oral rehydration therapy (ORS and appropriate feeding) and zinc. Indiscriminate use of antibiotics can worsen diarrhea and results in prolongation of the episode. Children with prolonged episodes of diarrhea should be screened for persistent gut infection or concomitant extraintestinal infection. Children with PD need to be identified early because unless the vicious cycle of continued mucosal injury/poor mucosal repair is broken with appropriate feeding with low lactose/lactose free/disaccharide free diet the consequences can be serious with high mortality.

CASE 2

A 9-month-old girl presented with severe diarrhea for 5 days. The child was well 10 days ago when she started passing 4–5 loose watery stools a day with occasional vomiting. She was initially treated with ciprofloxacin, antiemetics, and intravenous fluids. Ciprofloxacin was stopped after 5 days. The volume and frequency of loose stools decreased over first 5 days but worsened afterwards. From Day 6, she started passing more frequent, large, and frothy stools which the mother described as explosive with a lot of flatus. The child was irritable sometimes presenting with abdominal discomfort and was feeding poorly. The frequency and volume of stools decreased while the child was not fed and managed with intravenous fluids but got worse after feeding. On examination, the child had some dehydration, distended abdomen with exaggerated bowel sounds, and perianal area was excoriated with some superficial ulcers. Perianal excoriation extended to buttocks. The child was on animal milk given with a feeding bottle, and her weight for age was 8.5 kg and measured 73 cm in length. Systemic examination was normal.

Q1. What is differential diagnosis?

Ans. This child started with acute watery diarrhea which initially got better over 2–3 days but after Day 6 of the illness it got worse. The description of frequent, large, watery, and frothy stools with lot of flatus, abdominal distension with exaggerated bowel sounds and severe perianal excoriation strongly suggest secondary lactose intolerance in this case. Rotavirus diarrhea also results in frequent, large, and watery stools but the onset is generally abrupt and children continue to pass large volume of watery stools irrespective of type of feeding. Cow's milk allergy can also result in severe diarrhea, but is unlikely in this child as she had been taking animal milk for a long time. Even though the child did not fulfill the clinical criteria of PD, she could still be a potential case. Ciprofloxacin can cause antibiotic-associated diarrhea as a result of alteration in gut flora and usually manifests a week or so after starting the antibiotics. Zinc deficiency can result in perianal lesions similar to lactose intolerance, but those children generally have signs of severe acute malnutrition (SAM) and/or lesions at mucocutaneous junctions or skin.

Q2. What investigations would your consider?

Ans.
- Complete blood counts and C-reactive protein (CRP)—neutrophilic leukocytosis and positive CRP would suggest infective etiology.
- Stool examination for reducing substances and pH would help in making a diagnosis of lactose intolerance.
- Stool examination for presence of blood, RBCs/pus cells, ova, cyst, and fat globules can help to rule out parasitic infections and malabsorption. Stool culture can help in identifying organisms causing persistent gut infection.

Laboratory Test Results for Case 2

- Complete blood count—mild anemia with normal total and differential leukocyte count, CRP normal
- Stool examination for reducing substances was +++ with acidic pH.
- No ova or cyst, pus cells or fat globules seen in the stool. Stool culture did not grow any organism.

Q3. What further test would you like to do?

Ans. The clinical picture of this child supported by presence of reducing substances and acidic pH of the stools strongly suggests secondary lactose intolerance. Therefore a therapeutic trial with lactose free diet is a better approach than conducting further investigations for evidence of malabsorption. In occasional cases, one may need to conduct investigations such as lactose tolerance test or hydrogen breath test to confirm the diagnosis. In most of the cases, a strong clinical suspicion and feeding with lactose free formula/food is enough to manage these cases.

Final Diagnosis

The final diagnosis is secondary lactose intolerance.

Take Home Message

History of worsening of diarrhea with increase in frequency and volume of stools, passing large, frothy and explosive stools, abdominal distension with exaggerated bowel sounds and perianal excoriation strongly suggest secondary lactose intolerance. Feeding the child with lactose free milk formula/food results in remarkable decrease in frequency and volume of stools.

CASE 3

A 3-year-old boy presented with history of passing frequent loose stools without any visible blood or mucus over last 3 weeks. He had been having episodes of passing semi-solid or loose, sometimes bulky, often watery stools off and on over last 2 years. During this period, the child had been seen by several doctors including pediatricians who prescribed antibiotics, antiprotozoals and probiotics. The child was exclusively breastfed for first 4 months when animal milk was introduced. Complementary feeding was introduced after 6 months of age. The child was presently taking normal family food and generally had good appetite, but was not gaining weight adequately. On examination, the child was well hydrated, had some pallor and abdominal distension. His weight for age was 9 kg, height for age 90 cm, and weight for height was less than –3 SD.

Q1. What is differential diagnosis?

Ans. This child has history of chronic diarrhea with growth failure (underweight with stunting). "Toddler's diarrhea" is one of the common conditions in this age group which presents with periods of frequent, heterogeneous, often mucus containing, foul smelling stools, and often alternating with periods of normal stools. However, these children generally have a normal state of nutrition. Chronic diarrhea due to impaired intraluminal digestion (cystic fibrosis and other exocrine pancreatic deficiencies, and selective fat or protein malabsorption due to specific deficiencies of digestive enzymes), intraluminal fermentation (carbohydrate malabsorption), and intestinal malabsorption (celiac disease, food protein sensitivity, *Giardia lamblia* infestation, etc.) can be considered in the differential diagnosis of this child. The description of stools does not suggest diarrhea due to exocrine pancreatic insufficiency (loose and pasty stools, greasy, pale, and floating on the surface of water) or due to intraluminal fermentation (liquid and acidic stools with lot of flatus). Possibility of chronic diarrhea due to variable severity of intestinal malabsorption appears to be more likely possibility.

Q2. What investigations would your consider?

Ans.
- Complete blood counts and CRP—neutrophilic leukocytosis and positive CRP would suggest infective etiology.

- Stool examination for presence of blood, RBCs/pus cells will rule out gut infection. Stool examination for reducing substances and pH would help in making a diagnosis of lactose intolerance. Repeated stool examination will be helpful to rule out giardiasis.
- Fecal fat excretion studies, D-xylose test, anti-tissue transglutaminase antibodies (tTG), anti-endomysial antibodies (EMA), and endoscopic duodenal biopsy.

Laboratory Test Results for Case 3

- Complete blood count—moderate anemia (dimorphic type) with normal total and differential leukocyte count, CRP normal.
- No ova or cyst, pus cells or fat globules seen in the stool.
- tTG level raised. Endoscopy findings suggestive of celiac disease. Duodenal biopsy suggestive of villus atrophy with hyperplasia of the crypts.

Q3. What further test would you like to do?

Ans. In this child, the clinical picture raised tTG levels and characteristics findings of duodenal biopsy support a diagnosis of celiac disease (gluten-induced enteropathy). However, in some cases who are immunoglobulin A (IgA)-deficient, serological markers based on IgA such as tTG and EMA may be negative in celiac disease. In such cases, serum IgA level need to be estimated and IgG-based antigliadin tests performed.

In case celiac disease is ruled out, other investigations such as sweat chloride test for cystic fibrosis, hydrogen breath test for carbohydrate malabsorption, and genetic studies may need to be undertaken.

Final Diagnosis

The final diagnosis is celiac disease.

Take Home Message

History of normal bowel movements till the age of 1 year and repeated episodes of diarrhea following introduction of complementary feeding which included wheat and wheat products, with poor weight gain should arouse suspicion of celiac disease. tTG is the most commonly used serological test which should be used along with a duodenal biopsy to make a diagnosis. In cases with strong suspicion of celiac disease and with a negative tTG, EMA can be performed. If IgA deficiency is suspected, then serum IgA level need to be estimated and IgG-based antigliadin tests performed.

SUGGESTED READING

1. Bandsma RHJ, Sadiq K, Bhutta ZA. Persistent diarrhoea: current knowledge and novel concepts. Paediatr Int Child Health. 2019;39(1):41-7.
2. Sibal A, Patwari AK, Anand VK, et al. Associated infections in persistent diarrhea: another perspective. J Trop Pediatr. 1996;42(2):64-7.
3. Harvey L, Ludwig T, Hou AQ, et al. Prevalence, cause and diagnosis of lactose intolerance in children aged 1-5 years: a systematic review of 1995–2015 literature. Asia Pac J Clin Nutr. 2018;27(1):29-46.
4. Glissen Brown JR, Singh P. Coeliac disease. Paediatr Int Child Health. 2019;39(1):23-31.
5. Poddar U, Thapa BR, Singh K. Clinical features of celiac disease in Indian children: are they different from the West? J Pediatr Gastroenterol Nutr. 2006;43(3):313-7.
6. Patwari AK. Management of diarrhea: changing trends in last 50 years. Indian Pediatr. 2018;55(1):63-5.

Chapter 14

An Infant with Microcephaly with Recurrent Seizures

Rekha Mittal, Ridhimaa Jain

INTRODUCTION

Microcephaly is defined as head circumference that measures more than 3 standard deviations below the mean, or less than the 3rd centile for age and gender.

It is essential to document head circumference at each visit to monitor head growth. If previous records of head circumference are available, they should be reviewed to differentiate between congenital and acquired microcephaly to delineate the onset of microcephaly. The presence of microcephaly in a child presenting with recurrent seizures limits the differential diagnosis.

CASE SCENARIO

A 9-month-old child was referred with seizures and small head size.

Q1. What are the possibilities?

Ans. Before proceeding with clinical evaluation and workup, it is important to formulate the possible causes, as many of the advanced tests would have financial implications (Box 1).

Box 1: Causes of microcephaly with seizures in infancy.

Antenatal/perinatal insult:
- Hypoxic–ischemic encephalopathy
- Neonatal hypoglycemia
- Perinatal stroke

Structural malformations:
- Lissencephaly
- Pachygyria

Intrauterine infections:
- Cytomegalovirus (CMV)
- Rubella
- Toxoplasmosis
- Zika virus

Contd...

Contd...

Inborn error of metabolism:
• Phenylketonuria
• Congenital defects of glycosylation
• Molybdenum cofactor deficiency
• Sulfide oxidase deficiency
• Glutamine synthetase deficiency
• Glucose transporter defects
Chromosomal disorders:
• Down syndrome
• Edwards syndrome
• Wolf–Hirschhorn syndrome (4p- or monosomy 4p)
• Angelman syndrome
• Miller–Dieker syndrome
• 18q syndrome
• Other microdeletion/duplication syndromes
Genetic syndromes (nonmetabolic and nonchromosomal):
• Cornelia de Lange syndrome
• Smith–Lemli–Opitz syndrome
Post neonatal insult:
• Infantile stroke
• Meningitis/encephalitis
• Head injury
Craniosynostosis

*This list is not exhaustive

CASE 1

A 9-month-old male child presented with episodes of abnormal movements for 3 months and a small head size. Abnormal movements were in the form of sudden vacant stare, tightening of all four limbs and drooling from mouth lasting for 2–3 minutes after which child was drowsy for 15–20 minutes. Initially episodes occurred every 7–10 days, but now frequency has increased to once every 2–3 days.

Antenatal period was uneventful. Child was born at term gestation through vacuum-assisted vaginal delivery. Baby did not cry immediately after birth and required resuscitation after which he was shifted to the neonatal intensive care unit. Baby required mechanical ventilation for 3 days and had seizures on Day 2 (semiology not known). Was shifted to mother side on Day 7 of life and discharged on Day 9 on oral phenobarbitone. Baby was accepting breastfeeds and moving all limbs, though mother felt that his activity was less than that of the previous child.

Developmentally, he was globally delayed. He started head holding at 5 months, sitting with support at 8 months and now approaches objects with both hands. He had monosyllables at 8 months, social smile and recognition of the mother by 3 months, and smiles when sees his own image in mirror, but there is inconsistent response to own name, does not wave bye. He turns head to sound or when spoken to.

Family history revealed that he was the second child born to non-consanguineous healthy parents. No history of any abortions, fetal death, and early sibling deaths. No history of seizures, developmental delay, and neurological illness in family.

Physical examination revealed microcephaly with head size of 40 cm (expected 44 cm, which is below 3rd centile for age), no dysmorphism, organomegaly or neurocutaneous markers. Child was alert, visual tracking was present, cranial nerves normal, spasticity with brisk deep tendon reflexes and scissoring of lower limbs.

Q1. What is differential diagnosis?

Ans. A detailed history is the first step in evaluation of the child. This child has presented with tonic seizures with a small head size. The child had a significantly adverse perinatal course suggestive of perinatal asphyxia with hypoxic–ischemic encephalopathy (HIE). Following the neonatal period, the child is showing a global delay in achieving milestones, though he continues to gain milestones with time and there has been no regression. The most likely possibility in this child is thus of a static brain injury due to perinatal asphyxia and he is now experiencing its sequelae.

The absence of consanguinity, early neonatal/infantile deaths, similar history in family and the fact that the child was symptomatic on Day 1 of life without any history of recurrent vomiting, worsening on feeds or neuroregression makes the possibility of an inborn error of metabolism unlikely.

The antenatal history can give a clue to intrauterine infections, maternal illness, drug or radiation insult. Perinatal history is imperative as it is the most common cause of microcephaly with seizures in infancy. This may include perinatal asphyxia, metabolic derangements in neonatal period (neonatal hypoglycemia), or a perinatal stroke. The onset of symptoms is very helpful. A period of apparently good health after birth prior to neonate becoming sick is an indicator of possible inborn error of metabolism.

The other possibilities in this child can be structural defects such as congenital malformations of brain with perinatal asphyxia secondary to the malformed brain.

Q2. How will you investigate this child?

Ans.
Magnetic Resonance Imaging (MRI) Brain
This is the first-line investigation in the evaluation of a child with microcephaly and recurrent seizures. In this case, history is suggestive of a perinatal hypoxic–ischemic injury and MRI brain is indicated because the pattern of injury on MRI (Table 1) helps to corroborate the clinical diagnosis, predict the deficits and long-term sequelae in a given child, and also excluding other conditions which may present with failure to initiate respiration at birth, and follow a similar course. MRI may show structural defects of brain or indicators of TORCH infections. Perinatal metabolic insults may show specific patterns such as posterior (parieto-occipital) cerebral cortex and subcortical white matter injury in neonatal hypoglycemia.

A child having microcephaly with recurrent seizures but a normal MRI, possibility of an inborn error of metabolism is highly likely and one should consider workup for the same.

TABLE 1: MRI patterns of injury in perinatal asphyxia and its clinical correlates.

Pattern of injury	Neonatal period	Long-term sequelae
Neuronal injury—cerebral cortex, basal ganglia, thalamus, reticular formation, brainstem nuclei, and cerebellum	• Stupor and coma • Seizures • Hypotonia/hypertonia-dystonia • Oculomotor disturbances • Disturbed sucking swallowing—feeding difficulties	• Cognitive deficits • Spastic quadriparesis • Choreoathetosis • Dystonia • Epilepsy • Ataxia • Bulbar/pseudobulbar palsy
Parasagittal cerebral injury—parasagittal cerebral cortex and subcortical white matter (posterior > anterior)	• Proximal limb weakness upper > lower	• Spastic quadriparesis • Specific intellectual deficits (language and visuospatial)
Periventricular leukomalacia (involves the descending motor tracts, optic radiations, and association fibers)	• Possible lower limb weakness	• Spastic diplegia • Cognitive deficits • Visual deficits • Behavioral/attention deficits
Unilateral cerebral cortex and subcortical white matter in vascular distribution	• Focal seizures • Hemiparesis	• Spastic hemiparesis • Epilepsy • Cognitive deficits

Electroencephalogram (EEG)
An EEG helps in classifying the types of seizures (e.g. hypsarrhythmia/modified hypsarrhythmia in West syndrome), identifying particular syndromes (e.g. early myoclonic epilepsy/Ohtahara syndrome), and determining prognosis by background assessment (e.g. burst suppression).

Results of Investigations
- The MRI brain showed multicystic encephalomalacia, and EEG showed epileptiform discharges from right frontal region.
- Since the history and clinical examination, and the MRI brain all pointed to HIE as the cause of microcephaly and seizures, no further investigations were done to find the etiology.
- The EEG showed that the child was having focal onset seizures, and the child was started on Carbamazepine.

Any other Evaluations?
Evaluation is also required to test hearing, any loss of visual acuity and squint. Hence, brainstem evoked response audiometry (BERA) and vision assessment should also be done. The BERA and ophthalmic evaluation was normal.

Final Diagnosis
- Spastic quadriplegic cerebral palsy
- Focal epilepsy
- *Etiology*: Hypoxic–ischemic encephalopathy.

Q3. How can we manage this child?

Ans.
- Antiepileptics for treating the seizures
- Multidisciplinary management including occupational therapy, physiotherapy, anti-spasticity drugs, etc.

Take Home Messages

Detailed antenatal and birth history, measurement of head size at birth and on follow up, and clinical evaluation are essential to find the etiology. MRI brain is important to confirm the diagnosis and EEG for determining the type of seizures and the antiseizure medication. Evaluation of comorbidities must also be done to institute early intervention. The diagnosis must mention comorbidities as well as the etiology, if known.

CASE 2

A 9-month-old female presented with status epilepticus with history of recurrent multifocal seizures and a small head size since birth. She was the first child born to nonconsanguineous healthy parents. There was no family history of epilepsy or other neurological disorders. Antenatal period was uneventful. She was born vaginally at 36 weeks gestation with a birth weight of 1,360 g (−3.5 standard deviations), cried immediately after birth. At 2 months of age, she had clonic seizures involving her right arm. She was started on phenobarbital to which the seizures responded. At 7 months, she again started having seizures. Initially, clonic seizures of the right arm lasting 3–5 minutes, then clonic and tonic–clonic seizures involving sometimes the entire right side and sometimes the left side of the body. Despite 2 antiepileptics her seizures continued to worsen in frequency and duration. She was admitted in status epilepticus at 9 months.

On examination, she had severe microcephaly, abnormal craniofacial features (hypertelorism, micrognathia, low-set ears, and prominent glabella), broad short fingers, no neurocutaneous markers, and no organomegaly. Neurological examination revealed hypotonia with preserved reflexes. Ophthalmic examination was normal.

Q1. What is differential diagnosis?

Ans. This child had a normal antenatal and perinatal history, but was severely growth retarded at birth with recurrent multifocal seizures and dysmorphic facial features. The most likely diagnosis in this child is of a chromosomal disorder. The clinical features do not fit exactly into any particular syndrome.

Structural disorders or malformations of the brain are also likely in view of recurrent and difficult to control seizures. Several of the chromosomal syndromes can have structural abnormalities of the brain as part of the syndrome. Severe growth retardation at birth suggests antenatal onset of the disorder and one must consider other antenatal infections (TORCH), drug or radiation exposure.

Q2. How will you investigate this child?

Ans. Complete blood count (CBC), serum electrolytes, blood sugar, calcium ionized, magnesium, and blood gas: as child presented in status epilepticus are required. Normal blood sugars at the time of seizures help to rule out recurrent hypoglycemia as a cause for the seizures.

Electroencephalogram: Many of the chromosomal syndromes (such as Angelman syndrome) can give specific patterns on EEG. The location of epileptiform discharges helps in identifying the focus of the seizures and thereby in analyzing the MRI and guide treatment. Structural abnormalities of brain can give rise to certain patterns (e.g. Frontal beta activity in anterior lissencephaly). Presence of patterns such as burst suppression indicate graver prognosis and need for evaluation for metabolic disorders. EEG can also help in identifying ongoing electrographic seizures, especially in a sedated and ventilated child, indicating the need for further antiepileptics.

MRI Brain: To identify brain malformations, structural abnormalities or indicators of intrauterine infection.

Echocardiography, ultrasonography (USG) abdomen, and skeletal survey: As part of dysmorphology evaluation.

Results of Investigation:
- Laboratory investigations were unremarkable.
- EEG showed epileptiform discharges at multiple foci.
- Magnetic resonance imaging was normal.
- Echocardiography revealed an atrial septal defect.
- USG abdomen and skeletal survey were normal.

Q3. What further investigations will you order?

Ans. *Genetic Studies*: In a dysmorphic child with severe growth retardation at birth with microcephaly, recurrent seizures, congenital heart disease, normal ophthalmologic examination, no organomegaly, and a normal MRI, the most likely possibility is a chromosomal anomaly. Hence genetic studies may be required for confirming diagnosis. Types of genetic studies include:
- *Karyotyping*: If chromosomal abnormalities are suspected such as trisomies, large rearrangements, and translocations. It will not pick up very small changes in the chromosomes.
- *Fluorescence in situ hybridization (FISH)*: It is done if the clinical phenotype fits into a particular syndrome.
- *Chromosomal microarray*: It can detect microdeletion and duplications, and is indicated if results of karyotyping and/or FISH do not reveal any

abnormality; one may go straight for it if the dysmorphism does not clearly point to a syndrome.

TORCH titers in mother and child: Though a normal ophthalmic examination, absence of organomegaly and a normal MRI brain make the possibility of a congenital TORCH infection less likely, they cannot be definitely ruled out.

Results of Investigations:
- TORCH titers in mother and baby were negative.
- Karyotyping revealed a normal 46XX. Since the clinical features did not fit any particular syndrome, chromosomal microarray was sent which revealed microdeletion in the short arm of chromosome 4.

Final Diagnosis:
The final diagnosis is microdeletion syndrome (4p-).

Q4. How can we manage this child?
Ans.
- Symptomatic treatment and early intervention with neurodevelopmental therapy are important.
- Counseling is very important. Possibility of recurrence is low if the deletion is de novo. *Testing of the parents is also important once a microdeletion is detected.*

Take Home Messages

Significant dysmorphic features point to a chromosomal abnormality. Evaluation for cardiac, skeletal, and visceral abnormalities is also important. Karyotyping may be done initially, but further testing depends on whether a known syndrome is suspected. Genetic counseling is important.

CASE 3

A 9-month-old male child presented with recurrent focal seizures, sudden body contractions, and a small head. He was the second child born of third degree consanguineous healthy parents. Mother had low-grade fever with cough and coryza for 3-4 days during the second month of pregnancy. At term gestation mother developed pre-eclampsia and baby was delivered through cesarean section. He cried immediately, but had to be shifted to neonatal intensive care unit in view of respiratory distress. He did not require mechanical ventilation, developed jaundice requiring phototherapy on Day 3.

At 3 months, the child experienced clonic seizure of left leg lasting 1-2 minutes. He continued to have repeated episodes of clonic movement of left leg, left hand, and right leg lasting for 1-2 minutes every few days. A week ago, the child had vomiting and diarrhea for 3 days after which he started having jerks in the form of sudden contractions of his arms lasting a few seconds, 3-4 times per day.

The development is delayed globally; he started recognizing his mother at 4 months, head holding at 6 months, cooing at 6 months, sitting with support at 8 months, and rolling over 15 days back.

On physical examination, the patient had microcephaly, with an upturned nose, high-arched palate, retrognathia, a short neck and hepatomegaly. Bilateral chorioretinitis was determined at the ophthalmological examination. The patient had impaired neuromotor development, visual tracking was present but there was inconsistent head turn towards sound.

Q1. What is differential diagnosis?

Ans. An intrauterine infection seems highly likely owing to the presence of microcephaly, with hepatomegaly, chorioretinitis, and hearing loss.

An inborn error of metabolism may also be considered as there is third degree consanguinity, respiratory distress at birth, multifocal seizures, global development delay, probable hearing deficit, and recent onset myoclonic jerks with acute illness.

Perinatal asphyxia sequelae is also possible owing to history of maternal pre-eclampsia with baby having respiratory distress at birth followed by global developmental delay and seizures.

Q2. How will you investigate this child?

Ans. Complete blood count (CBC) with peripheral smear and liver function tests—as there is organomegaly. TORCH titers of mother and baby—as a congenital infection is the most likely diagnosis.

MRI brain—to identify structural defects, patterns suggestive of perinatal hypoxic–ischemic insult or intrauterine infections. Pointers of congenital TORCH infection include microcephaly, migrational abnormalities (lissencephaly, pachygyria, and schizencephaly), parietal or posterior white matter involvement with spared rim in immediately periventricular and subcortical white matter, ventriculomegaly and subarachnoid space enlargement, delayed myelination and periventricular and temporal pole cysts. Intracranial calcification may be identified on CT brain or susceptibility weighted MRI.

Role of EEG as discussed in previous cases.

Metabolic workup: As an inborn error of metabolism is probable blood gas, blood sugar, blood ammonia, lactate, urine for glucose/ketones, tandem mass spectrometry (TMS), and gas chromatography-mass spectrometry (GC-MS) should also be sent as sometimes the picture of intrauterine infections and some inborn errors of metabolism (IEM) may be very similar.

BERA: To assess hearing.

Results of Investigations:
- CBC revealed mild anemia with normal counts. Liver function tests were normal.
- Brain MRI showed pachygyria, dilated lateral ventricles, thin corpus callosum, and periventricular subependymal hyperintensities.
- Brain CT scan revealed periventricular subependymal calcifications.

- EEG showed epileptiform activity.
- Toxoplasmosis, Epstein-Barr virus, herpes simplex virus types 1 and 2, rubella, and human immunodeficiency virus (HIV) serologies were negative. Serum CMV immunoglobulin M (IgM) and IgG were positive. Mother's serum CMV IgM was negative and IgG was positive.
- BERA showed bilateral sensorineural hearing loss.
- Metabolic workup was normal.

Q3. What further investigations will you order?

Ans. Urine CMV deoxyribonucleic acid (DNA) polymerase chain reaction (PCR) was ordered to confirm diagnosis, which was very high (3,303 million copies/mL).

Final Diagnosis:
The final diagnosis is congenital CMV infection.

Q4. How can we manage this child?

Ans.
- Ganciclovir 10 mg/kg/day for 6 weeks to treat CMV infection
- Anti-epileptics drugs to control seizures
- Multidisciplinary neurodevelopmental therapies.

Take Home Messages

Subtle clues of congenital infection such as fever/rash during pregnancy, preeclampsia, and neonatal jaundice on history are important. Chorioretinitis, sensorineural hearing loss, and organomegaly are suggestive of an intrauterine infection. Neuroimaging abnormalities can guide further workup. Serology is easily available for diagnosis, though further confirmatory tests may be needed if positive. If correctly diagnosed, treatment is available for toxoplasmosis and cytomegalovirus infections, which can significantly improve outcomes.

CASE 4

A 9-month-old girl presented with recurrent seizures and small head size. She was first child born to third degree consanguineous but healthy parents. There was history of one spontaneous abortion previously. There was no family history of developmental problems, learning deficits, birth defects or genetic syndromes. Antenatal and perinatal periods were uneventful.

First seizures were noticed at 5 months in the form of tonic-clonic seizures lasting for 5-10 minutes every 15-20 days. She also had episodes of unresponsiveness and head bobbing.

Developmental delay was present—she had attained head holding and roll over, but could not sit, approached objects with both hands, spoke "ah-goo" but no monosyllables. Physical examination revealed microcephaly, mild hypotonia, and reduced spontaneous motor activity with brisk deep tendon reflexes.

Q1. What is differential diagnosis?
The differential diagnosis in this child includes structural malformations of brain and IEM. Urea cycle defects, fatty acid oxidation defects, and organic acidurias often present with epilepsy in infancy with developmental delays and episodic worsening. Though most of them do not fit the classical definition of microcephaly, many of them have a head size at the lower limit of the distribution curve. In addition, recurrent hypoglycemic/metabolic insults can result in microcephaly as is often seen with fatty acid oxidation defects.

Q2. How will you investigate this child?

Ans.
MRI: To look for structural defects and myelination patterns. It may be normal in many IEM. Hypoglycemic insult results in posterior cortical and subcortical white matter injury.

EEG: To look for the type of seizures and the background changes of any encephalopathy, especially during an episode of altered sensorium.

Metabolic Workup: In any acute seizure, blood sugar should be documented; serum sodium, ionized calcium, and magnesium levels should be measured.

If an inborn error of metabolism is probable blood gas, blood ammonia, lactate, urine for glucose/ketones, TMS, and (GC-MS) should be sent.

If clinical features suggest a congenital glycosylation defects isoelectric focusing for serum transferrin for should be sent.

Investigation Results:
- EEG showed epileptiform discharges in bilateral parieto-occipital regions and generalized slow spike wave discharges.
- MRI of the brain was normal.
- Metabolic investigations were also within normal limits.

Q3. What further investigations will you order?

Ans. Lumbar puncture revealed normal counts and protein, low glucose levels. Gene sequencing revealed point mutation in glucose transporter gene which was then confirmed by Sanger's sequencing.

Final Diagnosis
The final diagnosis is glucose transporter disorder [glucose transporter type 1 (GLUT1) deficiency syndrome].

Q4. How can we manage this child?

Ans.
- Special diet—ketogenic diet
- Antiepileptic drug—levetiracetam
- Neurodevelopmental therapy
- Genetic counseling.

Take Home Messages

- Consanguinity, positive family history, and episodic worsening are indicators of IEM but their absence does not rule out a metabolic disorder. A normal MRI indicates the need for evaluation for a metabolic disorder.
- Valproate should be avoided in children with suspected IEM.
- In case the diagnosis is not clear after MRI and metabolic screening on blood and urine, cerebrospinal fluid (CSF) examination must be done.
- Genetic confirmation of diagnosis should be attempted to enable genetic and prenatal counseling.

SUGGESTED READING

1. Abdel-Salam GM, Halasz AA, Czeizel AE. Association of epilepsy with different groups of microcephaly. Dev Med Child Neurol. 2000;42(11):760-7.
2. Ashwal S, Michelson D, Plawner L, et al. Practice parameter: Evaluation of the child with microcephaly (an evidence-based review): report of the Quality Standards Subcommittee of the American Academy of Neurology and the Practice Committee of the Child Neurology Society. Neurology. 2009;73(11): 887-97.
3. Delan D, Bamford A, Ferreira MU, et al. Infectious causes of microcephaly: epidemiology, pathogenesis, diagnosis and management. Lancet Infect Dis. 2018;18(1):e1-13.
4. Hanzlik E, Gigante J. Microcephaly. Children (Basel). 2017;4(6):E47.
5. Jayaraman D, Bae B, Walsh CA. The genetics of primary microcephaly. Annu Rev Genom Human Genetics. 2018;19:177-200.
6. Seregni F, Parker PJA. How to assess and support the child with microcephaly. Paediatr Child Health. 2018;28:468-73.
7. van Karnebeek CD, Stockler S. Treatable inborn errors of metabolism causing intellectual disability: a systematic literature review. Mol Genet Metab. 2012; 105:368-81.
8. von der Hagen M, Pivarcsi M, Liebe J, et al. Diagnostic approach to microcephaly in childhood: a two-center study and review of the literature. Dev Med Child Neurol. 2014;56:732-41.
9. Woods CG, Parker A. Investigating microcephaly. Arch Dis Child. 2013;98:707-13.
10. Yang Y, Muzny DM, Reid JG, et al. Clinical whole-exome sequencing for the diagnosis of mendelian disorders. N Engl J Med. 2013;369:1502-11.

CHAPTER 15

Neurocysticercosis in Children

RK Sabharwal

INTRODUCTION

Cysticercosis and neurocysticercosis (NCC) diseases caused by the parasitic tapeworm *Taenia solium* are distributed worldwide where contaminated food and unsupervised pork are eaten, and hygiene and sanitation are poor. The disease is being seen in the more developed countries as a result of increasing migration. Parenchymal NCC presents commonly as seizures as a result of inflammation caused by a dying cyst. Calcified cysts are an important cause of epilepsy. Parenchymal cysticercosis in children is generally benign.

CASE 1

A 6-year-old school-going girl was sitting in the classroom, when the teacher observed her head turning to one side with distortion of the face. She fell of the chair and had generalized convulsive movements lasting a couple of minutes, following which she became unresponsive. She was rushed to the school medical room where she was examined by the doctor and transported to our hospital. In the hospital, she was drowsy and confused. The examination revealed her to be afebrile. The pulse was 92/min and BP was 100/70 mm Hg. No rash, lymphadenopathy, bite marks, and purpuric spots were detected. Pupillary reactions were intact and fundus examination revealed no papilledema. Systemic examination was unremarkable. There was no discharge from the ears. Examination, an hour later, revealed a left pronator drift.

Her parents stated that the girl had been complaining of headache off and on for the past week, which they ascribed to impending examinations. No past history of epilepsy was forthcoming and the girl had not been on any medications. No history of Koch's disease existed in the family.

Q1. What do you think happened to the girl? What investigations would you consider?

Ans. This school-going girl had an unprovoked generalized tonic–clonic seizure with a focal onset. A pronator drift is a subtle sign of motor weakness and indicates Todd's palsy. One can infer that the ictal discharge is from the right cerebral hemisphere.

The investigations would include a complete blood count, calcium studies, and glucose estimation to exclude hypoglycemia or significant hypocalcemia. A 16-channel EEG (at least) and an urgent contrast-enhanced CT of the brain should be done to look for a hemorrhage, arteriovenous malformation (AVM), NCC, or other mass lesions. The CT is preferred as an urgent test because of the ease and brief time it takes to be performed.

Investigation results:
- The blood tests were normal.
- Electroencephalogram (EEG) (Fig. 1)

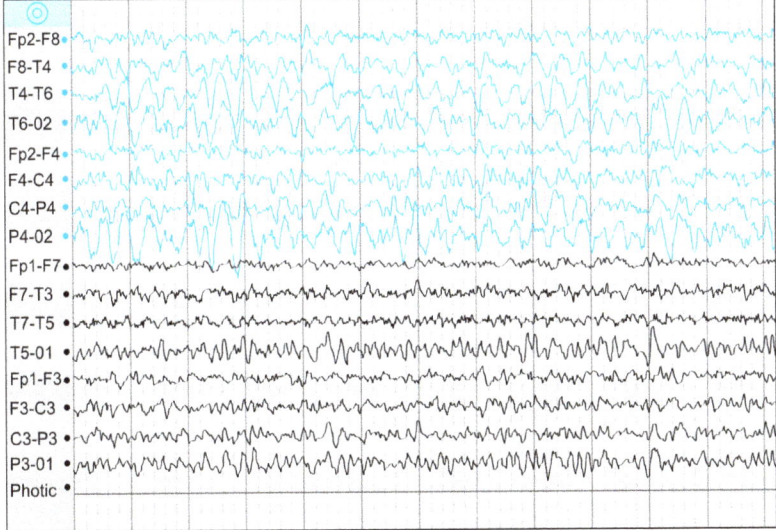

Fig. 1: The electroencephalogram shows moderately high-voltage sharp waves; theta and delta waves slowing over the right parietal and temporal regions (tracings in blue), indicating the location of epileptiform activity, and also suggesting the possibility of an inflammatory pathology because of the high voltage.

- *CT Scan (Fig. 2)*

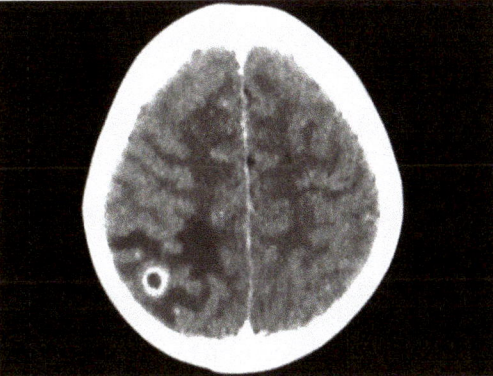

Fig. 2: CT scan shows a contrast-enhancing ring lesion with surrounding cerebral edema, located in the right high parietal lobe.

- Subsequently, a chest X-ray and Mantoux test were done and they were normal.

Q2. What is the diagnosis and what differential diagnosis would you consider in this child?

Ans. CT shows a lesion which has come to be described as "single, small, enhancing CT lesion" (SSECTL). The advent of CT had the medical community in a quandary as to the etiology of these cysts. These lesions were thought to be tuberculomas by Bhargava and Tandon while Sethi et al. proposed that focal encephalitis could be the likely cause. A number of authors attributed these lesions to be microabscesses, postictal state phenomenon, etc. The credit for resolving the issue rested with Rajshekhar (1991) who showed histopathological evidence of NCC in biopsy samples from 15 specimens. He proposed CT radiological criteria that favored NCC as the cause of the SSECTL:

- Single, small, <1 cm and well-defined lesion
- Contrast enhancing, the enhancement could be peripheral ("ring") or uniform ("disk" or "nodular")
- With or without surrounding edema
- Associated with minimal mass effect and no midline shift. The size of the lesion was subsequently amended to be not greater than 2 cm.

One may add that finding the presence of scolex in the cyst on neuroimaging is considered pathognomonic of NCC.

Ring-enhancing lesions of this nature in children are degenerating NCC in overwhelming majority of the cases. Singhi et al. found 82% of children with NCC had a solitary ring-enhancing lesion. Murthy et al. found SSECTL to be the cause of acute symptomatic seizures in 61% of 2,500 patients of different age groups from a tertiary care center in southern India.

A variety of infectious, neoplastic, inflammatory, or vascular diseases can manifest with a single ring-enhancing lesion of the brain, and differential diagnosis may be challenging.

Causes of single-enhancing lesions:
- *Common*:
  - Neurocysticercosis
  - Tuberculoma
- *Uncommon*:
  - Glioma
  - Larva migrans
  - Cryptic AVM
  - Brain abscess
- *In immunocompromised patients*:
  - Toxoplasmosis
  - Central nervous system (CNS) lymphoma
  - Fungal granuloma
  - Secondaries

- Sarcoidosis
- Small infarct
- Focal encephalitis.

A pyogenic abscess goes through stages of early and late cerebritis and capsule formation. It would be associated with a duration of illness, systemic signs, source of infection, leukocytosis, and more cerebral edema. Toxoplasma and fungal granulomas tend to occur in immunocompromised patients (e.g. AIDS and post-transplant). Only about 15% of toxoplasma lesions are solitary. Toxoplasmosis may generate focal brain lesions, mostly localized to the basal ganglia, but also in other brain regions. Magnetic resonance imaging (MRI) delineates them most clearly, sometimes revealing hemorrhagic zones.

The diagnostic dilemma, when it arises, is often between NCC and tuberculomas. Rajshekhar et al. observed the following features that favored the diagnosis of tuberculoma:

- Signs of increased intracranial pressure (ICP)
- Focal deficits
- CT showing a size of granuloma >2 cm
- Irregular, thick margins
- Significant perilesional edema.

Tuberculomas are common in children and often have an infratentorial location in contrast to adults. Systemic signs of Koch's disease and presence of subcutaneous nodules in NCC can also assist in diagnosis. Multiple calcifications on neuroimaging, or more than one cyst in different stages of involution would favor NCC while exudates would go in favor of tuberculosis.

Our patient thus had a SSECTL, namely a transitional colloidal NCC.

Q3. How was the child treated?

Ans. The child had received emergency treatment for the seizure with parenteral midazolam in the school sick bay. She had received a loading dose of fosphenytoin. At our hospital, she received maintenance doses of fosphenytoin and 7 days of oral steroids. Her antiepileptic drug (AED) was changed to oxcarbazepine, and fosphenytoin was gradually stopped. We are not in favor of using phenytoin because of its erratic pharmacokinetics, and cognitive and cosmetic side effects in children. Phenytoin dose/kg adjustment is generally more difficult than that of other AEDs and is even more difficult in a pediatric population. We find subtherapeutic phenytoin levels in children commonly.

Q4. In case the diagnosis cannot be established on CT scan, what is the role of: (a) Immunodiagnosis, and (b) Neuroimaging?

Ans.
Immunodiagnosis:
The presence of specific antibodies does not necessarily indicate current infection in a patient who resides in an endemic area. Of the antibody

detection tests available today, the enzyme-linked immunotransfer blot (EITB) is the immunodiagnostic test of choice for confirming a presumptive diagnosis of NCC.

Enzyme-linked immunosorbent assay (ELISA) has much less sensitivity as compared with EITB for serum as well as CSF samples, for both intraparenchymal and extraparenchymal NCC. Immunodiagnosis is often not helpful in the patients with single lesions. Seropositivity has ranged from 15% to 31% with ELISA in India.

Neuroimaging:

CT scan:

CT is a good screening procedure and can demonstrate calcification that could be missed by an MRI. A combination of calcified lesions and transitional lesions may obviate the need to obtain an MRI and thus save time and expenses. The cysts may appear as single or multiple, rounded lesions of variable size and low density, with a small, hyperdense, eccentric mural nodule representing the scolex. Edema is seen around the degenerating, enhancing granulomas (colloidal stage and granular-nodular stage). When multiple, the cysts may sometimes be grouped together like grapes.

MRI:

MRI is far superior to CT for identifying the cysts, their number, location, and their stage of involution. Cysts in the brainstem, orbit, ocular cysts, subarachnoid cysts, posterior fossa, small cysts, and intraventricular and intrasellar cysts can be identified by the MRI. Identification of the scolex on the different sequences, fluid-attenuating inversion recovery (FLAIR) and proton density images being ideal, becomes a primary goal as it confirms the diagnosis of NCC.

Use of sequences in magnetization transfer imaging (MTI), diffusion-weighted imaging (DWI), MR spectroscopy, fast-imaging employing steady-state acquisition sequence (FIESTA), constructive interference in steady state (CISS), or balanced-fast field echo (BFFE) protocols help in identifying the NCC and differentiating tuberculomas, abscesses, toxoplasma, lymphoma, metastasis, etc. with more certainty.

CASE 2

A 15-year-old boy was brought with a 4-day history of left frontal and orbital pain. Two days later, he noted drooping of his left upper eyelid and double vision. There were no vomiting, rash, pustular lesions on the face, vesicles, and purulent nasal or ear discharge.

On examination, there was a left-sided ptosis; the left eye was exotropic. On looking to right, the left eye did not cross the midline. The pupil was dilated as compared to the opposite side and reacted sluggishly to light.

Visual acuity was preserved and fundoscopy was normal. Other cranial nerves were normal. There was no proptosis, orbital cellulitis, or sinus tenderness.

Q1. What is the neurological dysfunction and what would be differential diagnosis?

Ans. This boy has developed an acute third-nerve palsy accompanied by headache. Even though the headache was not severe and there is no accompanying neck stiffness or subhyaloid hemorrhages, we would like to exclude a posterior communicating artery aneurysm. The other differentials we would consider would be intracavernous carotid artery aneurysm, cavernous sinus thrombosis, tumors of the pituitary, parasellar region, vasculitis, orbital pseudotumor, Tolosa–Hunt syndrome, etc.

Q2. What would be your investigation of choice?

Ans. Neuroimaging in the form of a gadolinium MRI brain with MR cerebral angiography with special attention to the orbit and sella regions should be performed on a priority basis.

Q3. What was the result of the neuroimaging?

Ans. The MRI studies revealed a ring-enhancing lesion in the tegmentum of the midbrain on the left side with significant surrounding edema suggestive of a degenerating colloidal NCC (Fig. 3).

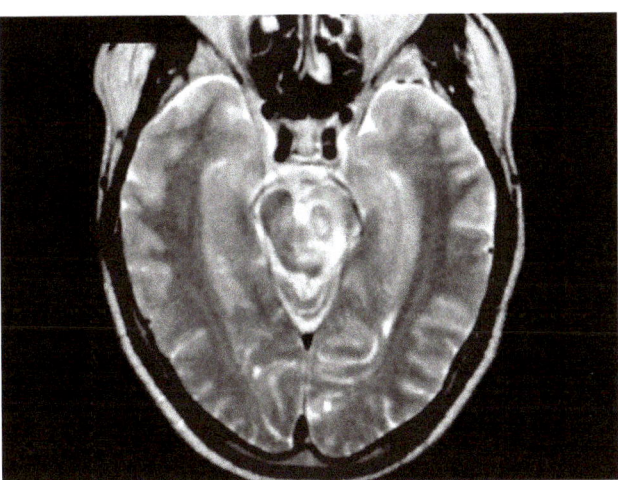

Fig. 3: T2W image showing a degenerating midbrain neurocysticercosis with surrounding edema.

Q4. How common is isolated brainstem neurocysticercosis?

Ans. Isolated brainstem NCC is considered to be distinctly rare. We feel that it is uncommon but is underreported. We have seen midbrain NCC presenting as bilateral ptosis due to third-nerve nuclear involvement; internuclear ophthalmoplegias (INO), sixth-nerve paralysis due to isolated pontine NCC. Del Brutto (2013) reviewed 29 cases of isolated brainstem NCC that had been reported till 2012, of whom five were children and adolescents. Clinical presentations included ocular nerve palsies or gaze palsies (INO).

Q5. What are the other clinical presentations of NCC?

Ans.
- *Seizures* are the most reported symptom in 70–90% of patients. These usually occur when a cyst is degenerating or because of a chronic, calcified granuloma. In the series reported by Singhi et al., 94.8% children had seizures at presentation.
- *Focal deficits,* such as hemiparesis, dysphasia, and dysarthria, can result from degenerating NCC and the edema, which is strategically located over eloquent areas. NCC-related arteritis is distinctly rare in India and even more so in children.
- Migraine-like headaches and ictal headaches
- Increased intracranial pressure/cysticercus encephalitis:

Increased ICP in patients with NCC can result from various mechanisms. It may be related to potentially life-threatening presentation where numerous degenerating NCC contribute to a picture of diffuse cerebral inflammation, cerebral edema, intracranial hypertension, drowsiness, cranial nerve palsies, seizures, etc., in varying combinations; a presentation termed cysticercus encephalitis or meningoencephalitis. *Cysticercotic encephalitis* occurs more frequently in children and young women, and reflects an intense immune response from the host. Use of antiparasitic treatment in these cases may aggravate symptoms and lead to the death of the patient. The treatment involves use of optimum doses of steroids and decongestive therapy. If necessary, drastic decompressive surgical measures may be required to save life and sight.

The other mechanism of raised ICP and headaches can result from intraventricular NCC; the children can present acutely with intense headache, vomiting, and neck stiffness simulating a subarachnoid hemorrhage or meningitis. The intraventricular form has a rapidly progressive clinical course and demands prompt action. The oncosphere reaches the ventricle through the choroid plexus.

Intraventricular cysticercosis is uncommon in India. The ideal treatment of intraventricular cysts is excision. As most of them are viable, albendazole is not recommended prior to surgery as the death of the cyst is likely to cause ependymitis, scarring, obstruction, and ventriculitis. An emergency ventriculostomy may be required in case of acute hydrocephalus.

Other deficits can include orbital NCC, myositis, trismus, movement disorders, spinal cord NCC (rare in children), ataxia, behavior disorders, etc.

Q6. What is the role of cysticidal therapy?

Ans. Criteria for the diagnosis of NCC have been proposed by Del Brutto et al. We have not found them useful in clinical practice. The criteria are not useful in a country where NCC is endemic, but may have a role in nonendemic countries. Concerns of their validity have been raised while some have criticized them for the complexity and difficulties in clinical and epidemiological application. Carpio (1999) has proposed a classification system that corresponds to the viability of the parasite: (a) *Active* (viable or live cyst, the cyst is usually asymptomatic, and on CT appears as a rounded, hypodense area, or with CSF-like signal on MRI), (b) *transitional* (cyst is degenerating and shows up with diffuse hypodense appearance and irregular border on CT, enhancing with contrast; colloidal, granular/nodular), and (c) *inactive* (calcified nodule or speck).

The bone of contention is the use of cysticidal drugs, with two schools of thought proposing and opposing their use vehemently.

In 1991, Rajshekar made the following observations in reference to SSECTL, the most common presentation of NCC: (1) Cysticercosis is the etiology of a majority of the lesions; (2) Most lesions are benign and resolve spontaneously; (3) No specific medical therapy is required; (4) Serological tests for cysticercosis with present techniques are useful in confirming the diagnosis in less than one-third of the patients, and (5) Surgical excision is only occasionally required to confirm the diagnosis. Most pediatric patients have a single transitional cyst that resolves spontaneously over a few months. Studies from Chandigarh and New Delhi groups have attempted to *show the benefits of albendazole* therapy in transitional NCC.

A large number of studies have *shown no benefit of cysticidal* therapy in the management of NCC, either in the form of resolution of cyst, reducing the rate of calcification, or late onset seizure, e.g. Garg and Nag, Talukdar et al., Carpio et al., Gogia et al., and Rajshekar. A recent MRI-based study of 81 patients, in whom 50% were less than 18 years and each underwent 4–5 serial MRI scans over 2 years, revealed no significant difference in the resolution of the albendazole-treated versus control patients (de Souza, 2010).

We feel that degenerating or transitional NCC is a benign condition in children, and cysticidal drugs are not indicated in the majority. The proponents of cysticidal therapy quote the evidence-based guideline: Treatment of Parenchymal NCC: Report of the American Academy of Neurology in support of their argument. Experts criticized the report stating that the meta-analysis was misleading and inaccurate.

A higher rate of calcification has been in many studies that have used cysticidal drugs in live NCC or degenerating NCC. Calcified cysts are a risk for later epilepsy.

Q7. If albendazole is used, then how long should it be administered?

Ans. Albendazole is used in a dose of 15 mg/kg/day in two divided doses, usually for 28 days particularly in multiple lesions. The studies have shown that 15-day albendazole courses, then 7-day courses, and now 3-day courses are almost as effective as the long-duration courses (Kaur et al., 2010; Singhi, 2003) in cyst reduction in children. The authors prime the patients with steroids, prednisone 2 mg/kg/day starting 2 days before administering the first dose of albendazole, and continuing it for a total period of 7 days to counteract the inflammatory response and edema.

Q8. When should you not use albendazole?

Ans. Avoid using albendazole in children with: (1) multiple cysts with significant edema and elevated intracranial pressure; (2) cysticercus encephalitis; and (3) ophthalmic cysticercosis due to the risk of inducing an inflammatory response and clinical worsening. A number of experts avoid using cysticidal drugs in ventricular cysts.

We would advise caution in using albendazole if cysts are located in the medulla and the pons.

Take Home Message

- NCC is the most common parasitic infection (involving the CNS) in developing countries.
- NCC presents with seizures and a solitary enhancing cerebral cyst in the majority of the children; some children may have more than one cyst.
- Live or viable cysts are generally asymptomatic and can survive for years because of immunoprotective mechanisms.
- A variety of infectious, neoplastic, inflammatory or vascular diseases can manifest with a single ring-enhancing lesion of the brain, and differential diagnosis may be challenging at times.
- Clinical symptoms develop due to immune and inflammatory reactions resulting from seepage of cyst fluid into the parenchyma, when the cyst begins to degenerate.
- The diagnosis is established by neuroimaging. Advanced MRI techniques help in differentiating NCC from other mimics.
- NCC in India is different from that in Latin American countries.
- Use of cysticidal drugs is controversial. Some, but not all, experts favor their use
- It is universally accepted that NCC in Indian children is benign.
- Too large and too highly significant reports may actually be more likely to be signs of large bias in most fields of modern research (John PA Ioannidis, 2005)

SUGGESTED READING

1. Baird RA, Wiebe S, Zunt JR, et al. Evidence-based guideline—treatment of parenchymal neurocysticercosis: report of the Guideline Development Subcommittee of the American Academy of Neurology. Neurology. 2013;80(15): 1424-9.
2. Baranwal AK, Singhi PD, Khandelwal N, et al. Albendazole therapy in children with focal seizures and single small enhancing computerized tomographic lesions: a randomized, placebo-controlled, double-blind trial. Pediatr Infect Dis J. 1998;17(8):696-700.
3. Battino D, Estienne M, Avanzini G. Clinical pharmacokinetics of antiepileptic drugs in paediatric patients. Part II. Phenytoin, carbamazepine, sulthiame, lamotrigine, vigabatrin, oxcarbazepine and felbamate. Clin Pharmacokinet. 1995; 29(5):341-69.

4. Bhargava S, Tandon PN. CNS Tuberculosis-lessons learnt from CT studies. Neurology India. 1980;28:207-12.
5. Bhargava S, Tandon PN. Intracranial tuberculomas: a CT study. Br J Radiol. 1980; 53(634):935-45.
6. Carpio A, Escobar A, Hauser W. Cysticercosis and epilepsy: a critical review. Epilepsia. 1998;39(10):1025-40.
7. Carpio A, Kelvin EA, Bagiella E, et al. Ecuadorian Neurocysticercosis Group. Effects of albendazole treatment on neurocysticercosis: a randomized controlled trial. J Neurol Neurosurg Psychiatry. 2008;79(9):1050-5.
8. Carpio A, Romo ML. The relationship between neurocysticercosis and epilepsy: an endless debate. Arq Neuropsiquiatr. 2014;72(5):383-90.
9. Carpio A. Diagnostic criteria for human cysticercosis. J Neurol Sci. 1999; 161(2):185-8.
10. de Souza A, Nalini A, Kovoor JME, et al. Natural history of solitary cerebral cysticercosis on serial magnetic resonance imaging and the effect of albendazole therapy on its evolution. J Neurol Sci. 2010; 288: 135-141.
11. Del Brutto OH, Del Brutto VJ. Isolated brainstem cysticercosis: a review. Clin Neurol Neurosurg. 2013;115(5):507-11.
12. Del Brutto OH, Rajshekhar V, White Jr AC, et al. Proposed diagnostic criteria for neurocysticercosis. Neurology. 2001;57:177-83.
13. Del Brutto OH, Wadia NH, Dumas M, et al. Proposal of diagnostic criteria for human cysticercosis and neurocysticercosis. J Neurol Sci.1996;142(1-2):1-6.
14. Garg RK, Nag D. Single enhancing CT lesions in Indian patients with seizure: clinical and radiological evaluation and follow up. J Trop Pediatr. 1998;44(4): 204-10.
15. Gogia S, Talukdar B, Choudhury V, et al. Neurocysticercosis in children: clinical findings and response to albendazole therapy in a randomized, double-blind, placebo-controlled trial in newly diagnosed cases. Trans R Soc Trop Med Hyg. 2003;97:416-21.
16. Gonzalez-Duarte A. Comments on evidence-based guideline—treatment of parenchymal neurocysticercosis: report of the Guideline Development Sub-committee of the American Academy of Neurology. Neurology. 2013;81(16): 1474-5.
17. Gulati S, Jain P, Sacchan D, et al. Seizure and radiological outcomes in children with solitary cysticercous granulomas with and without albendazole therapy: a retrospective case record analysis. Epilepsy Res. 2014;108(7):1212-20.
18. Gupta RK, Jena A, Sharma A, et al. MR imaging of intracranial tuberculomas. J Comput Assist Tomogr. 1988;12(2):280-5.
19. Ioannidis JPA. Why most published research findings are false? PLoS Medicine. 2005;2(8):e124.
20. Kalra V, Dua T, Kumar V. Efficacy of albendazole and short-course dexamethasone treatment in children with 1 or 2 ring-enhancing lesions of neurocysticercosis: a randomized controlled trial. J Pediatr. 2003;143(1):111-4.
21. Kaur P, Dhiman P, Dhawan N, et al. Comparison of 1 week versus 4 weeks of albendazole therapy in single small enhancing computed tomography lesion. Neurol India. 2010;58(4):560-4.
22. Machado Ldos R. The diagnosis of neurocysticercosis: a closed question? Arq Neuropsiquiatr. 2010;68(1):1-2.
23. Murthy JM, Yangala R. Acute symptomatic seizures-incidence and etiological spectrum: a hospital-based study from South India. Seizure. 1999;8(3):162-5.

24. Puri V, Sharma DK, Kumar S, et al. Neurocysticercosis in children. Indian Pediatr. 1991;28:1309-17.
25. Rajshekhar V, Chandy MJ. Validation of diagnostic criteria for a solitary cerebral cysticercus granuloma in patients presenting with seizures. Acta Neurol Scand. 1997;96(2):76-81.
26. Rajshekhar V, Haran RP, Prakash GS, et al. Differentiating solitary small cysticercus granulomas and tuberculomas in patients with epilepsy. Clinical and computerized tomographic criteria. J Neurosurg. 1993;78(3):402-7.
27. Rajshekhar V. Etiology and management of single small CT lesions in patients with seizures: understanding a controversy. Acta Neurol Scand. 1991:84(6): 465-70.
28. Rajshekhar V. Rate of spontaneous resolution of a solitary cysticercus granuloma in patients with seizures. Neurology. 2001;57(12):2315-7.
29. Rangel R, Torres B, Del Brutto O, et al. Cysticercotic encephalitis: a severe form in young females. Am J Trop Med Hyg. 1987;36:387-92.
30. Sahu PS, Seepana J, Padela S, et al. Neurocysticercosis in children presenting with afebrile seizure: clinical profile, imaging and serodiagnosis. Rev Inst Med Trop Sao Paulo. 2014;56(3):253-8.
31. Sethi PK, Kumar BR, Madan VS, et al. Appearing and disappearing CT scan abnormalities and seizures. J Neurol Neurosurg Psychiatry. 1985;48(9):866-9.
32. Singhi P, Dayal D, Khandelwal N. One week versus four weeks of albendazole therapy for neurocysticercosis in children: a randomized, placebo-controlled double blind trial. Pediatr Infect Dis J. 2003;22(3):268-72.
33. Singhi P, Jain V, Khandelwal N. Corticosteroids versus albendazole for treatment of single small enhancing CT lesions in children with NCC. J Child Neurol. 2004;19(5):323-27.
34. Singhi P, Ray M, Singhi S, et al. Clinical spectrum of 500 children with neurocysticercosis and response to albendazole therapy. J Child Neurol. 2000;15: 207-13.
35. Talukdar B, Saxena A, Popli VK, et al. Neurocysticercosis in children: clinical characteristics and outcome. Ann Trop Paediatr. 2002;22(4):333-9.
36. Tripathi M, Vibha D. Solitary small enhancing CT lesion. Medicine Update-2011; 2011;21:248-52.

CHAPTER
16

A Child with Recurrent or Nonresolving Pneumonia

Vimlesh Soni, Sanjay Verma

INTRODUCTION

Assessment of children with repeated respiratory tract infections requires recognition of factors to differentiate acute respiratory tract infection from recurrent/persistent pathology. Emphasis should be given on detail of each episode including feeding and family history with meticulous clinical examination. The aim of this article is to provide a case-based guide to a systemic approach for diagnosis of recurrent or nonresolving pneumonia.

CASE 1

A 13-month-old girl admitted with cough for 7 days, fever, and rapid breathing for 5 days. The child required hospitalization three times in the past with the similar complains at 2, 5, and 8 months of age and diagnosed as a case of pneumonia every time. She was managed with oxygen support and intravenous antibiotics during all those hospitalizations. Child never required nebulization in the past. There was no significant family history. Birth history was uneventful and development was normal. There was no exposure to smoke. Mother gave very peculiar details of coughing during feeding since beginning and episodic choking and vomiting also. On physical examination, her weight was 6 kg and length was 65 cm. There was pallor but no clubbing or cyanosis. On chest examination, intercostal and subcostal retractions were present and crepitations were heard over right infraclavicular and left axillary area. Other system examination was normal.

Q1. Does this illness is acute, recurrent or persistent?

Ans. When assessing children who present with repeated respiratory tract infections, it is important to recognize certain factors to ascertain whether it is simple acute respiratory tract infection or recurrent/persistent pathology. To identify this, one must go into the details of each episode, age of onset, history of prematurity, treatment details of previous episodes, status between the episodes, feeding details, and growth and development of the child. If the child is growing and developing normally, with no extrapulmonary infections, no family history of severe infections, physical examinations, and chest

X-ray between the episodes are normal; then they are unlikely to have any underlying structural malformation or defect in respiratory defense/immune system. These patients simply lie at one end of the normal distribution of acute respiratory infections, often because of their age or environment. As the index child had relation of respiratory symptoms with feeds, age of onset is quite early and child was not thriving well too. All these points indicate towards recurrent nature of significant underlying illness which requires further evaluation.

Q2. What is the working diagnosis?

Ans. This patient needs evaluation for recurrent pneumonia. Recurrent pneumonia is defined as at least two pneumonia episodes in 1 year or more than three at any time, with radiographic clearing between episodes. As child had coughing and choking episodes during feeding one should ask in detail about history of worsening of symptoms/irritability after feeds or in lying down position, frequent posseting with occasional cyanosis post feeds. All these indicate aspiration or gastroesophageal reflux (GER). Onset of symptoms since immediate postneonatal period arises another possibility of congenital malformation of lung. Focal clinical as well as radiological finding in the same area in every episode signifies congenital malformation such as pulmonary sequestration, cystic adenomatoid malformation, bronchogenic cysts, and aberrant vessels.

Q3. What investigations would you consider?

Ans. Diagnosis of recurrent/persistent pneumonia is based on abnormalities in chest X-ray. It also helps in localization of the involved lobes of lung. Further workup in cases of recurrent pneumonia depends upon unilobar or multilobar involvement. In cases of recurrent or persistent symptoms, when associated with unilobar involvement, it requires bronchoscopy. The differential diagnosis of single lobe involvement may be due to intra- or extraluminal bronchial obstruction and structural malformation of the bronchus, with the intraluminal obstruction being the most common. In children, the most important cause of intraluminal obstruction is a foreign body. If bronchoscopy is normal, then a chest computed tomography (CT) should be performed to identify presence of extraluminal obstruction. Multilobar involvement is either associated with normal or impaired immunity. Further workup of multilobar pneumonia depends upon clinical examination and chest X-ray of the patient. Aspiration is considered to be the most common cause of recurrent pneumonia in developed countries. Aspiration can be due to tracheoesophageal fistula, gastroesophageal reflux disease (GERD) or due to oropharyngeal incoordination. There is strong clinical suspicion of aspiration or GER in index patient too. Confirmation of reflux should be done by esophageal pH study, while video fluoroscopy should be used to confirm dyscordination. Technetium milk scan, esophagoscopy, and biopsy may be used if pH study is not conclusive, although in many cases the history would be sufficient to make the diagnosis.

Laboratory Test Results of the Index Patient
In this patient chest X-ray films of all the previous episodes were available. First chest X-ray showed right upper lobe consolidation, second had left lower lobe infiltrates, and third had right-sided upper and middle lobe infiltrates. Recurrent pneumonia was diagnosed on clinical details and radiological pictures. Multilobar involvement was found on serial chest X-rays. On the basis of clinical possibility of GERD, technetium milk scan was performed which showed significant reflux into the esophagus.

Final Diagnosis
- Recurrent pneumonia
- Gastroesophageal reflux disease.

Child is on antireflux measures and regular follow-up showing improvement in clinical symptoms.

Take Home Message

While managing recurrent pneumonia, one must understand first that which children should undergo a detail diagnostic workup. Relation of respiratory symptoms with feeding is very important to diagnose GER.

CASE 2

A 2.5-month-old boy admitted with cough and progressive increasing respiratory distress since birth. There was no history of forehead sweating, interrupted feeding, discoloration of skin, and worsening of symptoms or choking following feeding. Child required hospitalization at 22 days of life and got treated as pneumonia with intravenous antibiotics. Chest X-ray of that episode showed right upper lobe consolidation/collapse. His birth history was uneventful and family history was noncontributory. On examination, his anthropometry was appropriate for age; his respiratory rate was 60 breaths/minute. His chest was hyperinflated, chest movements were reduced, and bilateral wheeze was present.

Q1. What is the working diagnosis?

Ans. As child is symptomatic since birth, diagnosed as pneumonia at 22 days of life and there was no resolution of symptoms after treatment of first episode, possibility of nonresolving or persistent pneumonia is likely. Confirmation of nonresolving pneumonia requires repeated chest X-ray. Persistent pneumonia is defined as persistence of symptoms and radiological changes for 6 weeks or more despite adequate treatment. For etiology of nonresolving pneumonia, congenital malformation was the first possibility because the onset of symptoms was in neonatal period.

Other important possibilities were cystic fibrosis (CF) and immunodeficiency disorders. Common associated symptoms in CF are delayed passage of meconium, oily stools, failure to thrive, and presence of similar family history. Immunodeficiency disorders usually present with multisystem involvement, chronic malnutrition, and similar complains in the family or previous unexplained sibling losses. Absence of other system involvement, normal anthropometry, and no significant family history made the possibility of CF and immunodeficiency disorders unlikely.

Q2. What investigations would you consider?

Ans. Chest X-ray is the first recommended investigation and that showed left upper and right middle lobe hyperinflation with tracheal shift towards right (Fig. 1). The similar involvement was seen in previous chest X-ray which was done at 22 days of life. Similar lobar involvement with hyperinflation strengthens the possibility of congenital lobar emphysema (CLE), and CT scan of chest was performed. Bronchoscopy helps to demonstrate intrinsic airway compression but is often not necessary to make the diagnosis of CLE.

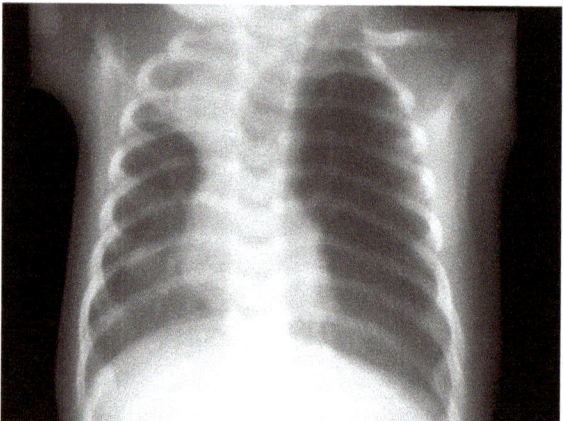

Fig. 1: Chest X-ray showing left upper and right middle lobe hyperinflation with tracheal shift towards right.

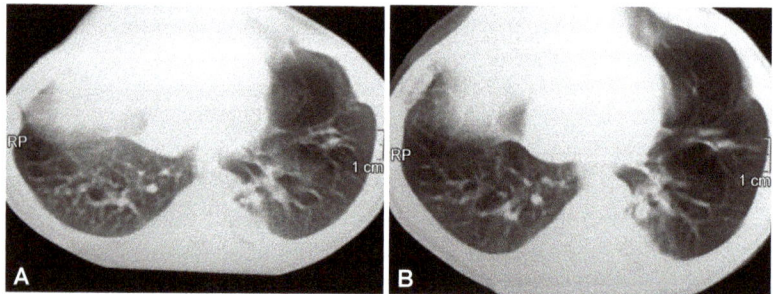

Figs. 2A and B: Contrast enhanced CT chest showing left upper lobe including lingula and right middle lobe hyperinflation with compressive atelectasis involving bilateral basal segments posteriorly.

Laboratory Test Results of the Index Patient
Contrast-enhanced CT chest showed left upper lobe (including lingula) and right middle lobe hyperinflation with compressive atelectasis involving bilateral basal segments posteriorly (Figs. 2A and B).

Final Diagnosis
- Persistent/nonresolving pneumonia
- Congenital lobar emphysema involving left upper lobe and right middle lobe.

Lobectomy was performed in two stage surgery. Patient is in regular follow-up and doing well.

Take Home Message

In case of recurrent and persistent pneumonia repeated similar lobe involvement indicates towards the possibility of either foreign body or congenital malformation. In very young children possibility of foreign body in unlikely. Investigation of choice for congenital malformation is CT scan of chest. Early diagnosis and management is lifesaving in such cases.

CASE 3

A 1-year-old boy admitted with history of fever, cough, and rapid breathing for 2 days. There was no recent change in feeding, activity and urine output. There was no history of bluish discoloration, seizure, altered sensorium, and loose or oily stools. Earlier also this child got admitted twice with the similar complains, first at 6 months and second at 8 months of age. Both the episodes were treated as pneumonia with intravenous antibiotics. But there was no requirement of nebulization in the past and no family member had asthma and atopy. On detail history, mother told that child had interrupted feeding and forehead sweating while feeding. On examination, his weight and length both were below −3 Z-score, he had pallor but no lymphadenopathy, clubbing or cyanosis, his respiratory rate was 52 breaths/minute, subcostal and intercostal retraction was visible, and crepitation in bilateral axillary and left infrascapular area was present. On cardiovascular examination, a pansystolic murmur of grade 3 was noted in left fourth intercostal space in parasternal area. Other systems were normal.

Q1. What is the working diagnosis?

Ans. The child had chronic malnutrition, recurrent pneumonia with clinical features of increased pulmonary blood flow in form of suck-rest-suck cycle and forehead sweating. Patient had history of recurrent pneumonia and this time also clinical features suggested pneumonia. Chest examination indicated involvement of bilateral lower lobes. As child had associated chronic malnutrition so possibility of significant underlying organic pathology leading to recurrent chest infection is likely. Interrupted feeding, forehead sweating, and presence of murmur on cardiac examination indicated towards acyanotic congenital heart disease most commonly ventricular septal defect (VSD).

Q2. What investigations would you consider?

Ans. Patient had chest X-ray of previous episode of 8 months of age and that was showing left lower lobe consolidation with evidence of increase pulmonary blood flow with cardiothoracic ratio (CT) of 67%. Patient had one more chest X-ray at 9 months of age when he was asymptomatic and was on regular follow-up, which showed normal lung fields with CT ratio of 58%. This time chest X-ray of the patient showed infiltrates in bilateral perihilar area, pulmonary plethora with cardiothoracic ratio of 65% suggestive of cardiomegaly (Fig. 3). Possibility of heart disease with increased pulmonary blood flow was kept and echocardiography was planned.

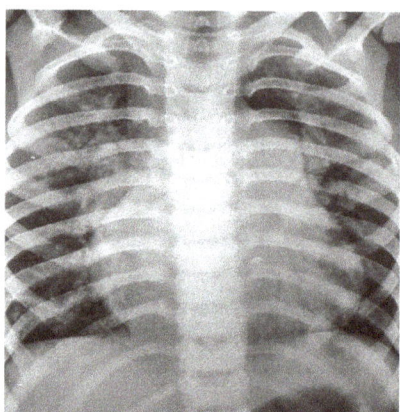

Fig. 3: Chest X-ray showing infiltrates in bilateral perihilar area, pulmonary plethora with cardiomegaly.

Laboratory Test Results of the Index Patient
Echocardiography showed membranous VSD 12 mm in size with left to right shunt with no evidence of pulmonary arterial hypertension.

Final Diagnosis
- Recurrent pneumonia
- Large VSD

Current episode was treated with intravenous antibiotics and patch closure surgery was performed for VSD 2 months later. Child is on regular follow-up, asymptomatic, and gaining weight.

Take Home Message

In case of multilobar recurrent pneumonia, important clinical clues for acute or chronic congestive cardiac failure in form of forehead sweating, interrupted feeding or preference for upright positions indicates towards congenital heart disease. Chest X-ray should be looked carefully for evidence of increase pulmonary blood flow and cardiomegaly to identify congenital heart disease.

CASE 4

A 9-month-old boy admitted with cough since 1 month of age, fever and rapid breathing for 4 days. There was also history of passing oily and loose stools 15–20 times per day since birth. Child did not have bluish discoloration, suck-rest-suck cycle or infections of any other site of the body. Child required hospitalization four times earlier with similar complains, each episode was managed as pneumonia with intravenous antibiotics and nebulization. Child was born out of third-degree consanguineous marriage, but there was no significant family history. On examination, weight was 6 kg and height was 65 cm. Chest was hyperinflated, wheeze was noted in bilateral axillary, and infrascapular area and crepitations were heard in right infraclavicular area. Other systems were normal.

Q1. What is the working diagnosis?

Ans. Child admitted with chronic cough and recurrent respiratory tract infections. There was associated complains of pancreatic insufficiency in form of loose and oily stools. Clue of some genetic illness most probably autosomal recessive in nature was obtained by history of consanguineous marriage of parents. Child was not thriving well on examination. All clinical details were indicating towards chronic respiratory pathology, genetic in nature so possibility of CF was considered.

Q2. What investigations would you consider?

Ans. Child already had three previous chest X-ray, two of symptomatic period and one was done at symptom-free duration. X-rays of symptomatic period were showing bilateral heterogeneous opacities and it was normal when child was asymptomatic. This time chest X-ray showed bilateral heterogeneous opacities predominantly in perihilar area (Fig. 4) with right upper lobe consolidation. Arterial blood gas was performed to look for respiratory as well as metabolic abnormalities. Stool for presence of fat globules was analyzed to identify pancreatic insufficiency. As CF was a strong possibility, sweat chloride was performed twice followed by genetic mutation analysis for CF. Bronchoscopy was also performed for isolation of any signature organism in bronchoalveolar lavage (BAL).

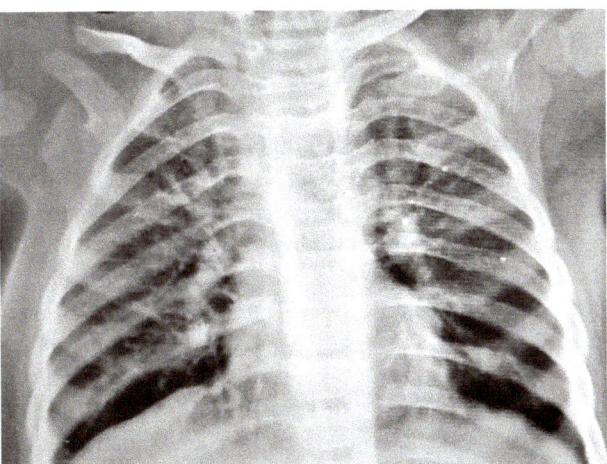

Fig. 4: Chest X-ray showing bilateral heterogeneous opacities predominantly in parahilar area.

Laboratory Test Results of the Index Patient

Arterial blood gas showed metabolic alkalosis with respiratory acidosis with hypoxemia with hypochloremia. Stool examination showed 100 fat globules per high power field. Methicillin sensitive *Staphylococcus aureus* was isolated in BAL. Sweat chloride values were 84 and 76 mmol/L. Most common genetic mutation analysis (delta F508) for CF was sent and child was homozygous for delta F508 mutation. As absence of vas deferens is associated abnormality in CF patients so ultrasound was done to look for vas deferens and it was normal.

Final Diagnosis
- Recurrent pneumonia
- Cystic fibrosis

Patient was treated with intravenous antibiotics for current episode of pneumonia and nebulization with hypertonic saline was initiated. Chest physiotherapy was advised following nebulization. Supplementation of all fat soluble vitamins with double of their recommended daily allowance and other multivitamin and microminerals was done. High calorie and protein diet was started. Pancreatic enzyme supplementation in form of Creon capsules with the dose of 2,000–4,000 lipase units per feeding was also initiated. Parents were counseled regarding the disease, need for lifelong treatment, regular follow-up, and antenatal check-up during future pregnancy.

Take Home Message

One should always suspect CF in a case of recurrent pneumonia with failure to thrive. Presence of features of pancreatic insufficiency with hypochloremic metabolic alkalosis makes this possibility even more strong. Early initiation of supportive treatment with regular screen for infections is important for improving life-span and quality of life.

CASE 5

A 19-month-old boy admitted with fever, cough, and rapid breathing for 7 days. Child required hospitalization two times in the past. First time, he was admitted with fever and rapid breathing at 6 months of age and managed as a case of pneumonia. Second time, he got admitted with swelling over left side of neck and diagnosed as having lymph node abscess. Incision and drainage was done for the swelling, Approximately 10 mL of pus was drained which grew methicillin-resistant *S. aureus (MRSA)* on culture. His one brother died at age of 6 months with pneumonia and he had one living sister with normal health status. There was no other significant history in the family and the health of his parents was normal. On examination, his weight was 7.3 kg, height was 72 cm, his respiratory rate was 60 breaths/minutes and oxygen saturation on room air was 84%. He also had pallor, generalized lymphadenopathy, crepitation in right mammary, and axillary area and hepatosplenomegaly. Other systems were normal.

Q1. What is the working diagnosis?

Ans. This child admitted with second episode of pneumonia with previous chest X-ray suggestive of left lower lobe consolidation. Child also had one other episode of suppurative infection of lymph node in the past and significant family history of sibling loss indicating towards some genetic illness manifesting as recurrent multiple site infections. Physical examination also showed chronic malnutrition with multiple system involvement. With all this information, possibility of immunodeficiency disorder was considered since admission. Workup for human immunodeficiency virus (HIV) infection and primary immunodeficiency was planned.

Most common primary immunodeficiency disorders which present in infancy with suppurative infections and recurrent pneumonia, selectively affects males are Wiskott–Aldrich syndrome (WAS) and chronic granulomatous disease (CGD).

Q2. What investigations would you consider?

Ans. Child admitted with clinical presentation of pneumonia so chest X-ray was done at admission which showed right upper and middle lobes consolidation (Fig. 5). Complete blood count was planned as basic investigation for pediatric immunodeficiency workup; as normal total leukocyte count rules out leukocyte adhesion defect, normal absolute lymphocyte count rules out severe combined immunodeficiency disorders, normal absolute neutrophil count rules out congenital neutropenia syndromes, and normal platelet count and size rules out WAS.

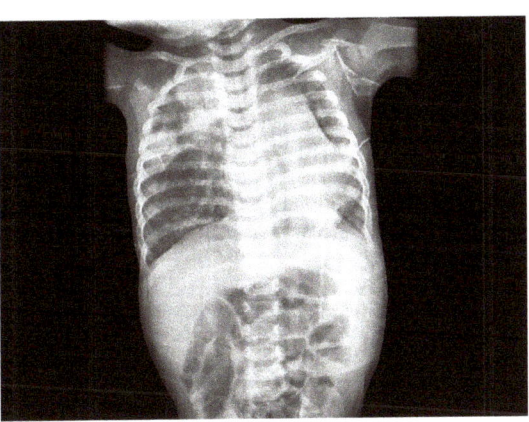

Fig. 5: Chest X-ray showing right upper and middle lobes consolidation.

Human immunodeficiency virus (HIV) enzyme-linked immunosorbent assay (ELISA) was sent as reported incidence of HIV, especially in developing countries more when compared to primary immunodeficiency diseases (PID). Other tests for PID such as immunoglobulin (Ig) levels, nitroblue tetrazolium test, dihydrorhodamine (DHR) test, and mutation analysis were planned after getting reports of initial workup. Bronchoscopy was also planned for obtaining BAL to isolate signature organism.

Laboratory Test Results of the Index Patient
Hemoglobin was 9 g/dL, total leukocyte count was 36,000/mm^3 with 60% neutrophils, 38% lymphocytes, and platelet count was 1,044,000/mm^3. HIV ELISA test was nonreactive. Isolation of MRSA was done in BAL fluid. Ig profile was suggestive of increase Ig levels of IgG (1,820 mg/dL), IgA (185 mg/dL), and IgM (272 mg/dL). Recurrent pneumonia and history of suppurative infection in the index patient with thrombocytosis and increased globulins levels are indicators of chronic granulomatous disease (CGD). On nitroblue tetrazolium test, no reduction was seen in this case as compared to 95% reduction in control indicated towards positive screen test for CGD. DHR, which is a flow cytometry screen test for CGD, was also done for this patient and showed positive result. Later mutation analysis was done for *CYBB* gene, seen in X-linked variant of CGD. The index patient was found to have mutation of *CYBB* gene.

Final Diagnosis
- Recurrent pneumonia
- Chronic granulomatous disease—X-linked.

The patient was treated for current episode of MRSA pneumonia with intravenous antibiotics. After proving the diagnosis of CGD, oral cloxacillin prophylaxis was initiated at discharge. Parents were counseled about the chances of recurrent infections in the child, need for regular prophylaxis and follow-up of index patient, and antenatal counseling in future pregnancies.

Take Home Message

Recurrent infections in a child, especially in association with poor physical growth, should always alarm the physicians for immunodeficiency disorders. Timely diagnosis and early antibiotic prophylaxis significantly reduces frequency of infections and morbidity in CGD.

SUGGESTED READING

1. Brand PL, Hoving MF, de Groot EP. Evaluating the child with recurrent lower respiratory tract infections. Paediatr Respir Rev. 2012;13:135-8.
2. Couriel J. Assessment of the child with recurrent chest Infections. Br Med Bull. 2002;61:115-32.
3. Lodha R, Puranik M, Natchu UC, et al. Recurrent pneumonia in children: clinical profile and underlying causes. Acta Paediatr. 2002;91:1170-3.
4. Montella S, Corcione A, Santamaria F. Recurrent pneumonia in children: a reasoned diagnostic approach and a single centre experience. Int J Mol Sci. 2017; 18(2):E296.
5. Singh M. Recurrent lower respiratory tract infections in children. Indian J Pediatr. 1999;66:887-93.
6. Wald ER. Recurrent and nonresolving pneumonia in children. Semin Respir Infect. 1993;8:46-58.
7. Yousif TI, Elnazir B. Approach to a child with recurrent pneumonia. Sudan J Paediatr. 2015;15:71-7.

Chapter 17

A Case of Recurrent Jaundice

Shrish Bhatnagar

INTRODUCTION

Etiological diagnosis and management of recurrent jaundice is very diverse, and hence challenging in children. The spectrum of causes includes hematologic, anatomical, biochemical, inflammatory, and infective which may be benign to life threatening. In this chapter, we have tried to discuss important hepatobiliary causes of recurrent jaundice in children.

CASE 1

A 7-year-old boy initially presented to his local hospital with mild fever, vomiting, and anorexia for 1 week followed by jaundice with high colored urine. At this point, fever had subsided but jaundice progressively increased. They received symptomatic treatment. Parents noticed clearance of jaundice, improvement in appetite, and some improvement in liver function test (LFT) were also observed (though still not normal). However, after 3 weeks jaundice increased along with worsening of LFTs but no clinical deterioration. There was no history of recent travel/blood transfusion/jaundice in family members recently. No history of recent drug intake, e.g. antitubercular therapy (ATT) or any other hepatotoxic drugs. Physical examination showed weight 20 kg, height 120 cm, icterus, and no palmar erythema/spider nevi. Liver was palpable 3 cm below costal margin, soft in consistency, no splenomegaly or ascites. Other systems were normal on examination.

Q1. What is differential diagnosis?

Ans. The child has presented with jaundice of acute onset with prodromal symptoms of fever, anorexia, and vomiting. High-colored urine indicates it to be conjugated hyperbilirubinemia and not unconjugated. Soft hepatomegaly, with no stigmata of underlying chronic liver disease, normal anthropometry is pointer towards acute onset liver illness. Enlarged liver with no change in clinical condition makes possibility of liver failure unlikely. Subsidence of fever in few days makes malaria or typhoid unlikely as etiology. No purities, fever or pale stools makes obstructive jaundice unlikely. Absence of anemia, lymphadenopathy, bone pain, weight loss, and conjugated jaundice makes hemolysis as an unlikely cause. Hence the differential diagnosis would be acute hepatitis (viral/bacterial/protozoal). Drug-induced hepatitis should be suspected if history of hepatotoxic drugs, especially ATT intake is present. Leptospirosis should be suspected in a patient with high-grade fever, jaundice, and decreased urine output. However in this case, worsening of LFTs after initial improvement suggests relapse of initial, which is seen with hepatitis A.

Q2. Which investigation would you consider?

Ans. *Complete blood count (CBC), erythrocyte sedimentation rate (ESR), peripheral smear, malarial parasite smear (MP Smear), and blood culture*: To rule out hemolysis, malaria, and typhoid.

LFT, prothrombin time/international normalized ratio (PT/INR): To look for rise in alanine aminotransferase/aspartate aminotransferase (ALT/AST) (which may be in thousands); however rise in PT, INR is more bothersome as it may indicate acute liver failure.

Ultrasonography (USG) abdomen: To look for ascites and pericholecystic edema (associated findings seen in acute hepatitis).

Viral serology: For immunoglobulin M (IgM), hepatitis A virus (HAV), IgM hepatitis E virus (HEV), and hepatitis B virus surface antigen (HBsAg)

Leptospiral serology: To rule out leptospirosis.

Laboratory Results
- LFT showed AST/ALT 1,600/2,440, normal PT/INR, and IgM HAV positive.
- IgM HEV, HBsAg, and leptospiral serology was negative.

Q3. Why did child have relapse of jaundice? Explain the management.

Ans. Studies from Indian subcontinent on acute viral hepatitis A, observe a double peak of jaundice or relapsing hepatitis in 11% of patients. The mean time to relapse was 3.4 weeks with a range of 2–6.7 weeks. Management of relapse of acute hepatitis remains symptomatic treatment.

Take Home Message

Relapse in HAV is seen in a subset of patients and management remains the same.

CASE 2

A 3-year-old girl presented with high-grade fever with jaundice, irritability, and pale stools for 1 week. She had similar episode of jaundice 6 months back lasting 2 weeks requiring hospitalization and intravenous (IV) antibiotics. No history of total parenteral nutrition or antibiotics for prolonged period in infancy. Physical examination revealed weight 15 kg, height 90 cm, deep icterus, and itch marks on skin. No hepatosplenomegaly or ascites. Systemic examination was normal.

Q1. What is differential diagnosis?

Ans. This young child presented with two distinct episodes of cholangitis (jaundice, fever, and pain abdomen). Jaundice, pale stools, and itch marks suggest obstructive pattern of jaundice rather than hepatocellular. Such young age of presentation hints at congenital defect in biliary system such as choledochal cyst (CDC) or choledocholithiasis. Similar presentation of obstructive jaundice can be seen in biliary ascariasis in endemic areas (Jammu and Kashmir). In cases with biliary atresia, there is persistent jaundice since neonatal period with pale stools and decompensate very early within a year short of Kasai portoenterostomy.

Q2. What investigation would you consider?

Ans. *CBC and ESR:* Neutrophilia and raised ESR suggest cholangitis/sepsis.

LFT, gamma-glutamyl transpeptidase (GGT), and PT/INR: Liver function tests will show direct hyperbilirubinemia with disproportionate increase in GGT and alkaline phosphatase (ALP) compared to transaminases is suggestive of obstruction in biliary system.

Serum amylase and lipase: To rule out pancreatitis, this may be one of the complications of CDC.

Ultrasound abdomen: Dilated common bile duct with or without stones can be seen. Worms in bile duct can be seen in cases of biliary ascariasis.

Laboratory Results
- *LFT*: Showed total bilirubin 15 mg/dL with direct bilirubin 13 mg/dL.
- AST/ALT 134/145, GGT 1,120, and ALP 990. PT INR normal.
- CBC: Hemoglobin (Hb) 11 g/dL, total leukocyte count (TLC) 15,000/mm^3, differential leukocyte count (DLC) neutrophils 90%, and ESR 48 mm.
- *USG abdomen*: Showed dilated common bile duct of 12 mm.
- *Further investigation*: Magnetic resonance cholangiopancreatography (MRCP) was done which confirmed the findings of ultrasound and showed type 1 CDC with upstream intrahepatic biliary duct dilatation.

Management
Surgery is the definitive treatment. It involves *radical cyst excision and reconstruction by hepaticoenterostomy*. It aims for restoration of normal bile flow by bilioenteric anastomosis and reduction of the risk of malignancy by removing the most common sites of malignant transformation (i.e. the cyst wall and the gallbladder). Timing of surgery in a case presenting with acute cholangitis is 4–6 weeks after cholangitis resolves.

Treat cholangitis with IV antibiotics ± endoscopic retrograde cholangiopancreatography (ERCP) for biliary drainage. Antibiotics of choice are piperacillin/tazobactam, third-generation cephalosporins, and quinolones. Meropenem and imipenem are resorted in case of nonresponse to above antibiotics.

Take Home Message
Recurrent attacks of jaundice in young child with fever and pale stools, one needs to rule out obstructive causes especially congenital defects in biliary system.

CASE 3
A 15-year-old boy presented with history of yellowness of eyes noticed once every year since 3 years of age. This yellowness subsided with or without treatment in 15–20 days and mostly observed during summers. Urine color during these episodes was always normal. There was no history of anemia, blood transfusions, bone pains or itching. No family history of anemia or hemoglobinopathy. On examination, weight 50 kg, height 168 cm, and mild icterus. No hepatosplenomegaly and other systemic examination was normal.

Q1. What is differential diagnosis?
Ans. Important thing to note here is urine color being normal in presence of yellow sclera which is suggestive of unconjugated hyperbilirubinemia.

This distinction is important for making correct list of differentials. In summary, this boy has self-limiting episodes of jaundice without any blood transfusion requirement/bone pains since young age. Thus possibility of hemolytic episodes causing jaundice as in sickle cell disease is unlikely here. Infectious etiology with recurrent episodes without any complications with early onset is unlikely. Other differential diagnosis could be Gilbert syndrome, where such episodes are seen and is commonly seen in general population (prevalence 3–7%). It is a heterogeneous condition in which bilirubin UDP glucuronosyltransferase gene (*UGT1A1*) is defective, and hence problem in bilirubin conjugation.

Q2. Which investigation would you consider?
Ans. *CBC, blood film, and reticulocyte count*: To look for anemia or hemolysis.

LFT: To look for unconjugated or conjugated hyperbilirubinemia and transaminases.

Lactate dehydrogenase (LDH): High LDH may indicate ongoing hemolysis.

Hb electrophoresis: In presence of anemia and unconjugated hyperbilirubinemia, it should be done to rule out hemoglobinopathies.

Ultrasound abdomen: To rule out cholelithiasis seen in hemolytic disorders.

Laboratory Results
Hb 13 g/dL, total bilirubin 6 mg/dL, direct bilirubin 0.8 mg/dL, indirect bilirubin 5.2 mg/dL, AST/ALT 22/23, and reticulocyte count 0.4%.

Further Testing
Genetic testing for Gilbert's polymorphism for *UGT1AI* gene to confirm the diagnosis of Gilbert's syndrome.

Take Home Message
- In case of jaundice, urine color is important factor to distinguish conjugated and unconjugated hyperbilirubinemia.
- In a child with recurrent unconjugated jaundice and normal liver enzymes think about disorder in bilirubin conjugation such as Gilbert's syndrome.

CASE 4

A 9-year-old girl presented with three episodes of jaundice in 2 years with dark urine. She also developed gross abdominal distension and pedal edema in the last episode. Previous two episodes lasted 2–3 weeks and were managed symptomatically at the local hospital. She had lost weight and appetite in 2 years. No history of encephalopathy, pruritus, bleed or melena. She had family history of hypothyroidism. Physical examination revealed weight 22 kg, height 120 cm, icterus, palmar erythema, and vitiligo patch on forehead. On abdominal examination, liver was palpable 2 cm below costal margin, firm in consistency, and spleen 1 cm below costal margin with shifting dullness present.

Q1. What is differential diagnosis?

Ans. The given case represents a case of recurrent jaundice, hepatocellular in nature with recent decompensation as ascites. Differentials in such a case should consider causes of chronic liver disease in a young girl. Though the first differential for chronic liver disease in a 9-year-old child would be Wilson's disease but here a young girl with family history of autoimmune disease and vitiligo and recurrent jaundice, autoimmune hepatitis (AIH) is more likely. Wilson's disease must be ruled out, which may present in a similar fashion. Budd–Chiari syndrome is other differential which may present as ascites alone. Hepatitis B and C are causes of chronic liver disease but they do not usually present as decompensated liver disease in <10 year of age.

Q2. What investigation would you consider?

Ans. *LFT and PT/INR*: Increase in liver enzymes (AST/ALT) suggests hepatocellular jaundice. AST elevation may be more than ALT suggestive of chronicity. Reversal of albumin globulin ratio may indicate AIH.

USG abdomen and Doppler for liver (size and nodularity) and portal vein diameter and collaterals: Shrunken liver, nodularity of liver with splenomegaly indicate cirrhotic liver with portal hypertension.

Upper gastrointestinal tract (UGI) endoscopy: To look for varices which signify portal hypertension.

Laboratory Results:
- *LFT*: Total bilirubin 5 mg/dL, direct bilirubin 3 mg/dL, AST/ALT 840/536, serum albumin 2.8, total protein 7.1, serum globulin 4.3, and PT INR 1.7.
- *USG abdomen* showed coarse liver echotexture with liver size of 7 cm, mild splenomegaly, and moderate ascites. Hepatic veins and inferior vena cava patent and portal vein diameter of 12 mm.
- UGI endoscopy showed small esophageal varices.

Further Investigations
- *Autoimmune markers*: Antinuclear antibody (ANA), smooth muscle antibody (SMA) (1:20 dilution), and anti-liver kidney microsomal (LKM) (1:10 dilution) to establish diagnosis of AIH.
- *Serum ceruloplasmin, Kayser–Fleischer (KF) ring by slit-lamp examination, and 24-hour urine copper estimation* to rule out Wilson's disease.
- *Immunoglobulin G (IgG), C3, C4 levels*: High IgG levels >1.5X normal and low C3, C4 indicate AIH.
- *Liver biopsy*: Interface hepatitis with dense plasma cell infiltrate is characteristic finding of AIH.

Laboratory Results and Management:
Anti-smooth muscle antibody (ASMA) and ANA were strongly positive suggestive of type 1 AIH.

Liver biopsy done later after correction of coagulopathy and resolution of ascites confirmed the diagnosis of AIH. She was initially managed with steroids for induction, and then switched to azathioprine and low-dose steroids for maintenance. Her liver function tests normalized and ascites resolved.

Take Home Message
- Chronic liver disease in a female child who presents with recurrent jaundice and reversal of albumin/globulin (A/G) ratio suggest AIH.
- Wilson's disease should always be ruled out by doing serum ceruloplasmin; KF ring, and 24-hour urinary copper estimation (2/3 criteria should be present).

SUGGESTED READING
1. Berk PD, Noyer C. The familial unconjugated hyperbilirubinemias. Semin Liver Dis. 1994;14:356-85.
2. Dhawan A, Taylor RM, Cheeseman P, et al. Wilson's disease in children: 37-year experience and revised King's score for liver transplantation. Liver Transpl. 2005;11:441-8.
3. Gregorio GV, Portmann B, Reid F, et al. Autoimmune hepatitis in childhood: a 20-year experience. Hepatology. 1997;25:541-7.
4. Joseph VT. Surgical techniques and long-term results in the treatment of choledochal cyst. J Pediatr Surg. 1990;25:782-7.

5. Kumar A, Yachha SK, Poddar U, et al. Does coinfection with multiple viruses adversely influence the course and outcome of sporadic acute viral hepatitis in children? J Gastroenterol Hepatol. 2006;21:1533-7.
6. Owens D, Evans J. Population studies on Gilbert's syndrome. J Med Genet. 1975;12:152-6.
7. Samanta T, Das AK, Ganguly S. Profile of hepatitis A infection with atypical manifestations in children. Indian J Gastroenterol. 2010;29:31-3.
8. Stringer MD, Dhawan A, Davenport M, et al. Choledochal cysts: lessons from a 20 year experience. Arch Dis Child. 1995;73:528-31.
9. Vergani D, Alvarez F, Bianchi FB, et al. Liver autoimmune serology: a consensus statement from the committee for autoimmune serology of the International Autoimmune Hepatitis Group. J Hepatol. 2004;41:677-83.
10. Watson KJ, Gollan JL. Gilbert's syndrome. Baillieres Clin Gastroenterol. 1989;3:337-55.
11. Yamaguchi M. Congenital choledochal cyst: analysis of 1,433 patients in the Japanese literature. Am J Surg. 1980;140:653-7.

CHAPTER
18

Case-based Scenarios in Rickettsial Infection

Atul Kulkarni, Vikram Hirekerur

INTRODUCTION

Rickettsial disease is classically divided into three groups, viz. "typhus group," the "spotted fever group," and "Others". Of these, scrub typhus from the typhus group is endemic all over Asia (including India). Indian tick typhus, a subspecies "indica" of species *Rickettsia conorii* from the spotted fever group is found in southern India, especially in Maharashtra, Karnataka, and Tamil Nadu. Other rickettsial diseases are sporadically reported in India.

CASE 1

A 5-year-old girl from a rural area in Karnataka state presented with fever of 8 days' duration. The child was well prior to onset of fever. Fever was high grade, remittent, and was not relieved by antipyretics. She was treated with oral chloroquine, amoxicillin, and cefpodoxime. She also had rash on extremities and trunk that appeared on the 4th day of fever. She had lost appetite, had generalized body ache, and headache 4 days prior to presentation. She also complained of pain in legs and hence was not able to walk.

On physical examination, the child was conscious and alert. Fever was 101°F. Heart rate was 120/min. Respiration was normal and blood pressure was 98/60 mm Hg. Weight was 15 kg and height was 108 cm.

There was no pallor, icterus, or significant lymphadenopathy. The child appeared moderately dehydrated. There was edema over both lower limbs.

Rash was generalized, nonpruritic, discrete, and maculopapular in nature. It extended over face and extremities, including palms and soles. Liver was palpable 2 cm below the costal margin and was soft in consistency. Spleen was just palpable.

The child was conscious and well oriented but irritable. She had pain in legs and hence did not want to walk. Power in all four limbs and deep tendon reflexes were normal. There were no meningeal signs.

Other systems were normal.

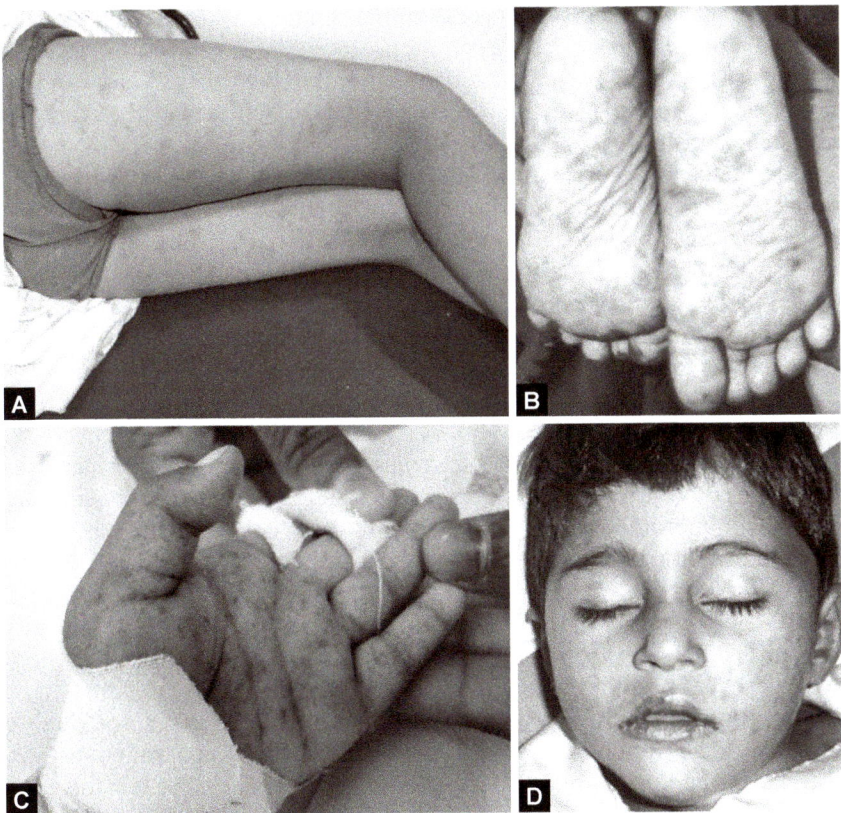

Figs. 1A to D

Q1. What is differential diagnosis?

Ans. Child presented with an acute febrile illness and rash. The following would be considered as differential diagnosis:
- Scarlet fever
- Dengue fever
- Measles
- Rickettsia
- Typhoid fever
- Immune thrombocytopenia/hemolytic-uremic syndrome (ITP/HUS)
- Infectious mononucleosis
- Drug rash
- Kawasaki disease.

In scarlet fever, fever and pharyngitis are the presenting complaints. The characteristic rash appears within 48 hours of fever. The typical features of scarlet fever are sandpaper rash and strawberry tongue.

The rash of dengue fever is a diffuse erythematous rash (erythroderma) or petechial/purpuric rash. The rash sometimes has a typical appearance of "white islands in red sea". Fever disappears after Day 5 or 6. Serositis, i.e. pleural effusion, and ascites are common.

In measles, there is a characteristic prodrome (i.e. cough, cold, running nose, and watering of eyes), Koplik's spots, and the typical pattern of measliform rash.

Rickettsial fever is a classic triad of fever, headache, and rash. Rash usually appears on the 3rd or the 4th day of fever. Initially rash is discrete pale rose red, blanching, and macular or maculopapular in nature. Characteristically, it starts on the extremities and spreads rapidly to involve the entire body including palms and soles. Rash is seen in more than 90% of cases of Indian tick typhus and clinches the diagnosis. Eschar is uncommon in Indian tick typhus. Hepatosplenomegaly may be seen.

Typhoid fever presents with a low-to-high grade fever. Rash of typhoid fever appears in the second week of illness, appears on lower chest and abdomen, and lasts for 2–3 days. In typhoid, the severity of fever increases with time. There are associated features such as sick look, coated tongue, and mild splenomegaly.

Immune thrombocytopenia/hemolytic uremic syndrome (ITP/HSP) presents with petechiae, purpura, or ecchymosis that are unmistakable. In ITP, there is no fever and the patient does not look ill. HSP prominently presents with joint pain, pain in abdomen, hematuria, and vasculitic purpura typically over lower limbs and buttocks.

Infectious mononucleosis comes into differential diagnosis due to fever and rash in an older child. It is characterized by pharyngotonsillitis, generalized lymphadenopathy, and splenomegaly that are absent in this case.

Drug rash can be in the form of erythema multiforme (EM) or Stevens–Johnson syndrome. Apart from a history of a potentially offending drug, EM rash presents peripherally on palms and soles. Iris lesion is the hallmark of EM. Stevens–Johnson syndrome will have involvement of two or more mucosal surfaces.

Kawasaki is a differential diagnosis but does not fulfill the standard criteria.

Hence, rickettsial fever appears to be the closest differential diagnosis.

Q2. What investigation would you like to do in this patient?

Ans.
- Complete blood count (CBC) for leukopenia, thrombocytopenia and hemoconcentration in dengue fever, and leukopenia, thrombocytopenia and anemia in rickettsia
- Urine routine to rule out urinary tract infection
- Dengue NS1, IgM, Weil–Felix test, and enzyme-linked immunosorbent assay (ELISA) for spotted fever/scrub typhus
- Blood culture to rule out sepsis and typhoid fever.
 The results were as follows:
- *CBC*: Hb 10 g%, TC 14,500, and platelets 140,000.
- *Dengue IgM*: Negative

- *Blood culture*: Sterile
- Weil–Felix test: OX 1:160, OX19 1:320, OXK negative
- *ELISA for spotted fever*: Positive
  The investigations point to the diagnosis of rickettsial fever.

Q3. How would you manage the case?

Ans. Appropriate intravenous (IV) fluids would be administered. Oral intake would be encouraged.

Tablet doxycycline would be the mainstay of treatment and was promptly instituted.

Within 24 hours fever subsided, patient began to walk and oral intake improved. This dramatic response to doxycycline definitely supports the diagnosis of rickettsia.

Take Home Message

- Spotted fever disease or the "Indian tick typhus" should be considered as a differential diagnosis in a case of fever with rash.
- Patients coming from endemic area and with history of contact with pets such as dogs and tick bite should be suspected to have rickettsial infection.
- In rickettsia, the classical triad of symptoms consists of fever, rash, and headache. Rash typically involves palms and soles.
- Doxycycline is the drug of choice for uncomplicated rickettsial infection and clinical response is usually dramatic.
- Weil–Felix test or ELISA are not the confirmatory tests but are the only available tests. Indirect fluorescent antibody (IFA) and PCR are the confirmatory tests but are not easily available.
- Rising titer/high titers of Weil–Felix test can be taken as a supportive evidence of rickettsia.

CASE 2

A 4-year-old boy was referred by a pediatrician with fever of 6 days' duration. Child was well prior to the onset of fever. Fever was high grade, continuous, and was not relieved by antipyretics. Patient also had rash of 3 days' duration. Rash appeared on the extremities and later spread to involve the entire body including palms and soles. Patient had convulsions which were generalized and tonic-clonic in nature. The patient had altered sensorium since 2 days prior to presentation.

On physical examination, the child was unconscious, pale, and had sick look. Fever was 103°F. Heart rate was 160/min. Respiration was irregular, BP was 90/70 mm Hg, and oxygen saturation was 60–70%.

The child was not responding to verbal stimuli and had decerebrate posturing.

Weight was 15 kg and height was 110 cm.

Rash was generalized, discrete, and maculopapular in nature. Also, there was necrotic rash over upper and lower limbs, face, and buttocks. There was gangrene of both ear lobes and of four digits of left hand. Liver was enlarged 5 cm below the costal margin and was firm in consistency. Spleen was palpable 2 cm below the costal margin.

The respiratory system examination revealed irregular respiration, reduced breath sounds and bilateral conducted sounds. The CNS examination revealed an unconscious child with Glasgow Coma Scale (GCS) of 7, decerebrate posturing, and Babinski's sign.

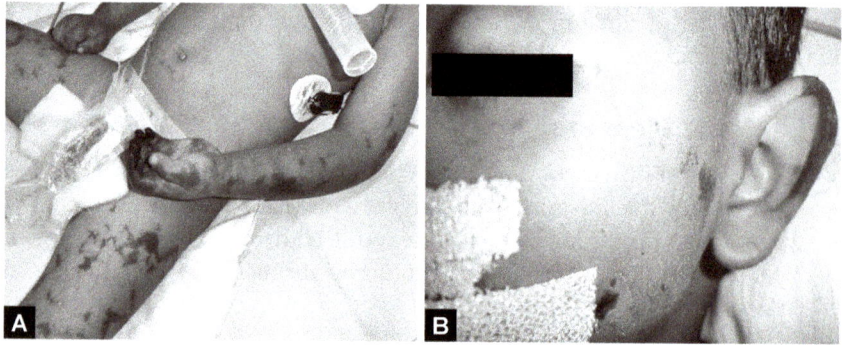

Fig. 2A and B

Q1. What is differential diagnosis?

Ans. The child presented with febrile illness of acute onset with necrotic rash, gangrene of fingers, altered sensorium, convulsions, and sick look. This can mimic the following:
- Meningococcemia
- Rickettsia
- Thrombotic thrombocytopenic purpura
- Purpura fulminans.

Acute meningococcal septicemia is indistinguishable in early stage of illness but is often associated with septic shock. Rash in meningococcemia is usually present in the territory of inferior vena cava. Rash may be petechial, purpuric, or necrotic. Rash is more necrotic in the center of the lesion. At times, there can be gangrene of the digits. Once rash appears, child rapidly goes in hypotension, coma, and disseminated intravascular coagulation (DIC).

The pathological hallmark of rickettsial infection is microvasculitis. This may lead to complications such as encephalitis, acute respiratory distress syndrome (ARDS), pneumonia, myocarditis, hepatitis, and renal failure. Similarly, skin manifestations can be in the form of necrotic rash, gangrene of digits, gangrene of earlobes, and scrotal skin gangrene. Severe vascular obstruction may lead to gangrene of the entire limb.

Thrombotic thrombocytopenic purpura (TTP) is a rare disorder in childhood albeit possible. It presents with microangiopathic hemolytic anemia, fever, renal failure, neurological symptoms, and purpuric or necrotic rash.

Purpura fulminans due to other bacterial infections should be thought of in such a scenario. Blood culture is needed for confirmation of the causative organism. Rickettsial fever with encephalopathy appears to be the closest differential diagnosis.

Q2. What investigations would you like to do in this patient?

Ans.
- CBC for leukocytosis and thrombocytopenia for bacterial infection and rickettsial fever.
- Weil–Felix Test and ELISA for spotted fever.
- Serum electrolytes, creatinine, ALT (alanine transaminase), PT (prothrombin time), aPTT (activated partial thromboplastin time), and chest X-ray as part of evaluation of a critically ill child.
- Lactate dehydrogenase (LDH), reticulocyte count, and peripheral smear for Burr cells for TTP.
- Blood culture and CSF (cerebrospinal fluid) examination to rule out sepsis and meningitis, respectively.
- CT head would be asked at an appropriate time.

The results were as follows:
- *CBC*: Hb 8 g%, WBC 24,000, and platelets 86,000
- Weil–Felix done positive OX 1:160, ELISA for spotted fever—positive
- Serum sodium 119 mEq/L, serum potassium 3.8 mEq/L, and ALT 84 mg%
- Creatinine 0.4 mg%, and PT/APTT—within normal limits
- Chest X-ray suggestive of ARDS
- LDH 110 units/L, reticulocyte count 0.7%, and peripheral smear for Burr cells for TTP negative
- CSF: Cells 32 , P 30%, L 70%, sugar 54 mg%, protein 62 mg%, Cl 95, and culture—sterile
- Blood culture—sterile
- CT head showed minimal cerebral edema.

The investigations point to the diagnosis of rickettsial fever with ARDS with encephalopathy.

Q3. How would you manage the case?

Ans. Patient was in unconscious state and convulsing. Attention to "ABC" took precedence. The child was intubated and taken on ventilator.

He was given anticonvulsants (injection lorazepam and injection phenytoin) and cerebral decongestants (injection mannitol).

Injection methylprednisolone is given to reduce cerebral edema in rickettsial encephalitis.

The ARDS-restricted fluids (two-thirds of maintenance) were administered because of possibility of aggravation of ARDS or cerebral edema due to excessive fluids.

Tablet doxycycline was administered by nasogastric route and injection chloramphenicol 100 mg/kg/day by IV infusion.

RBC transfusion was given to keep hemoglobin (Hb) more than 10 g%.

Standard care of an unconscious child was ordered.

Take Home Message

- Spotted fever disease is prevalent throughout the world. In India, it is known as "Indian tick typhus." It is prevalent in the southern part of the country. It should be considered as a differential diagnosis in a case of fever with rash.
- In a patient coming from an endemic area with a complaint of fever and with a history of contact with pets such as dogs and tick bite, rickettsial infection should be strongly suspected.
- Classical triad of symptoms consists of fever, rash, and headache
- Clinical features include fever, rash extending over palms and soles, palpable purpura, necrotic rash, gangrene, non-pitting edema over body and on legs, and hepatosplenomegaly.
- Meningoencephalitis, ARDS, acute respiratory failure (ARF), DIC, and myocarditis are the usually seen complications.
- Doxycycline and chloramphenicol are the drugs recommended to effectively treat rickettsial infection.

CASE 3

A 5-year-old male child was brought by parents with complaints of fever of 7 days' duration, headache, irritability, and pain in legs of 4 days' duration.

The child was apparently fine 7 days back. Since then he had fever which was acute in onset, high grade, and not relieved by antipyretics. Parents consulted a private practitioner and was treated with some antibiotics. However, symptoms persisted. The boy also had headache, irritability, and pain in legs since 4 days prior to presentation. There was no history of convulsions. There were no other complaints.

On physical examination, child was sick and irritable.

Weight of child was 20 kg and height was 110 cm.

The patient was febrile on admission (101°F). There was mild pallor. There was significant generalized nontender lymphadenopathy and bilateral pedal pitting edema.

Liver was palpable 3 cm below the costal margin. Spleen was palpable 3 cm below the costal margin. There were no other significant findings.

Differential diagnosis: In a 5-year-old child who presents with acute-onset and high-grade fever and is not relieved by antipyretics and antibiotics with generalized lymphadenopathy and hepatosplenomegaly, the following conditions should be considered:
- Typhoid
- Malaria
- Scrub typhus
- Leptospirosis
- Infectious mononucleosis.

Typhoid fever presents with a low-to-high grade fever. There is a typical pattern of fever called "step-ladder fever" though rarely seen. Though splenomegaly is a common feature, lymphadenopathy is not seen in typhoid fever. Toxic look and coated tongue are common features.

Malaria commonly presents with splenohepatomegaly and anemia. Significant lymphadenopathy is not common.

Scrub typhus can present with fever without focus, generalized lymphadenopathy, and hepatosplenomegaly. Painless eschar is seen in only 7–40% of cases and maculopapular rash is present in less than 30% cases. Both can be absent. Gastrointestinal symptoms such as abdominal pain, diarrhea, and vomiting are seen in up to 40% of cases.

The septicemic phase of anicteric leptospirosis can present similarly but is characterized by conjunctival suffusion, chemosis, purulent exudates, photophobia, or orbital pain.

Infectious mononucleosis presents with tonsillopharyngitis, lymphadenopathy, and hepatosplenomegaly. Spleen is very soft on palpation.

Hence, rickettsial fever appears to be the closest differential diagnosis.

Q1. What investigations would you like to do in this patient?
Ans.
- CBC for leukopenia, eosinopenia, and thrombocytopenia for enteric fever. In rickettsial fever, there is anemia, leukocytosis, and thrombocytopenia. Thick smear for malaria.
- Widal test for typhoid fever. Weil–Felix test and ELISA for spotted fever. Rapid diagnostic test (RDT) for malaria antigen.
- Leptospira IgM
- Blood culture for typhoid fever.

  The results were as follows:
- *CBC*: Hb 8 g%, TC 17,500, P 40 L 60, and platelets 1,05,000. Peripheral smear for malaria—negative
- Widal—negative. Weil-Felix Test—positive —1:160 (OXK). ELISA—scrub typhus strongly positive. RDT for malaria—negative
- Leptospira IgM—negative
- Blood culture—sterile.

  The investigations point to the diagnosis of rickettsial fever.

Q2. How will you treat this child?

Ans. The drug of choice for scrub typhus is tetracycline/doxycycline.

Doxycycline: 2.2/kg/dose BD for 5–7 days

Tetracycline: 25–50 mg/kg/day PO in 4 divided doses for 5–7 days

Chloramphenicol: 50–100 mg/kg/day IV/PO in 4 divided doses for 5–7 days

Azithromycin, rifampicin, and fluoroquinolones are the alternative drugs.

Supportive measures include maintenance of fluids and electrolyte balance and nutrition.

Take Home Message

- Scrub typhus is caused by *Orientia Tsutsugamushi* species of genera *Rickettsia*. Infection occurs through the bite of infected chiggers, the larval stage of trombiculid mite (rat mite). The entire region of Asia is an endemic zone for scrub typhus.
- Clinically, the disease presents as acute febrile illness without focus. It may also present with lymphadenopathy and hepatosplenomegaly. Rash and eschar may be present in few cases.
- High index of suspicion for the disease is helpful in early diagnosis and treatment. Fever without focus and painless eschar points toward scrub typhus.
- Leukopenia in early stages and leukocytosis in later stages as well as anemia and thrombocytopenia are associated features.
- Positive ELISA test is the most feasible test. Though IFA and PCR are the confirmatory tests, they are not the easily available tests.
- Tetracycline (doxycycline) is the drug of choice.

SUGGESTED READING

1. Baldwin K, Rathi N. Rickettsial Disease. In: Robert L, Daniel T, William M (Eds). International Neurology, 2nd edition. UK: Wiley Blackwell; 2016. pp. 291-5.
2. Kulkarni A. Rickettsial infections. IAP Textbook of Infectious Diseases, 1st edition. New Delhi: Jaypee Brothers Medical Publishers; 2013. pp. 376-85; 6-85.
3. Kulkarni A. Spotted Fevers. PG Textbook of Pediatrics. New Delhi: Jaypee Brothers Medical Publishers; 2013. pp. 1309-12.
4. Rahi M, Gupte MD, Bhargava A. DHR-ICMR Guidelines for Diagnosis and Management of Rickettsial Diseases in India. Indian J Med Res. 2015;141(4): 417-22.
5. Rathi N, Kulkarni A, Yewale V. IAP guidelines on rickettsial diseases in children. Indian Pediatr. 2017;54(3):223-9.
6. Rathi N, Maheshwari M, Khandelwal R. Neurological manifestations of rickettsial infections in children. Pediatric Infectious Disease. 2016;7(3):64-6.
7. Reller ME, Dumler JS. Rickettsial infection. In: Kliegman RM, Bonita, Stanton, St Geme J, Schor NF (Eds). Nelson's Textbook of Paediatrics, 20th edition. USA: Elsevier Health Sciences; 2015. pp. 1497-511.

CHAPTER 19

Case Scenarios on Rational Antibiotic Usage

Dhanya Dharmapalan

INTRODUCTION

The misuse of antibiotics has been the biggest driving force for antibiotic resistance. Rational antibiotic usage involves avoidance of both unnecessary use and suboptimal antibiotic therapy.

An antibiotic therapy can be optimized by choosing the right antibiotic, in the correct dose, route, duration, and taking into account the host morbidity factors. The pharmacokinetic/pharmacodynamic properties of the drug help to guide these decisions and are different for every antibiotic.

- In every patient suspected to be harboring an infection, the first question that a physician needs to find an answer to is if an antibiotic is required in first place. This requires the art of clinically differentiating a viral infection from a bacterial infection on the basis of history and examination. For example, antibiotics can be easily avoided in a viral setting such as well-looking child with fever, coryza, cough, or another child with vomiting and watery loose stools. The family history of similar illness also points toward a viral etiology. Antibiotics have no role to play in any of the viral illnesses. The only place if there is complication with a secondary bacterial infection, for example as in a child with measles who develops a bacterial pneumonia as a complication.
- Once a clinician is certain that the infection is bacterial and not viral, antibiotics can be started either empirically (before confirmation by laboratory investigations) or as definite therapy (after confirmation by laboratory investigations).
- Empirical therapy is usually started urgently when a child is sick or immunocompromised, e.g. in neonates, waiting to start an antibiotic can be dangerous. The other setting where an empirical antibiotic is started is when it is reasonably a bacterial infection on clinical grounds, for example, otorrhea and abscess.
- Before starting an empirical therapy with an antibiotic, it is important to find the answers to the five golden questions: (1) What is the causative bacteria? (2) What is the site of infection? (3) What is host comorbidity? (4) What is suspicion of drug resistance? (5) What is severity of illness?

- If the infection is mild-like impetigo, a probability of a cure rate of 70% is acceptable; if moderately severe like end-organ damage (e.g. pyelonephritis), a cure rate of around 80–90% should be targeted; if severe infection such as sepsis/meningitis, we need to target 100% cure rate as failure to initiate the right treatment early is dangerous.
- Take relevant microbiological samples for cultures, for example, blood, urine, and pus, before starting the empiric antibiotic.
- After 24–48 hours of starting the empiric antibiotic, reassess the patient and follow the options given below:
  - Stop antibiotics, if there is evidence of a nonbacterial infection, for example, dengue and malaria. Change antibiotic to narrow-spectrum antibiotic as per culture sensitivity report.
  - Switch to oral antibiotics, if there is clinical improvement and the child can accept orally.
  - If no improvement or worsening is seen, review diagnosis and treatment, check for complications, and review again.

Let us look at few case scenarios of rational empiric therapy:

CASE 1

A 3-year-old boy is brought with fever and cough since 5 days. On examination, the child is lethargic, tachypneic, and has crepitations on the right side of chest. Rest of the examination is normal.

This case scenario is that of clinical community-acquired pneumonia. In a lethargic child with localized respiratory symptoms, one must consider a bacterial cause and start an antibiotic. Now, let us go through the exercise of the five golden questions which are as follows:

Q1. What are the causative bacteria?

Ans. In children, the leading bacterial causes of community acquired pneumonia as per age are gram-negative organisms in the neonatal period. *Streptococcus pneumoniae, Haemophilus influenzae B* and *Staphylococcus* in children upto 5 years of age. And in above 5 years of age—*Streptococcus pneumoniae, Mycoplasma* and *Staphylococcus aureus*.

Q2. What is the site of infection?

Ans. Respiratory tract: Both the drugs have a reasonably good penetration in the respiratory tract.

Q3. What is host comorbidity?

Ans. This child otherwise has no host comorbidity. Situations where this factor may influence the decision, for example a child with cystic fibrosis, are known to be colonized with *Pseudomonas* bacteria.

Q4. What is the suspicion of drug resistance?

Ans. No. Upfront cover for community-acquired methicillin-resistant *Staphylococcus aureus* (MRSA) or any suspected drug-resistant *Streptococcus pneumoniae* is not required as the child is otherwise hemodynamically stable and there is always scope for upgrading antibiotics, if required.

Q5. What is the severity of illness?

Ans. This child, though hemodynamically stable, is lethargic and warrants a parental antibiotic. Therefore, the choice of antibiotic was either IV (intravenous) ceftriaxone or IV co-amoxiclav.

The reports are as follows: CBC (complete blood count)—Hb 9.8 mg/dL, TLC (total leukocyte count) 24,000 N 82%, L 10%, E 2%, M 0%, platelets 2.25 lacs, CRP (C-reactive protein) 46 mg/dL, blood culture sent (awaited). X-ray chest showed right lower zone haziness.

At the end of 48 hours, it was found that the child continued to have high-grade fever and air entry was reduced further on the right side.

Q6. What next? Do we escalate antibiotic?

In a case of pneumonia, when there is no improvement in 48 hours post-antibiotic administration, one must look for possibility of any collection before considering any escalation in antibiotic.

A repeat X-ray showed pleural effusion. USG chest was suggestive of tappable fluid with septae. Fluid was tapped and found to be exudates. An intercostal drainage (ICD) tube was inserted and pus was drained (Fig. 1). The same antibiotic was continued. There was a fever defervescence in the next 48 hours.

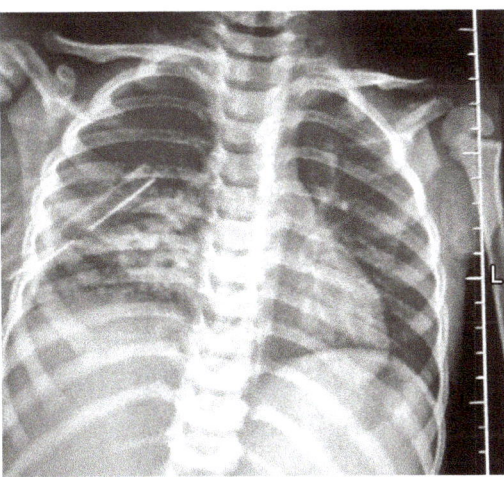

Fig. 1: In case of pneumonia, if there is no clinical improvement after 48 hours of antibiotics, always rule out a collection in the pleura before stepping up the antibiotic. Simple drainage of pus may bring about the required clinical improvement rather than escalation of antibiotics.

After removal of ICD on the 6th day of admission, the discharge was planned for the patient. The child was afebrile, accepting orally with a significant improvement in air entry. Both pus culture and blood culture grew *S. pneumoniae* sensitive to all penicillins.

The decision to shift from IV to oral and to step down to most narrow antibiotic was taken—in this case, oral amoxicillin. The duration of antibiotic in a case of empyema is 3–4 weeks. The child was discharged and prescribed oral amoxicillin for 3 weeks. The child showed complete resolution after therapy.

Suppose, in this child, the repeat X-ray had not shown any collection for trial of drainage or the child had deteriorated hemodynamically with negative cultures; then, antibiotics should be empirically escalated to cover any resistance such as MRSA. So addition of clindamycin/vancomycin/linezolid would be considered. Vancomycin being bactericidal would be preferred, if there is hemodynamic compromise. Renal function tests need to be monitored on vancomycin. Clindamycin and linezolid both have an additional property of antitoxin effect (may be needed in severe pneumonia such as necrotizing pneumonia). One must remember that daptomycin should not be used in treatment of MRSA pneumonia as the surfactant in the lungs makes it ineffective. Rarely *Mycoplasma pneumoniae* can be a cause for empyema, irrespective of the age of the child and should be kept as a differential for nonresponding empyema.

CASE 2

A 4-year-old girl was admitted with status epilepticus and required intubation. She was started empirically on ceftriaxone. She started spiking high after 2 days on ventilator, secretions became purulent. X-ray chest which was normal on admission now showed left zone haziness.

A diagnosis of ventilator-associated pneumonia was made. Endotracheal secretions were sent for culture.

Now let us look at the antibiotic choice.

Q1. How does this case differ from the earlier?

Ans. Though the age group of the child is the same as well as the site of infection and the severity, the causative pathogens differ (includes gram-negative organisms) and suspicion of drug resistance will be high.

Since the pneumonia occurred while on ceftriaxone, one needs to cover the extended-spectrum beta-lactamase (ESBL) producers, such as resistant *Klebsiella, Acinetobacter,* and *Pseudomonoas*, and also look at the local antibiotic susceptibility pattern of the ICU (intensive care unit). Also, there is fairly good chance of it being a resistant gram-positive bug-like MRSA. Vancomycin is required especially where the prevalence of MRSA is higher than 10%. The combination of piperacillin-tazobactam plus vancomycin has been found to be associated with kidney injury in children and should be avoided as far as possible. This child was started on combination of meropenem and vancomycin. The cultures showed growth of *Klebsiella* only sensitive to carbapenem and colistin. Vancomycin was stopped and meropenem continued.

Meropenem being a beta-lactam antibiotic follows time-dependent killing; therefore, timely administration of the drug is important to maximize its efficacy. Extended/continuous infusions can be tried for severe gram-negative organisms with high minimum inhibitory concentration (MIC) levels.

An important point to note is that in these conditions, when the causative organism has been established as a resistant *Klebsiella*, there is no role of the co-administered antibiotic, and it should be stopped as soon as possible. The antibiotics need to be continued at least for 10–14 days depending on the clinical status.

Stricter infection control measures and ventilator-associated pneumonia (VAP) bundles need to be reinforced in the ICU.

CASE 3

A 10-month female baby was admitted with high fever, vomiting, and intermittent irritability since 2 days. There was no other symptoms. Systemic examination revealed no abnormalities. Anterior fontanelle (AF) was normal. CBC showed Hb 9.8 g%, TLC 24,000 N 78% L 20% E 2%, platelets 2.6 lakhs/cumm. Urine routine showed plenty of pus cells suggestive of UTI (urinary tract infection).

Now, if we apply the principles of choosing antibiotic therapy here:

Q1. What is the site of infection?

Ans. Urinary tract is the site of infection.

Q2. What are the causative organisms?

Ans. The causative organism are usually gram-negative organisms.

Q3. Is there any suspicion of resistance?

Ans. No (suspicion will be higher if the child has received antibiotics in the preceding 3 months).

Q4. Is there any host comorbidity present?

Ans. No, renal function derangement should caution one to avoid or modify nephrotoxic drugs as per creatinine clearance.

Q5. What is the severity of illness?

Ans. It requires parenteral administration.

The choice of antibiotic in this regard was IV ceftriaxone/IV cefotaxime as in the treatment of community-acquired complicated UTI.

While treating a suspected case of UTI, it is extremely important to send urine culture before starting antibiotics. The method of collection of urine is a crucial step for interpretation of urine culture. Many times, for ease of collection, a plastic urine bag is used for an infant as it becomes tedious for a caretaker to wait and watch for the infant to pass urine. Ideally, the urine should be collected either by catheterization or by suprapubic catheterization. If either of the two is not feasible, collect urine by a clean-catch sample. For this method, the child is held by the arms after half an hour of a feed when it is expected that the bladder might be full. One assistant rubs in circular fashion the lumbar area while other taps in front on the suprapubic area at a speed of about 100 taps/min. With this method, within few minutes, by reflex action the infant voids out urine which can be collected in a sterile container. It is also important to ensure that the urine sample reaches the laboratory for processing within an hour. If any delay is anticipated, then urine sample should be refrigerated.

While interpreting any urine culture report in practice, it is important to ask the caretaker how the urine is collected. If it is by the bag method, then there is possible contamination by feces or skin flora, and hence should be disregarded.

Also pyuria on urine routine (>10 leukocytes per mm^3 in a fresh uncentrifuged sample, or >5 leukocytes per high-power field in a centrifuged sample) is considered as hallmark for diagnosis of UTI and can differentiate true UTI from asymptomatic bacteriuria. Asymptomatic bacteriuria does not require treatment.

As per the urine collection method, the culture can be interpreted as significant colony count for UTI as follows:
- *Suprapubic/catheterization*: Colony count of 50,000 or more
- *Clean-catch sample*: Colony count of 1 lakh or more

The child clinically responded with defervescence of fever after 48 hours of antibiotics. USG abdomen was normal. Urine culture grew *Escherichia coli* > 1 lakh colony count, ESBL.

When an organism is ESBL, it is generally not amenable for treatment for cephalosporins. But here this child was started on ceftriaxone and showed clinical improvement with ceftriaxone. This in vivo discrepancy occurs due to urinary concentration of beta-lactam antibiotics where the drug concentration is much higher than MIC of the organism than compared to when tested in laboratory conditions. In such a situation, it is advisable to continue the same antibiotic and switch to oral antibiotic such as cefixime after 24–48 hours of fever defervescence.

Suppose this child had not clinically responded to ceftriaxone. Then we should change the antibiotics as per the culture sensitivity pattern, i.e. with injection piperacillin-tazobactam or injection meropenem.

The total duration of treatment for complicated UTI is at least 10–14 days.

Nitrofurantoin, a bacteriostatic drug, should be avoided for treatment of UTI even if the culture report shows sensitivity. One must not forget to put this child on UTI prophylaxis until further test reports are available like micturating cystourethrogram (MCUG) done after 3 weeks of UTI.

As seen in the earlier case scenarios, microbiological diagnosis aids in rational antibiotic therapy. But it should be interpreted with caution and depends strongly on the method of collection.

Clinical improvement should be given higher consideration when deciding about changing/escalating antibiotics.

CASE 4

A 10-year-old girl presented with fever since 3 weeks and weight loss of 3 kg. There was no history of cough/loose motions. There was no history of cattle contact/consumption of pasteurized milk/travel. There was no contact with TB (tuberculosis). The child had received multiple courses of antibiotics before referral.

Systemic examination was unremarkable. Counts, urine routine, liver enzymes, X-ray chest, and USG abdomen, all were normal. Computed tomography chest done as part of pyrexia of unknown origin (PUO) workup was suggestive of necrotic mediastinal lymph nodes. A lymph node present just below the skin in the supraclavicular area was aspirated and sent for GeneXpert, histopathology, and MGIT culture. The sample showed caseous necrosis while GeneXpert came positive for mycobacterial TB, rifampicin sensitive. Four-drug AKT was started (isoniazid, rifampicin, pyrazinamide and ethambutol).

While counseling about AKT, attention was given to counsel caretakers about the importance of taking drugs on empty stomach in the morning. The caretakers were also counseled about the side effects of the drugs.

Q1. Could we have started AKT emperically based on the clinical scenario and CT suggestive of necrotic mediastinal lymph nodes?

Ans. No. Emperical treatment of TB should be avoided and attempts must always be made to make a tissue and microbiological diagnosis of tuberculosis in view of the rising multidrug resistance in tuberculosis.

It is important to understand the limitations of tests such as erythrocyte sedimentation rate (ESR), Mantoux, and nonspecific shadows on X-ray chest.

In spinal TB, bone TB, and TB meningitis, the continuation phase is to be extended to 10 months, on a case-to-case basis for delayed response and as per discretion of the treating pediatrician.

Take Home Message

- Rational antibiotic usage starts with the question whether an antibiotic is necessary in the patient.
- Once a decision to start an antibiotic is taken, an empirical choice is made by asking further questions such as the suspected causative organisms, the site of infection where the antibiotic should reach, if any drug resistance, any host comorbidity, and the severity of illness. Initiation of antibiotics should not be delayed in severely ill children/neonates.
- Attempts should be made for microbiological diagnosis by sending appropriate cultures. In many febrile conditions, cultures may not yield organism as in rickettsia, leptospirosis, etc. Other nonculture methods,

such as PCRs (polymerase chain reactions), and serological evidence can be resorted to for microbiological evidence.
- In case an alternative diagnosis which does not warrant antibiotics is made, for example, dengue, infectious mononucleosis, and malaria, then antibiotics should be stopped immediately. Alternative diagnosis like noninfectious cause of fever should be looked for if not responding to treatment after ruling out complications or reviewing current regimen.
- Antibiotics should be de-escalated based on the susceptibility results. Caution is to be taken while interpreting culture reports. Colonization and contamination should not be treated.
- National/International guidelines should be referred to implement the correct treatment regimens and duration.
- The antibiotic dose and route should be optimized considering the pharmacokinetic and pharmacodynamic properties of the drug. Timing of drug, for example, before food [Isoniazid (INH) and rifampicin]/with fatty meal (artemether-lumefantrine), helps to optimize the absorption of the drug.
- Proper prescription and communication to the caretaker are essential for completion of the course and rational use of antibiotic at their end.

SUGGESTED READING

1. Downes KJ, Cowden C, Laskin BL, et al. Association of acute kidney injury with concomitant vancomycin and piperacillin/tazobactam treatment among hospitalized children. JAMA Pediatr. 2017;171(12):e173219.
2. Indian Society of Pediatric Nephrology, Vijayakumar M, Kanitkar M, et al. Revised statement on management of urinary tract infections. Indian Pediatr. 2011;48(9):709-17.
3. Kumar A, Gupta D, Nagaraja SB, et al. Updated National Guidelines for Pediatric Tuberculosis in India, 2012. Indian Pediatr. 2013;50(3):301-6.
4. Patra PK, Thirunavukkarasu AB. Unusual complication of *Mycoplasma pneumonia* in a five-year-old child. Australas Med J. 2013;6(2):73-4.
5. Roberts KB. Revised AAP Guideline on UTI in Febrile Infants and Young Children. Am Fam Physician. 2012;86(10):940-6.

CHAPTER 20

Approach to a Case of Matted Lymphadenopathy

Vineet Saxena, Pranjali Saxena

INTRODUCTION

Lymphadenopathy may present alone as a symptom or may be associated with other symptoms. The pathology can be primarily of lymph nodes or it may associate with any underlying illness such as leukemia or malignancy. Human body has approximately 600 lymph nodes, submandibular, axillary, or inguinal regions which may normally be palpable in healthy people, and abdominopelvic are deep group of lymph nodes. Lymphadenopathy refers to nodes that are abnormal in size, consistency, or number.

Localized lymphadenopathy is more common than generalized in patients with lymphadenopathy. Lymphadenopathy is said to be generalized when lymph nodes are enlarged in two or more noncontiguous areas. It is localized, if only one area is involved. In pediatric age group, infections rather than malignancies are more common etiology.

CASE 1

A 3-year-old boy presented to clinician with complaint of multiple nodular painless swelling in neck below right jaw which the mother noticed 3 months back. The child otherwise has no documented fever, chills, cough, sore throat, and dental problem. She took a course of antibiotic for 14 days from another doctor but the swelling did not regress. Meanwhile, the child appetite also worsened and outdoor activities were reduced. On local examination, only right upper cervical lymph nodes are enlarged significantly, non-tender, matted, and fluctuant.

Hospital stay: Child examination was suggestive of matted, significant, non-tender upper cervical lymphadenopathy. Complete blood count suggests mild anemia with lymphocytosis. Tubercular workup was done. Purified protein derivative (Mantoux test) was positive. Fine-needle aspiration cytology (FNAC) was done suggestive of caseous necrosis with tubercular picture. Antitubercular therapy (ATT) was started and the patient improved with ATT.

CASE 2

A 13-year-old boy admitted to pediatric ward with complaints of multiple nodular painless swelling in neck below the jaw. It was associated with low-grade fever and night sweats from 8–9 months. There is no history of TB contact. Parents consulted few doctors and was prescribed antibiotic course every time. Now he was taking ATT from past 6 months advised from local doctor but swelling and other symptoms did not improve. In spite, the swelling outgrows with increasing size and fever, night sweats continue to persist. His appetite too worsens and looks lean and thin as per the mother.

Hospital stay: Child examination was suggestive of matted, significant, nontender generalized lymphadenopathy. Complete blood count showed neutrophilic predominance with moderate anemia. Tubercular workup was negative. FNAC was done suggestive of reactive hyperplasia. Excisional biopsy was then planned. Report of nodular sclerosis came. Immunohistochemistry markers, CD15 and CD30 were positive. Positron emission tomography-computed tomography (PET-CT) done for staging was suggestive of stage IIb. Then patient was managed on lines of Hodgkin lymphoma.

DIAGNOSTIC APPROACH TO MATTED LYMPHADENOPATHY

Q1. What are the specific history markers?

Ans.
- Localized tender lymphadenopathy responding to antibiotic usually suggest infections' cause.
- A triad of tender lymph nodes, fever, and pharyngitis, with or without splenomegaly characterizes classic infectious mononucleosis.
- In HIV infection, initially there is fever, fatigue, rash, pharyngitis, and malaise, and lymphadenopathy appears after 2–6 weeks.
- Cytomegalovirus, toxoplasmosis, and human herpes virus type 1 cause painless lymphadenopathy with mononucleosis-like syndrome.
- Gradually progressive, single or matted lymph nodes with or without discharging sinus may suggest *Mycobacterium* TB involvement
- Significant fever, night sweats, and unexplained weight loss (more than 10% in 6 months) are the "B symptoms" of lymphoproliferative disorders. Organomegaly causing abdominal distention may present in Hodgkin lymphoma (HL) or non-Hodgkin lymphoma (NHL). Generalized pruritus is often seen in lymphomas. CNS involvement is common, if NHL presents in early age of life. These symptoms may also present in TB or collagen vascular diseases.
- If the patient has associated petechiae, purpura, bony pain and/or splenomegaly, high index of suspicion should be there for acute leukemia.
- Lymphadenopathy with arthralgia, unusual rashes, muscle weakness and/or anemia points to autoimmune diseases such as rheumatoid arthritis, systemic lupus erythematous, and dermatomyositis.
- *Lymphogranuloma venereum*: History of unsafe sexual contact in adolescent patients with self-limited genital papules or ulcers. It includes HSV 2 (herpes simplex virus), syphilis, and chancroid (Table 1).

TABLE 1: Etiology of matted lymphadenopathy	
Malignancy	Hodgkin or non-Hodgkin lymphoma, acute lymphoblastic leukemia, acute promyelocytic leukemia, and metastasis.
Infection	Tuberculosis, cryptococcosis, HIV, sarcoidosis, lymphogranuloma venereum, and toxoplasmosis
Miscellaneous	May occur in storage disorders, Rosai–Dorfman disease (sinus histiocytosis)

Q2. What are the specific examination markers?

Ans. The physical examination of the node must include specific examination markers given in Table 2.

TABLE 2: Specific markers in examination.	
Location	• Localized or generalized (more than two noncontiguous lymphadenopathy) • The Virchow node, in the left supraclavicular area, suggests intra-abdominal malignancies (e.g. gastric carcinoma), while the right-sided supraclavicular suggests intrathoracic malignancies.
Size	The maximum diameter (in cm) Significant lymphadenopathy: Cervical >1 cm Inguinal >1.5 cm Epitrochlear >0.5 cm
Pain and tenderness	Acute bacterial infections usually cause pain
Consistency: Hard, firm, rubbery, solitary, or matted	• Matted lymph nodes are described when a group of nodes are conglomerated. Causes can be benign (mycobacterial infection and sarcoidosis) or malignant (lymphoma and metastatic carcinoma). Chronic inflammation leads to fibrotic changes, and thus the hard lymph node on palpation. • Stony-hard and painless nodes are usually signs of metastatic cancer or granulomatous disease. Firm and rubbery nodes are present in lymphoma.
Adherence to underlying structures	Malignancy-associated lymph nodes are often fixed to the skin or surrounding tissues.
Overlying skin erythema, sinuses, and discharge	Overlying erythema suggests some infective bacterial pathology. Discharging sinus and scrofuloderma are the cutaneous extensions of tubercular lymphadenitis

The American Academy of Otolaryngology System (2002) classification with respect to location of the lymph nodes (Table 3).

TABLE 3: Classification of lymph nodes.		
Levels	Lymph nodes	Regions
Level I	*Ia*: Submental	Floor of mouth, anterior oral tongue, anterior mandibular alveolar ridge, and lower lip
	Ib: Submandibular	Oral cavity, anterior nasal cavity, soft tissue structures of mid face, and submandibular gland

Contd...

Contd...

Levels	Lymph nodes	Regions
Level II	Upper jugular *IIa*: Anterior to SCM *IIb*: Superior and posterior	Oral cavity, nasal cavity, nasopharynx, oropharynx, hypopharynx, larynx, and parotid gland
Level III	Mid jugular	Oral cavity, nasopharynx, oropharynx, hypopharynx, and larynx
Level IV	Lower jugular	Hypopharynx, cervical esophagus, and larynx
Level V	*Va*: Spinal accessory (posterior triangle)	Nasopharynx, oropharynx
	Vb: Transverse cervical artery nodes	Thyroid gland
Level VI	Prelaryngeal Pretracheal Paratracheal	Thyroid gland, glottic and subglottic larynx, apex of piriform sinus, and cervical esophagus.
Level VII	Upper mediastinal	

Q3. What is the systematic approach to matted lymphadenopathy?

Ans. After obtaining a comprehensive history with physical, systemic, and local examination, matted lymphadenopathy can be approached with the diagnostic algorithm given in Flowchart 1.

Flowchart 1: Systematic approach to matted lymphadenopathy.

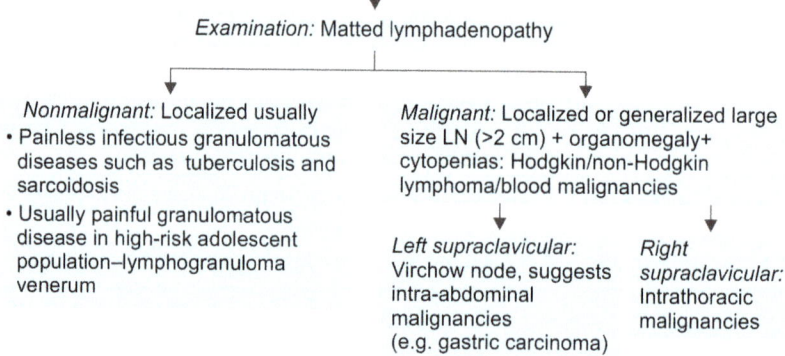

Q4. What are the contributory diagnostic tests?

Ans.
- *Hematological tests*: Complete blood count is done to see the differential counts and lymphocytosis in granulomatous diseases. Presence of atypical lymphocytes and/or cytopenias are pointers of leukemia. Anti-HIV antibodies test to be done to rule out HIV, especially in tubercular patients.
- *Imaging*: Ultrasound is a simple imaging technique to see the characteristics of malignant and benign LN. Borders are not sharp in case of

matted lymphadenopathy. Color Doppler ultrasound can evaluate the vascular pattern, displacement of vascularity, vascular resistance, and pulsatility index. A normal or reactive node is usually oval with a hilum, while metastatic and lymphomatous lymph nodes generally emerge as round lesions. A low long axis-to-short axis (L/S) ratio with hypoechocity and absent hilum of lymph nodes usually indicates lymphoma and metastatic cancer. The resistive index (>0.8) and pulsatility index (>1.5) are higher in malignancy as compared to reactive lymph nodes. Tubercular lymphadenitis has characteristic strong internal echoes, if calcification is present.

- *Histopathology*: Tissue diagnosis is the gold standard in lymphadenopathy evaluation. FNAC is a simple and safe procedure. The FNAC has certain limitation such as inadequate specimen and high rate of false-negative diagnoses in Hodgkin disease and incomplete classification of non-Hodgkin lymphoma. In these cases, excisional biopsy is the recommended gold standard test.
- *Investigations pertaining to specific disease pathology*: X-ray chest, PPD, cartridge-based nucleic acid amplification test (CBNAAT) for tuberculosis. Excisional biopsy especially in malignancy. The American College of Radiology recommends first imaging modality for cervical lymphadenopathy in <14 years' children as ultrasonography and computed tomography for persons older than 14 years.

Box 1: Key recommendations for practice.

Ultrasonography should be used as the initial imaging modality for children up to 14 years presenting with a neck mass with or without fever.	C
Computed tomography should be used as the initial imaging modality for children older than 14 years and adults presenting with solitary or multiple neck masses.	C
In children with acute unilateral anterior cervical lymphadenitis and systemic symptoms, empiric antibiotics that target *Staphylococcus aureus* and group A streptococci may be given.	C
Corticosteroids should be avoided until a definitive diagnosis of lymphadenopathy is made because they could potentially mask or delay histologic diagnosis of leukemia or lymphoma.	C
Fine-needle aspiration/excisional biopsy may be used to differentiate malignant from reactive lymphadenopathy.	C

A = consistent, good-quality patient-oriented evidence; B = inconsistent or limited-quality patient-oriented evidence; C = consensus, disease-oriented evidence, usual practice, expert opinion, or case series.

Note: For information about the SORT evidence rating system, go to http://www.aafp.org/afpsort.

Sources:
1. American College of Radiology. (2018). ACR Appropriateness Criteria: neck mass/adenopathy. [online] Available from https://acsearch.acr.org/docs/69504/Narrative. [Last accessed December, 2019].
2. Lioe TF, Elliott H, Allen DC, et al. The role of fine needle aspiration cytology (FNAC) in the investigation of superficial lymphadenopathy: uses and limitations of the technique. Cytopathology. 1999;10(5):291-7.
3. King D, Ramachandra J, Yeomanson D. Lymphadenopathy in children: refer or reassure? Arch Dis Child Educ Pract Ed. 2014;99(3):101-10.

Take Home Message

- Do not miss to examine all the groups of body lymph nodes to get the clue for etiology.
- Ultrasound is the simple screening modality to look for benign and malignant nature of lymph nodes.
- Tissue histopathology is the gold standard for diagnosis.
- Corticosteroid use to be avoided till a definitive diagnosis is made.

SUGGESTED READING

1. American College of Radiology. (2018). ACR Appropriateness Criteria: neck mass/adenopathy. [online] Available from https://acsearch.acr.org/docs/69504/Narrative. [Last accessed December, 2019].
2. Ferrer R. Lymphadenopathy: differential diagnosis and evaluation. Am Fam Physician. 1998;58(6):1313-20.
3. Gaddey HL, Riegel AM. Unexplained lymphadenopathy: evaluation and differential diagnosis. Am Fam Physician. 2016;94(11):896-903.
4. Jeffrey B. Neck dissection and sentinel lymph node biopsy. Grand Rounds Presentation, 2006.
5. King D, Ramachandra J, Yeomanson D. Lymphadenopathy in children: refer or reassure? Arch Dis Child Educ Pract Ed. 2014;99(3):101-10.
6. Lioe TF, Elliott H, Allen DC, et al. The role of fine needle aspiration cytology (FNAC) in the investigation of superficial lymphadenopathy: uses and limitations of the technique. Cytopathology. 1999;10(5):291-7.
7. Metzgeroth G, Schneider S, Walz C, et al. Fine needle aspiration and core needle biopsy in the diagnosis of lymphadenopathy of unknown aetiology. Ann Hematol. 2012;91(9):1477-84.
8. Morland B. Lymphadenopathy. Arch Dis Child.1995;73:476-9.
9. Mohseni S, Shojaiefard A, Khorgami Z, et al. Peripheral lymphadenopathy: approach and diagnostic tools. Iran J Med Sci. 2014;39(2 Suppl):158-70.
10. Thakkar K, Ghaisas SM, Singh M. Lymphadenopathy: differentiation between tuberculosis and other non-tuberculosis causes like follicular lymphoma. Front Public Health. 2016;4:31.
11. Tschammler A, Ott G, Schang T, et al. Lymphadenopathy: differentiation of benign from malignant disease: color Doppler US assessment of intranodal angio-architecture. Radiology. 1998;208:117-23.

Chapter 21

A Two-month-old Child with Acute Kidney Injury

Amit Agarwal

INTRODUCTION

Over the last one decade, there has been a lot of new understanding in the pathophysiology, incidence, prevalence, and long-term effects of acute kidney injury which earlier was denoted only by the rise of creatinine and known as renal failure. As we all know now that the renal failure is an arbitrary term and denotes only a stage in the development of kidney injury. Since the introduction of RIFLE (Risk, Injury, Failure, Loss, End stage) criteria and its pediatric modification (pRIFLE), we have been able to classify and diagnose kidney injury more often and it also led us to understand the consequences of even a mild derangement in biochemical parameters which often gets neglected earlier. Acute renal failure is equal to the stage 3 kidney injury (class failure—according to RIFLE). In 2012, Kidney Disease: Improving Global Outcome (KDIGO) comes up with a uniform definition of kidney injury which could be applied in all age groups.

Staging of Acute Kidney Injury

Table 1 shows the KDIGO Acute Kidney Injury Staging.

TABLE 1: Staging of acute kidney injury.		
Stage	**Serum creatinine**	**Urine output**
1	1.5–1.9 times baseline OR ≥0.3 mg/dL (≥26.5 mmol/L) increase	<0.5 mL/kg/hr for 6–12 hours
2	2.0–2.9 times baseline	<0.5 mL/kg/hr for ≥12 hours
3	3.0 times baseline OR Increase in serum creatinine to ≥4.0 mg/dL (≥353.6 mmol/L) OR Initiation of renal replacement therapy OR, in patients <18 years, decrease in eGFR to <35 mL/min/1.73 m^2	<0.3 mL/kg/hr for ≥24 hours OR Anuria for ≥12 hours

(eGFR: estimated glomerular filtration rate)

CASE 1

A 2-month-old child presented to you in outpatient department (OPD) with increased frequency of loose stools and vomiting for the last 3 days. The baby has become lethargic since last 8 hours and did not pass urine since then. There is no history of fever, abnormal movements, and rash over the body. On examination, the weight of the baby is 4 kg (at 6 weeks' vaccination, baby's weight was 4.5 kg), has feeble pulse, difficult to wake, skin turgor goes back slowly, oral mucosa is dry, and on catheterization of the urinary bladder, there is no urine.

Emergency—"Golden Hour" management
Secure an IV (intravenous) line and take a sample for kidney function test, serum electrolytes, blood gas, complete blood count, liver function test, blood culture, urine routine, urine culture, stool routine and stool culture, and stool for rotavirus antigen. Give an IV bolus of 20 mL/kg and repeat it till the child has passed urine or 60 mL/kg had been given. The first antibiotic shot must be given in the first hour of arrival in hospital in all patients suspected to have sepsis.

TABLE 2: Patient investigations during the stay in hospital.

Investigation	Day 1	6 hours	12 hours	18 hours	Day 2	Day 3
Hemoglobin	15	14			13.5	
PCV	48	42			37	
WBC count	18,000				11,500	
DLC	P65L35				P65L35	
Platelets	460,000				230,000	
Blood urea	100	88	60	55	40	
Serum creatinine	1.5	1.2	1.2	1.1	0.9	0.3
Serum sodium	160	156	154	152	150	144
Serum potassium	5.8	5.0	5.0	4.5	4.5	4.3
Uric acid	9.0				5.5	
Serum calcium	9.1				9.2	
Serum phosphate	6.7				5.2	
Serum albumin	3.2				3.2	
SGOT	55				35	
SGPT	75				42	
Blood pH	7.28	7.32	7.35	7.35	7.40	7.40
Serum bicarbonate	10	15	18	20	22	24
Urine protein	1+					
Urine WBC	Nil					
Urine bacteria	Nil					
Urine culture						Sterile
Blood culture						Sterile
Stool rotavirus					Positive	

(DLC: differential leukocyte count; PCV: packed cell volume; SGOT: serum glutamic oxaloacetic transaminase; SGPT: serum glutamic pyruvic transaminase; WBC: white blood cell)

Further management
Once the baby has become stable, fluids must be started as soon as possible while requesting the laboratory to process the sample at the earliest. Once we receive the renal function test and electrolytes report, formal calculation for fluids and electrolyte deficits must be done and recorded in the case file.

Q1. What will be the final diagnosis?

Ans. Hypernatremic dehydration with acute kidney injury.

Calculation for hypernatremic dehydration: We should target the 8–10 mEq/L/day fall in sodium, because rapid correction can cause cerebral edema and can have deleterious effect on the baby.

Basics of fluid management: In dehydration, there is a variable loss from the extracellular fluid (ECF) and intracellular fluid (ICF) compartments. The percentage deficit from these compartments is based on the total duration of illness.
- *Illness <3 days*: 80% ECF deficit and 20% ICF deficit
- *Illness ≥3 days*: 60% ECF deficit and 40% ICF deficit.

Normal concentration of sodium and potassium in ECF and ICF are as follows:
- Na^+ *ECF*: 133–145 mEq/L
- K^+ *ICF*: 150 mEq/L.

Total fluid deficit is measured by subtracting current weight from the preillness weight:

Fluid deficit (*liters*) = Preillness weight (kg) – Illness weight (kg)

Free water deficit (FWD) is estimated at 4 mL/kg which is needed to decrease serum Na^+ by 1 mEq/L.
Therefore,

FWD = 4 mL/kg × Body weight × (Concentration Na^+ present – Concentration Na^+ desired)

Solute fluid deficit (SFD) (mL) = Total fluid deficit (mL) – FWD (mL)

Solute Na^+ deficit = SFD (L) × Proportion of Na^+ lost from ECF × Na^+ concentration (mEq/L) in ECF

Solute K^+ deficit = SFD (L) × Proportion of K^+ lost from ICF × K^+ concentration (mEq/L) in ICF

Maintenance fluid: Calculate as per Holliday-Segar method.

Ongoing losses: Every significant loose stool should be replaced by 10 mL/kg isotonic fluid with maintenance potassium.

First 24-hour fluid: Replace half of FWD + all solute deficit + maintenance fluid + ongoing losses replacement.

Next 24-hour fluid: Half of FWD + maintenance fluid + ongoing losses replacement.

If serum sodium is >170 mEq/L, then FWD should be calculated using 3 mL/kg formula, and all the sodium should be corrected beyond 48 hours.

In our case, calculation of the fluid is as follows:
Fluid deficit = 4.5–4.0 = 0.5 L = 500 mL
Free water deficit: 4 × 4 × (160 − 145) = 240 mL
Solute fluid deficit: 500–240 mL = 260 mL = 0.26 L
Solute Na^+ deficit = 0.26 × (0.6 × 145) = 22.62 ≈ 23 mEq/L
Solute K^+ deficit = 0.26 × (0.4 × 150) = 15.6 ≈ 16 mEq/L
First 24-hour fluid: 120 mL + 260 mL + 400 mL = 780 mL
First 24-hour Na^+ requirement: 23 + 12* = 35 mEq
First 24-hour K^+ requirement: 16 + 8* = 24 mEq
*Daily requirement of sodium and potassium.

So, we need to administer the 780 mL of total fluid with 35 mEq of sodium and 24 mEq of potassium in it in the first 24 hours. Even though we meticulously calculate the sodium and potassium requirement of the fluid, the fall of sodium cannot be predicted, so it is very important to check the electrolyte levels periodically in the first 24 hours and then every 4-6 hours.

Next 24-hour fluid: 120 mL + 400 mL = 520 mL
Next 24-hour Na^+ requirement: 12 mEq
Next 24-hour K^+ requirement: 8 mEq.

Once the serum sodium is in the normal range, we need to continue with normal maintenance fluid along with any ongoing losses, if any. As our patient is suffering from rotaviral diarrhea, which is a self-limiting disease, once we maintain the hydration, the child becomes active and alert. Following this, the child can be put on oral feeds and oral rehydration solution (ORS) as required.

Q2. How will you follow-up on a long-term basis?

Ans. As this baby has suffered an acute kidney injury, he should be followed up in pediatric nephrology clinic for early detection and management of long-term sequelae [proteinuria, hypertension, and chronic kidney disease (CKD)] of acute kidney injury.

Take Home Message

Initial assessment of any infant presenting as renal failure is of utmost important because the golden hour management usually decides the outcome of baby, as too much fluid can lead to pulmonary edema and too little fluid can cause persistence of shock and further deterioration of renal function. Maintenance fluid and solute requirement must be calculated as mentioned, and recalculation must be done with every report of sodium, in case there is a too rapid and too slow fall of serum sodium.

CASE 2

A 2-month-old male child presented to the emergency department with complaints of fever for 4 days, not accepting oral feeds for 2 days, and fast breathing for the last 1 day. The child was also passing less urine since the last 2 days and passed the last urine around 12 hours back. There is a history of bilateral antenatal hydronephrosis and oligohydramnios which has not been evaluated postnatally. On examination, the child is having high-grade fever, severe respiratory distress, respiratory rate (RR) >60/min with subcostal and intercostal retractions, heart rate (HR) >160 beats/min, and weak and thready pulse. Abdomen is distended and on palpation, bilateral kidneys are large and ballotable, and liver size is enlarged. On auscultation, chest had bilateral decreased air entry at base and there are coarse crepitations. Heart sounds, S1 and S2, are normal, and S3 gallop is heard as well.

Q1. What will be the emergency management?

Ans. Secure two IV lines and catheterize the urinary bladder. Send complete blood count, kidney function test with electrolytes, liver function test, arterial blood gas, blood culture, urine routine microscopy, urine culture and sensitivity, chest X-ray and ultrasound of abdomen. Give IV fluid 10 mL/kg twice over next 1 hour, if child does not pass urine, then give 1 mg/kg of furosemide in 10 mL of normal saline as infusion over 10 minutes.

Q2. What will be the clinical diagnosis?

Ans. Sepsis with acute kidney injury.

TABLE 3: Patient investigations during the stay in hospital.

Investigation	Day 1	12 hours	Day 2	Day 3	Day 4
Hemoglobin	10				13.5
PCV	29				37
WBC count	28,000				15,000
DLC	P85L15				P60L40
Platelets	160,000				230,000
Blood urea	230	150	96	65	50
Serum creatinine	4.5	4.2	2.2	1.8	0.9
Serum sodium	125	130	134	138	137
Serum potassium	6.8	5.7	5.1	4.5	4.5
Uric acid	16.2	11.0	9.8	7.7	5.5
Serum calcium	9.1				9.2
Serum phosphate	6.7				5.2
Serum albumin	3.2				3.2
SGOT	105				35
SGPT	85				42
Blood pH	7.08	7.32	7.35	7.35	7.40
Serum bicarbonate	5	11	14	20	22
Urine protein	3+				
Urine WBC	80–100				
Urine bacteria	+++				
Urine culture					Proteus
Blood culture					Sterile

(DLC: differential leukocyte count; PCV: packed cell volume; SGOT: serum glutamic oxaloacetic transaminase; SGPT: serum glutamic pyruvic transaminase; WBC: white blood cell)

Q3. What will be the general management?

Ans. The child has passed only 10 mL of urine even after the furosemide infusion, which is sent for tests. The earliest report available in that scenario is arterial blood gas, which reveals severe metabolic acidosis with respiratory compensation and serum bicarbonate of 5 mEq/L. Chest X-ray was suggestive of cardiomegaly, bilateral pleural effusion, and pulmonary edema. Ultrasound abdomen revealed bilateral gross hydroureteronephrosis with flaking shadows in pelvis along with congestive hepatomegaly. While waiting for other reports, child has been put on mechanical ventilation and inotropes, given the first dose of non-nephrotoxic broad-range antibiotics and the preparation for starting peritoneal dialysis has been started.

Once the other reports came which suggested severe anemia, leukocytosis with neutrophilia, hyponatremia, hyperkalemia, hyperphosphatemia, and hyperuricemia with deranged urea and creatinine. Liver function tests showed mild elevation of enzymes.

Once the child is hemodynamically stabilized, peritoneal dialysis has been started with rapid cycles and target ultrafiltration according to the medication volume (maximum 5–7% of body weight per day).

Child started improving after 24 hours in the form of correction of metabolic acidosis, dyselectrolytemia, reduction in inotropic, and ventilation requirements. Peritoneal dialysis has been continued with same prescription for another 24 hours. On day 3 of admission, child is off inotropes and started passing cloudy urine and fever was less, but the child still required minimal settings of ventilation. And the child still had visible edema, peritoneal dialysis is continued with same prescription, but feeds had been started which the child was tolerating well. Urine culture showed proteus mirabilis >100,000 colonies, sensitive to third-generation cephalosporin. On Day 4 of admission, the child started passing large amount of clear urine and mechanical ventilation was taken off. As the child was accepting tube feeds well, off mechanical ventilation, peritoneal dialysis has been put on hold. Once the child started accepting orally and was afebrile for over 2 days, micturating cystourethrography (MCU) is planned. MCU showed bilateral grade 5 vesicoureteral reflux and dilated posterior urethra, which is suggestive of posterior urethra valve. Urine culture has been sent again which was sterile. Fulguration of posterior urethral valves (PUVs) was done, peritoneal dialysis catheter was removed once the child is stable postoperatively and started accepting feeds and passing urine normally. Total antibiotics was given for 14 days.

Q4. What will be the final diagnosis?

Ans. Posterior urethral valve with urosepsis with acute kidney injury stage 3.

Q5. How will you follow-up?

Ans. Once the child is discharged in stable condition and asked to follow-up in pediatric nephronurology clinic. The child with PUV requires lifelong follow-up with both pediatric nephrologist and pediatric urologist as 70–80%

patients with PUV have dysfunctional bladder and 40–50% end up with end-stage renal disease in the next 10 years.

Take Home Message

Early dialysis support saves the patient as dialysis rapidly corrects metabolic acidosis and dyselectrolytemia, which eventually leads to rapid correction of shock and lesser requirements of mechanical ventilation.

SUGGESTED READING

1. Hughes HK, Kahl LK (Eds). The Harriet Lane Handbook, 12th edition. Philadelphia: Elsevier, International Edition; 2018.
2. Sterns RH, Ingelfinger JR (Eds). Disorders of plasma sodium: causes, consequences, and correction. N Engl J Med. 2015;372:55-65.

CHAPTER 22

Pediatric Septic Shock

Vivek Saxena

INTRODUCTION

Pediatric septic shock is associated with high mortality, especially in low resource settings. Management of septic shock evolves around early recognition, aggressive fluid resuscitation, timely antibiotics, timely institution of vasoactive drugs, and intubation and ventilation. Recently, emphasis has shifted from protocolized care to individualized physiology-based care with more emphasis is on conservative approach on fluid therapy, noninvasive ventilation, and deresuscitation. Present article is a simplified attempt to incorporate basic issues in management of pediatric septic shock with key changes that are recommended now at various steps and can be successfully followed in low resource settings.

CASE 1

A 5-year-old girl presents to pediatric OPD. Her mother states that she is "not herself" and seems "lethargic." She had a fever and a cough for the last 3 days. Today she just seems different. She was brought straight into a resuscitation room and the charge nurse came to find you to tell you the child looks unwell.

Physical examination: Weight: 20 kg looks toxic and pale, temperature 102°F heart rate (HR) 140 beats/min, SaO_2 91% on room air, respiratory rate (RR) 40/min, subcostal retractions, and on auscultation rhonchi on right side of the chest. BP 90/50 mm of Hg, capillary refill time > 5 sec, she is lethargic and has staring gaze.

Q1. What is the diagnosis?

Ans. Before coming to diagnosis, one must consider few definitions:
- Systemic inflammatory response (SIRS) which is systemic response to burn, trauma, infection, and surgery and it manifests as tachycardia, tachypnea, hyper- or hypothermia, and leukocytosis or leukopenia.
- *Sepsis:* SIRS with suspected or proven infection.
- *Severe sepsis:* Sepsis with multiorgan failure or cardiovascular dysfunction or acute respiratory distress syndrome (ARDS).
- *Septic shock:* Sepsis with cardiovascular dysfunction.

- *Cardiovascular dysfunction:* It is defined as hypotension [<5th percentile of systolic blood pressure (SBP) for age or need for vasoactive drugs to maintain SBP] or unexplained metabolic acidosis. Raised lactate levels in the blood, capillary refill time >5 seconds, oliguria (urinary output <0.5 mL/kg /hour) and core to peripheral temperature difference >3°C.

Q2. Are there any risk factors for sepsis?

Ans. Extreme of age, malnutrition, asplenia, immunodeficiency disorders, chronic systemic steroid use, and recent antineoplastic drugs use.

Any condition that makes gastrointestinal (GI) tract permeable to Gram-negative bacteria such as burn, trauma, and pancreatitis.

Q3. How will you start initial management in this child?

Ans. Priorities in initial management of septic shock include:
- Early recognition of septic shock
- Early fluid resuscitation, early institution of vasoactive drugs to normalize disordered hemodynamics
- Early administration of appropriate antibiotics and identification of focus and source control (for example, drainage of abscess or laparotomy to seal an intestinal perforation).

Q4. How will you recognize septic shock clinically?

Ans. The inflammatory triad of fever, tachycardia, and vasodilation is common in children with benign infections.

Septic shock is suspected when children with this triad have a change in mental status manifested as irritability, inappropriate crying, drowsiness, confusion, poor interaction with parents, lethargy, or becoming unarousable.

The clinical diagnosis of septic shock is made in children who: (1) have a suspected infection manifested by hypothermia or hyperthermia, and (2) have clinical signs of inadequate tissue perfusion including any of the following:
- Decreased or altered mental status, prolonged capillary refill greater than 2 seconds, diminished pulse volume, mottled cool extremities, or flash capillary refill, bounding peripheral pulses and wide pulse pressure or decreased urine output less than 1 mL/kg/hr.
- Hypotension is not necessary for the clinical diagnosis of septic shock; however, its presence in a child with clinical suspicion of infection is confirmatory.
- Hypotension is a late feature in pediatric septic shock. Be very cautious of hypotension in a setting of tachycardia because this may be a prearrest scenario.
- Before onset of hypotension in pediatric septic shock, three changes are commonly seen, these are hypo- or hyperthermia, change in mental status and vasodilatation (warm shock) or vasoconstriction (cold shock).
- In warm shock, there will be bounding pulses, decreased capillary refill time and decreased tissue perfusion in form of decreased urinary output, altered mental status, and metabolic acidosis.

- In cold shock, patients will have cold extremities and prolonged capillary refill time, weak peripheral pulses and decreased tissue perfusion.

In present case, we have hyperthermia, altered mental status and capillary filling time > 2 seconds.

Clinical diagnosis: Septic shock (Table 1)

TABLE 1: Early recognition of shock.

Core temperature	Oral/rectal <98°F or >101.5°F
CNS	Change in mental status, decreased arousability, inconsolable, not recognizing parents.
Breathing	"Quiet" tachypnea or increased WOB.
HR (threshold)	<1 year: <100/min or > 180/min; >1 year: <80/min or >160/min
BP	Low systolic BP or mean BP (MAP preferred)
Peripheral perfusion	Cold peripheries, central + peripheral pulses feeble/absent with CFT >3 sec (cold shock) or warm extremities, bounding pulses with CFT <1 sec (warm shock)
Urinary output	Ask parent if urine output is normal or decreased in last 6 hours?
Metabolic acidosis	Base deficit >–5 or lactate >twice upper limit normal

(BP: blood pressure; CNS: central nervous system; CFT: capillary filling time; HR: heart rate; MAP: mean arterial pressure; WOB: work of breathing)

Heart rate increases by approximately 10 beats/min and RR by 5 breaths/min for every Celsius degree (1.8°F) of fever >38°C.

Normal Podiatric Vital Signs (Table 2)

TABLE 2: Normal pediatric vital signs.

Age	Heart rate (beats/min)	Blood pressure (mm Hg)	Respiratory rate (breaths/min)
Premie	120–170	55–75/35–45	40–70
0–3 months	100–150	65–85/45–55	35–55
3–6 months	90–120	70–90/50–65	30–45
6–12 months	80–120	80–100/55–65	25–40
1–3 years	70–110	90–105/55–70	20–30
3–6 years	65–110	95–110/60–75	20–25
6–12 years	60–95	100–120/60/75	14–22
>12 years	55–85	110–135/65/85	12–18

Q5. Once you have diagnosed your patient as septic shock, how will you manage?

Ans. Initial ABC should be addressed and 100% oxygen by nonrebreathing mask (NRM) should be delivered to all patients. After recognition of septic shock, each patient should be managed with first hour resuscitation phase followed by stabilization phase (Box 1).

Box 1: Summary—initial intervention.

- Assess and maintain airway
- By NRM, capillary glucose (correct if low)
- Insert two large bore peripheral IV cannulas (or intraosseous)
- *One IV line for rapid fluid boluses*: 20 mL/kg boluses of NS/RL until goals achieved.
  - If SBP/MAP low for age, infuse each bolus by push-pull technique/pressure bag over 5–10 min.
  - If SBP or MAP normal for age, infuse by free flow over 20 min (no pediatric burette)
- Insert 2nd line with aseptic precautions (sterile gloves, skin prep); send cultures × 2 sets (each 5–10 mL) at least 10 min apart; send CBC, ABG, and lactate.
- Administer first dose antibiotic
- Insert urinary catheter.

(ABG: arterial blood gas; CBC: complete blood count; IV: intravenous; MAP: mean arterial pressure; NRM: nonrebreathing mask; NS: normal saline; RL: Ringer's lactate; SBP: systemic blood pressure)

Resuscitation phase consists of (can be undertaken in emergency room):
- Intraosseous or intravenous (IV) access within 5 minutes
- Appropriate fluid resuscitation initiated within 30 minutes
- Initiation of broad-spectrum antibiotics within 60 minutes
- Blood culture, if it does not delay antibiotic administration
- Appropriate use of peripheral or central inotrope within 60 minutes.

The stabilization phase consists of [preferably done in pediatric intensive care unit (PICU)]:
- Multimodal monitoring to guide fluid, hormonal, and cardiovascular therapies to attain a normal perfusion pressure [Mean arterial pressure–central venous pressure (MAP-CVP) for age ($55 + 1.5 \times$ age in year)], and central venous oxygen saturation ($ScvO_2$) greater than 70% and/or cardiac index (CI) 3.3–6.0 L/min/m²
- Administration of appropriate antibiotic therapy and source control.

Q6. What fluids and how to give?

Ans. Early fluid resuscitation is the mainstay of management of septic shock. Venous access must be established in minutes and if not able to establish put an intraosseous line. There is no consensus on type of fluid hence normal saline remains the standard of care.

Initial bolus of 20 mL/kg of normal saline should be given over approximately 20 minutes followed up by reassessment of therapeutic end points.

If some end points are not met, reboluses up to 60 mL/kg in first hour can be given. Rate of transfusion depends on SBP of the patient. If patient is in hypotension, push method should be given till his SBP/MAP is normal for age. If patient is in compensated shock state, with normal SBP for age boluses can be given over 20 minutes. If underlying cardiac dysfunction suspected, then use smaller fluid aliquots of 10 mL/kg over 20–30 minutes. After the initial 40 mL/kg, consider colloid (starch easily available).

Correct hypoglycemia by a separate dextrose bolus followed by continuous infusion to maintain normoglycemia. Stop/slow down fluid rates if shock resolves or features of fluid intolerance develop.

Such an aggressive stand on fluid resuscitation in septic shock has recently been questioned by the Fluid Expansion as Supportive Therapy (FEAST) trial, which demonstrated increased mortality in children who received fluid boluses as compared to maintenance fluids, particularly in malnourished and anemic children.

This study inferred that rapid fluid resuscitation may not be the best therapeutic strategy across the board for all children, especially in resource-limited settings where facilities to provide advanced ventilation and hemodynamic support are inadequate.

Hence further research is required to know how much fluid is to be given before starting vasoactive drugs in patients of septic shock. Many patients will require stopping/restricting of fluids and use of diuretics to remove extra fluid given in resuscitation. This strategy being called as deresuscitation.

Continue to titrate fluids at a slower rate (10-20 mL/kg/hr) even after the first hour till shock resolves. Extra isotonic fluids may be required for initial 6-12 hours. It is important to remember that ARDS and multiorgan failure may be more common in patients with uncorrected hypovolemia and shock.

Q7. How to start antibiotics?

Ans. At least two sets of blood samples must be drawn for culture, one set from existing central lines (if present) and the second from a peripheral site with all aseptic precautions. Initially, the selection of antibiotics is empiric and should be broad spectrum.

Choice of empiric antibiotic should be based on a consideration of:
- The suspected site/focus of infection
- The suspected organism
- Whether the infection was acquired in the community or a hospital setting.

Hospital antibiotic resistance reports, patient's comorbid condition and immunity status are other factors which should be taken in to accounts before deciding about antibiotics.

Coming back to our index patient diagnosed as septic shock (cold), she was immediately taken to ER, two separate IV lines were put in including one central line, within few minutes samples for blood culture and other investigations were taken. Her blood sugar was normal. 400 mL of NS was transfused over 15-20 min. Repeat two doses were given as there was no response. A chest X-ray was also taken for her chest findings. X-ray chest was suggestive of right lower lobe pneumonia, she was started on injection vancomycin and ceftriaxone. She was shifted to PICU for further management.

Q8. What are the therapeutic end goals?

Ans. Capillary refill less than or equal to 2 seconds, normal pulses with no differential between the quality of peripheral and central pulses, warm extremities.

Urine output greater than 1 mL/kg/hr, normal mental status, and normal blood pressure for age.

Normal glucose concentration, normal ionized calcium concentration, and decreasing/normal lactate levels.

Q9. What is fluid intolerance, and how to manage?

Ans. Patients frequently show features of fluid overload/pulmonary edema during fluid resuscitation.

These may be in the form of new-onset or worsening crepts, hepatomegaly and increased O_2 requirement or work of breathing (WOB).

Causes of fluid intolerance:
- Capillary leak into lungs
- Cardiogenic pulmonary edema (due to septic myocardial dysfunction)
- Acute respiratory distress syndrome
- Fluid overload.

Capillary leak is the most common reason for fluid intolerance in septic shock.
- This may be seen even with uncorrected hypovolemia and normal cardiac function.
- Uncorrected hypovolemia may be documented by low CVP/ECHO features of underfilling.

Management of fluid intolerance:
- Slow down fluid rate, consider colloids, and consider vasoactive drugs and positive pressure ventilation (Box 2).
- An early CVP and or ECHO will clarify, if hypovolemia corrected. A normal/high CVP inpatients with uncorrected shock suggest need for inotrope and vasodilator.
- If CVP <8 mm Hg, continue colloids at slower rates with positive pressure.

Box 2: Vasoactive drugs in septic shock—summary.

- *Cold shock with narrow/normal pulse pressure (indicative of myocardial dysfunction with high SVR)*
  - *MAP low for age:* Commence dopamine @10 µg/kg/min or adrenaline @0.1–0.3 µg/kg/min
  - Add noradrenaline, if MAP remains low despite adrenaline up to 0.5 µg/kg/min or dopamine @10 µg/kg/min. Add dobutamine 10 µg or milrinone 0.25 µg/kg/min, if MAP better but shock not reversed or ECHO evidence of impaired LV/RV function.
- *Warm shock with wide pulse pressure (hyperdynamic circulation with low SVR):*
  - *Most need large volume fluid titrate fluids (aim CVP 10–12 mm Hg):*
    - *MAP low for age:* Commence noradrenaline @0.1 µg/kg/min, titrate up to 0.5–1.0 µg/kg/min to normal MAP.
    - Add dobutamine, if extremity perfusion worsens with noradrenaline, acidosis persists or $ScvO_2$ <70% or >80% despite adequate CVP/MAP/HCT, or ECHO evidence of impaired LV function
  - Early ECHO is helpful in monitoring fluid responsiveness or more fluid requirements and cardiac dysfunction to decide about addition of chronotrope-like dobutamine.

(CVP: central venous pressure; HCT: hematocrit; LV: left ventricular; MAP: mean arterial pressure; RV: right ventricular; $ScvO_2$: central venous oxygen saturation; SVR: systemic vascular resistance)

Q10. How to assess fluid responsiveness?

Ans. The clinical signs such as heart rate and SBP have been found to be poorly predictive of fluid responsiveness. Static variable like CVP is also poorly predictive of fluid responsiveness.

At the bedside; however, the hemodynamic changes induced during the passive leg raising (PLR) test have been reported to be good predictor of fluid responsiveness.

Additionally, these measurements are reliable irrespective of mode of ventilation, type of fluid, PLR starting position, and measurement technique.

Studies in children have demonstrated similar effect with the difference in CI/stroke volume with PLR (CI-PLR or SV-PLR) being good predictors of fluid responsiveness (Box 1).

Q11. What is fluid refractory shock?

Ans. This is shock that persists despite restoration of normovolemia as documented by a CVP of >12–15 mm Hg or by ECHO demonstrating adequate inferior vena cava (IVC) and cardiac chamber filling.

Causes are coexisting myocardial dysfunction or other morbidities.

Fluids may be stopped, if all therapeutic goals met or if features of pulmonary edema and hepatomegaly occur without further hemodynamic improvement OR a CVP (if present) is >12–15 mm Hg. A lower CVP is acceptable, if shock has resolved.

Enteral feeds should be started, if pulses have returned and perfusion has improved.

Q12. When will you intubate and start invasive ventilation?

Ans. Consider early intubation in fluid refractory septic shock (after 3 boluses of 20 mL/kg IV NS) or in any compromised airway.

Infants or neonates with severe sepsis may require early intubation. Intubation and mechanical ventilation increase intrathoracic pressure which reduce venous return and lead to worsening shock. Therefore, fluid resuscitation must be done first.

Anticipate worsening of hemodynamics when positive pressure ventilation is initiated. Continue fluid boluses at 10–20 mL/kg during and after intubation. Commence an inotrope/vasopressor infusion prior to intubation. Set up dopamine @10 µg/kg/min or nor-adrenaline 0.1 µg/kg/min prior to intubation.

Preoxygenate with 100% O, via NRM if not already initiated. A positive end-expiratory pressure (PEEP) device is helpful to maintain oxygenation in a child with hypoxemia.

Drugs: Sedative agents used for intubation can precipitate cardiovascular collapse.

Drug regimen for intubation in shock: Ketamine 1 mg/kg, atropine 0.01 mg/kg, muscle relaxation with succinylcholine 1 mg/kg, or vecuronium 0.1–0.2 mg/kg.

If patient has severe hypoxemia or decompensated shock, any IV sedation can precipitate cardiac arrest and no drugs are necessary except topical anesthetics. On occasion, low dose fentanyl at titrated boluses of 0.05 µg/kg may be used. Even subtherapeutic doses of midazolam can worsen the shock state.

If shock is not reversed despite 60 mL/kg of fluid, an inotrope and/or vasopressor infusion may be necessary.

Q13. How to choose different vasopressor-inotrope infusions?

Ans. Pediatric patients present usually with cold shock with low pulse pressure and low MAP. Other possibility is cold shock with low pulse pressure and normal MAP.

Other groups of patients are with warm shock with wide pulse pressure with either low MAP or normal MAP for age.

- *Cold shock with low pulse pressure with low MAP for age*:
  - *Choices:* Dopamine or Adrenaline
  - Dopamine at a starting infusion rate of 10 µg/kg/min is a usual first-line agent, though American College of Critical Care Medicine recommends adrenaline @0.05–0.3 µg/kg/min as a peripheral infusion. However, dopamine being the time-tested inotrope can be administered safely through a peripheral line in a resource-limited setting, it continues to be first-line inotrope to be used in day-to-day clinical practice.
  - If the hypotension is profound and the patient is unstable, initiate adrenaline at 0.3–0.5 µg/kg/min.
  - This is a more efficient inotrope and can also increase MAP due to its pressor effect.
  - If the MAP remains low despite dopamine of 10 µg/kg/min or adrenaline at 0.5–0.6 µg/kg/min, the addition of noradrenaline (NA) may be preferred rather than escalating the dose of dopamine/adrenaline in order to avoid undesirable tachycardia. NA will effectively increase the systemic vascular resistance (SVR) along with modest inotropy and minimal chronotropy. If MAP normalizes, but the patient remains in cold shock with hypoperfusion and persistent acidosis, add further inotropy with dobutamine at 5–10 µg/kg/min. Assess cardiac function with early ECHO.
- *Cold shock with low pulse pressure and normal MAP*:
  - Start dobutamine at 7.5–10 µg/kg/min. It is a reasonable initial agent.
  - Dobutamine will provide inotropy with moderate vasodilatation, both of which are beneficial for myocardial dysfunction, which is common.
  - Consider milrinone for documented myocardial dysfunction or pulmonary hypertension and/or if shock is unresolved despite standard inotropes such as dobutamine.
  - Milrinone, a phosphodiesterase inhibitor, has synergistic effect with catecholamine such as dobutamine. It is also effective when shock is catecholamine refractory.

- *Warm shock with wide pulse pressures and a low MAP for age*:
  - The best agent is nor adrenaline (NA) at 0.05–0.5 μg/kg/min, titrated to achieve normal MAP for age.
  - If the low MAP is refractory to NA at maximum doses (0.5–1 μg/kg/min), consider adding vasopressin (VP) or terlipressin infusion. VP infusion doses range from 0.0005 units/kg/min to 0.001 units/kg/min. Higher doses may result in significant splanchnic ischemia. If vasopressor infusions result in worsening indices of perfusion (cold extremities with poor peripheral pulses, etc.) despite improving MAP, underlying left ventricular dysfunction is likely. Early ECHO is helpful in this scenario.
  - Addition of dobutamine as an inotrope is beneficial in this scenario, combination of NA and dobutamine helps in maintaining splanchnic and vital organs perfusion.
- *Warm shock with wide pulse pressure and normal MAP*:
  - The mainstay of therapy in these patients is continuous aggressive fluid titration therapy as capillary leaks and vasodilatation are the causative factor.
  - If diastolic blood pressure (DBP) is low, NA is drug of choice.

Coming back to our patient her condition further deteriorated with SBP now was 70 mm of Hg, She was now put on dopamine infusion @10 μg/kg/min through central line. Measured CVP was 12 cm now. She is intubated under ketamine sedation and put under IMV mode of ventilation. Her MAP is now 50 mm of Hg but $ScVO_2$ is still 60 and capillary filling time still > 5 sec. An Echo was performed which revealed cardiac dysfunction with good filling pressures. Dobutamine was added @10 μg/kg/min with continuation of maintenance fluid.

Q14. When to give blood and components transfusion?

Ans. American College of Critical Care Medicine-Pediatric Advanced Life Support (ACCM-PALS) guidelines recommend a target hemoglobin of 10 g/dL to achieve adequate tissue oxygen delivery in children with septic shock. However, there is no consensus due to higher incidences of transfusion reactions and its morbidities. Many recent studies have concluded that improving hemoglobin to 10 g% does not show any difference in mortality, ischemic events, or use of life support.

It will be prudent to maintain a hematocrit of 30% in patients with persistent shock, $ScvO_2$ of <70%, and persistent metabolic acidosis indicating excessive tissue oxygen extraction in face of decreased cardiac output (CO).

Other components such as fresh frozen plasma (FFP) and platelet concentrate are indicated depending upon clinical scenario.

Q15. Can steroids be given in septic shock?

Ans. The utility of steroids in sepsis lacks definitive evidence and consensus. Though the pathophysiological basis for starting steroids such as sepsis-induced inotrope unresponsiveness, and the exaggerated inflammatory response is strong, it is not backed by strong evidence.

Despite this, the surviving sepsis campaign guidelines state that hydrocortisone should be considered for a catecholamine-resistant septic shock with suspected or proven adrenal insufficiency. Dose recommendations vary from a bolus of 1–2 mg/kg of hydrocortisone followed by 1 mg/kg Q6-8h.

Q16. How to manage acid base and electrolytes?

Ans. Hypoglycemia is common in septic child, serum glucose should be monitored and promptly treated. If persistent 10% D normal saline should be used as maintenance fluid.

If a child is found to have persistent hyperglycemia, dextrose-free fluids should be used and low-dose insulin therapy should be started (0.05–0.1 units/kg/hour). Infusion should promptly be stopped once capillary glucose levels show normalization.

Low ionized calcium levels (<0.8 mmol/L) must be corrected in a patient with refractory shock. Mild hypocalcemia should not be corrected.

Patients in septic shock usually have a wide anion gap acidosis from lactic acid. This is a marker of tissue ischemia and does not need bicarbonate correction. The best therapy is to restore normal perfusion.

Q17. What kind of monitoring is required in shock management?

Ans. Continuous monitoring of septic patient is essential component of management of shock. Each child should be monitored for hourly urinary output. Intake output monitoring and neurological monitoring are a must in any setting; however, monitoring in ER and low-resource settings may include pulse oximeter, continuous electrocardiogram (ECG), BP, and pulse pressure, temperature, glucose, ionized calcium.

In PICU settings, additional early central venous and invasive arterial monitoring will facilitate rapid and appropriate therapeutic responses to any hemodynamic changes.

Serial $ScvO_2$ monitoring, and lactate levels are an important component of ICU monitoring of septic shock in conjunction with hemodynamic and perfusion indices.

Monitoring of the $ScvO_2$ provides an indirect indicator of the adequacy of the CO. The $ScvO_2$ may be measured from an appropriate sited central venous catheter [SVC-right atrial (RA) junction of IVC-RA junction].

Normally, the tissues extract 25% of oxygen from the arterial blood such that, if the arterial saturation, is 100%, the $ScvO_2$ should be around 75%. $ScvO_2$ <70% indicates low CO.

Q18. What laboratory tests are necessary for shock management?

Ans. *At admission*: Arterial blood gas (ABG), lactate, capillary blood glucose, complete blood count, coagulation profile, electrolytes including ionized calcium, magnesium, renal, and liver function tests, blood and suspected source culture. Continue to check blood sugars hourly if not stable.

Arterial blood gas, $ScvO_2$, and lactate every 6 hours until patient is stable. Clinical history guides imaging such as chest X-ray.

Our patient's investigations revealed metabolic acidosis. Raised (2.5 times) lactate levels hemoglobin 10 g%, total leukocyte count (TLC) 24,300, P94L6. She gradually showed improvement in her hemodynamics over next 12 hours with recovery of BP as 100/60 mm of Hg and capillary filling time (CFT) <3 sec, and urinary output >1 mL/kg/hour.

Q19. What is refractory shock?

Ans. Children with refractory shock must be suspected to have unrecognized morbidities, including inappropriate source control of infection (remove nidus and use antibiotics with the lowest minimum inhibitory concentration possible, preferably <1, use IV immunoglobulin for toxic shock), pericardial effusion, pneumothorax, hypoadrenalism, hypothyroidism, ongoing blood loss, increased IAP, necrotic tissue, excessive immunosuppression, or immune compromise.

Address these potentially treatable causes in refractory shock.

Q20. What extracorporeal life support therapies are recommended in present day shock management?

Ans. Shock persisting despite optimization of preload, vasoactive, source control, appropriate antibiotics, and correction of identifiable factors may require extracorporeal membrane oxygenation (ECMO) therapy.

The utilization of extracorporeal therapies is indicated in those with multiorgan dysfunction syndrome (MODS).

Recent ACCM/PALS guidelines recommend use of either diuretics, peritoneal dialysis, or CRRT (continuous renal replacement therapy) in patients with fluid overload of more than 10% and impaired renal function.

Therapeutic plasma exchange (TPE) could be considered as a strategy to reverse MODS, especially in patients with significant coagulopathy, this modality should be used only after initial resuscitation.

The concept of "deresuscitation" is gaining momentum, as evidence has clearly shown that fluid overload acts as a "third hit" phenomenon resulting in increased mortality due to organ dysfunction. Therefore, after initial resuscitation and stabilization, transition to a negative fluid balance needs to be aggressively achieved with restricted maintenance fluid, targeted diuresis.

Our patient showed gradual recovery, MAP remained >70 mm throughout the Day 2, dobutamine was tapered off gradually on Day 3, her temperature started showing downward trend and normalized on Day 3, ABG now normal on Day 3, lactate levels showing downward trends with normal urinary output. She was continuously monitored and was weaned off the ventilator on Day 4 with tapering off dopamine, oral feeds started and was shifted from PICU on Day 6.

Take Home Message

- Early recognition and appropriate initial resuscitation are the mainstay of management of septic shock in children.
- Hypotension is late in septic shock and may represent prearrest situation.
- Optimal fluid resuscitation and early initiation of vasoactive drugs to achieve therapeutic endpoints with individualized targeted deresuscitation are key to success in management of septic shock.
- Dynamic variables (e.g. PLR test and changes in CO variables) of fluid responsiveness are more useful than static variables (e.g. CVP). Early ECHO is very useful tool in management and monitoring of septic shock.
- Adrenaline is gaining acceptance over dopamine as first-line inotrope.
- Lower hemoglobin levels are accepted now as they are noninferior to higher levels.
- Extracorporeal membrane oxygenation, CRRT, and TPE are now recommended in management of refractory shock with MODS.

SUGGESTED READING

1. Davis AL, Carcillo JA, Aneja RK, et al. American College of Critical Care Medicine Clinical Practice Parameters for Hemodynamic Support of Pediatric and Neonatal Septic Shock. Crit Care Med. 2017;45:1061-93.
2. Ismail J, Jayashree M. Advances in the Management of Pediatric Septic Shock: Old Questions, New Answers. Indian Pediatrics. 2018;55:319-25.
3. Nichols DG. Roger's Textbook of Paediatric Intensive Care, 4th edition. Broadway: Walters Kluwer; 2007.
4. Ranjit S. Manual of Paediatric Emergencies and Critical Care, 2nd edition. Hyderabad: Paras Publications; 2010.

CHAPTER 23

Unusual Skin Manifestations of Pediatric Tuberculosis

Rajesh Rai, Pallavi Gahlowt

INTRODUCTION

Skin tuberculosis (TB) is basically invasion of mycobacteria into the skin. The manifestations of these lesions may be very nonspecific which consists of erythematous papules, or vesicles or even pustular lesions as seen in cases of miliary TB as a result of hematogenous spread. Essentially, they also have very severe systemic symptoms and obvious clinical manifestations. On the other hand, there are other skin manifestations of skin TB which may pose a diagnostic difficulty. Here, we are discussing few less commonly seen manifestations which may be a diagnostic challenge for many of us. If we have some underlying tubercular pathology, it helps us reach a diagnosis because it may be as a result of lymphatic or hematogenous spread of underlying deeper tubercular focus, but skin lesions may evolve and persist for years together and sometimes spontaneous resolution may occur. Bacillus Calmette-Guérin (BCG) vaccination itself gives rise to a scar in the skin and at times additional skin tuberculides requiring antitubercular treatment (ATT).

In clinical practice, we may come across many skin rashes which were treated like psoriasis or a fungal infection to start with, only to find out later that it was something totally different.

Cutaneous TB continues to be one of the most elusive and more difficult diagnoses to make for dermatologists practicing in developing countries. Not only because they have to consider a wider differential diagnosis (leishmaniasis, leprosy, actinomycosis, deep fungal infections, etc.) but also because of the difficulty in obtaining a microbiological confirmation. Despite all the advances in microbiology including sophisticated techniques such as polymerase chain reaction, the sensitivity of new methods are no better than the gold standard, i.e., the isolation of *Mycobacterium tuberculosum* in culture. Even now, in the 21st century, we rely on methods as old as the intradermal reaction purified protein derivative (PPD) standard test and therapeutic trials as diagnostic tools. In this situation, it is important to recognize the many clinical faces of cutaneous TB to prevent missed or delayed diagnoses.

Cutaneous TB comprises only a small proportion (1-2%) of all cases of TB; nevertheless, bearing in mind, the high prevalence of TB in many developing countries, these numbers become significant.

Scrofuloderma and lupus vulgaris appear to be the most common forms with an increasing incidence of tuberculides being reported. Factors, such as HIV coinfection and migration, will ensure that cutaneous TB will remain a diagnosis that the dermatologist should always consider.

CASE 1

A 2-year-old child presented with fever and rashes since 15 days coupled with oronasal bleed since 4 days. Fever was mild, intermittent, and not associated with chills or rigors. Rashes appeared on the same day as fever and was erythematous, maculopapular, nonitching, noneczematous associated with crusting. They were present on the chest, trunk, and back. The child also had oronasal bleed which was spontaneous, small in quantity, intermittent and not associated with trauma. The child was pale, had multiple submandibular lymph nodes 1 × 1 cm, nonmatted, nontender, and mobile. He had a 2-cm palpable liver and a just palpable spleen. Respiratory system was essentially normal.

There was history of chickenpox in mother and sibling 20 days ago. Mother also suffered from tubercular lymphadenitis 6 years back and was cured with 6 months of ATT. The child was immunized till 9 months of age.

Q1. What are your first three differential diagnoses for this case of fever with rash?

Ans. In a child with fever and maculopapular rash, the most common differential diagnosis is a viral exanthematous disease. But neither the rash looked like that of measles/rubella, etc. nor the fever was associated with the typical cough, coryza, conjunctivitis, or diarrhea that a viral exanthem presents with. The oronasal bleed was atypical as well.

Dengue and dengue-like illnesses are another differential diagnoses which is to be kept in mind, especially with the history of oral and nasal bleed. The duration of fever and pattern of rash were not very convincing though.

Bacterial and rickettsial infections are the third category that is commonly seen with such a presentation. A special mention needs to be made about TB here because of the prolonged duration of fever. Though we do not come across skin lesions and bleeding manifestations in TB so often, it is still worth keeping in mind due to its high prevalence in India.

Drug hypersensitivity reaction is another very strong differential diagnosis owing to the rash and bleeding associated with fever. Most of them are mild and self-limiting but life-threatening eruptions can be seen in rare conditions such as toxic epidermal necrolysis (TEN) which has high mortality.

Last but not to forget, collagen vascular diseases can have a similar presentation but mostly in a higher age group of 6–9 years.

Q2. How will you approach this case? What basic investigations are warranted in this scenario?

Ans. The complete blood profile showed hemoglobin of 11.4 g/dL, leukocyte count of 5,000, and platelet count of 30,000/mm^3. In view of thrombocytopenia, a platelet transfusion was given. His chest radiograph showed hilar lymphadenopathy which was confirmed on CT scan. Lymph node biopsy suggested reactive lymphadenitis. Koch's workup was done which showed ESR of 80 mm and Mantoux test was strongly positive (15 × 14 mm). Coagulation profile was normal.

Q3. What is the confirmatory test which will guarantee the right diagnosis?

Ans. Skin biopsy of the lesion showed a solitary granuloma in superficial dermis and loose granuloma with epithelioid cells characteristic of Lichen scrofulosorum (Fig. 1).

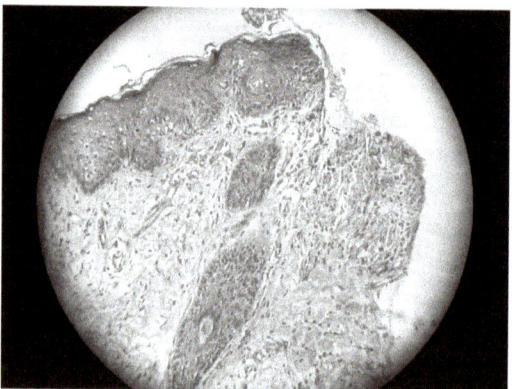

Fig. 1: Skin biopsy of the lesion.

Q4. What is the treatment for cutaneous TB and how long does it take for the rash to heal?

Ans. The child was started on anti-tubercular drugs and the skin lesions started diminishing after 2 weeks of therapy and showed complete healing after 6 weeks.

CASE 2

A 7-year-old girl presented with sore throat, fever, and coryza since 5 days. Fever was low grade, intermittent and was associated with itchiness of throat and watery nasal discharge. There was no significant past or family history. The child's appetite had reduced considerably since the onset of fever. General appearance of the child was dull. On physical examination, the child was averagely built, pale, and had multiple subcentimetric cervical lymph nodes. Tonsils were grossly enlarged, almost fused, and had numerous pustules. Chest was clear. Abdominal examination revealed a palpable spleen of 2 cm with span of 10 cm, no hepatomegaly. There were no other significant systemic findings.

Q1. Is it a case of upper respiratory tract infection or not?

At the onset, it looks like a simple case of upper respiratory tract infection of viral/bacterial origin. The child looked sick and had a splenomegaly so ruling out a systemic infection becomes significant. Kissing tonsils could be indicative of infectious mononucleosis.

Investigations
Complete blood count showed Hb of 9.4 g/dL and WBC count of 24,000 with neutrophilic predominance Throat swab was not very helpful in isolating the organism. USG abdomen showed few subcentimetric mesenteric lymph nodes.

Treatment
The child was given symptomatic treatment in form of antipyretic and povidone-iodine gargles and oral amoxicillin and asked to follow up in 5 days.

Q2. Was the follow-up indicated in this case?

The child came back to the OPD after a month with a discharging sinus and ulcers which were shallow and with undermined edges overlying a cervical lymph node (Fig. 2). An urgent chest X-ray was done showing Ghon's complex. Gastric lavage confirmed the diagnosis of scrofuloderma (Fig. 3). The child showed rapid improvement on antitubercular drugs over the next 1 month. Treatment was given for a period of 6 months. The ulcer healed with puckered scar.

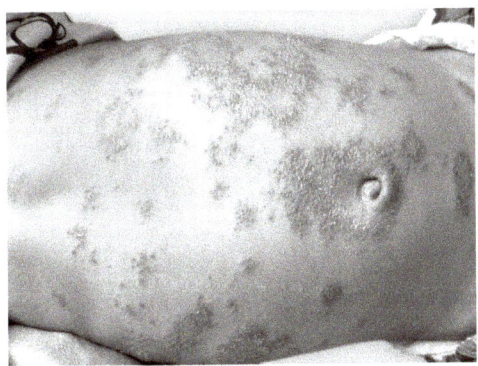

Fig. 2: Lesions of lichen scrofulosorum on chest and trunk.

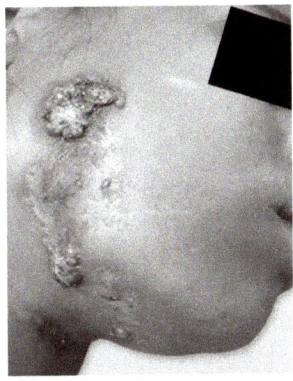

Fig. 3: Lesions of scrofuloderma overlying the cervical lymph node.

CASE 3

A 9-year-old immunized child presented with a 2-year history of pink plaques appearing and progressing slowly on the left buttock. Physical examination revealed a well-demarcated, irregularly bordered, slightly tender, pink, infiltrated plaques on the left buttock reaching the midline (Fig. 4). Diascopy examination indicated apple-jelly color appearance of the lesion classical of lupus vulgaris. There was no inguinal lymphadenopathy, and systemic examination was normal. No other family members had similar lesions. The child was diagnosed with pulmonary TB at 2 years of age and had taken antitubercular drugs for 6 months.

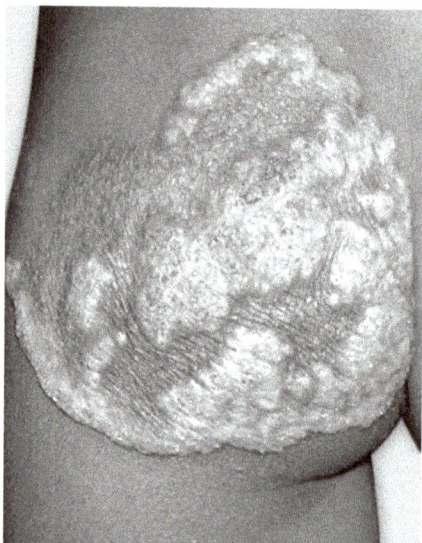

Fig. 4: Lupus vulgaris plaque over the buttock region.

DIFFERENTIAL DIAGNOSIS

Differential diagnosis of lupus vulgaris is difficult and unreliable purely on clinical grounds, and histopathological and microbiological examinations are required.

Investigations

Routine biochemical analysis, complete blood count, and urine microscopy were all normal, and the erythrocyte sedimentation rate was 8 mm/hour. HIV and venereal disease research laboratory (VDRL) tests were negative. Chest radiograph and computed tomography findings were normal, and there was no sign of pulmonary tuberculosis. The purified protein derivative test (Mantoux test) showed normal reactivity with a 10-mm induration after 48 hours.

Q1. Is it a medical negligence to rule out cutaneous TB based only on blood and radiological findings?

Ans. Histopathological examination of the incisional biopsy specimen showed normal epidermis with superficial focal parakeratosis, and non-caseating tuberculoid granulomas consisting of epithelioid histiocytes, plasmocytes, and Langhans giant cells in the papillary dermis. The tissue sections were negative for acid-fast bacilli (AFB) by the Ehrlich-Ziehl–Neelsen stain, and cultures of the biopsy material and blood were negative.

TREATMENT

Antitubercular therapy of 2HRZE + 4HR was started. Marked improvement of the lesions with atrophic scarring was seen by the end of 6 months treatment.

CONCLUSION

These are few of the cutaneous presentations of tuberculosis among the numerous forms detected so far. Though we do not come across them very often either due to delay in diagnosis or varied presentation, it does not imply that cutaneous TB is a rarity. We need to be very aggressive in diagnosing these cases and rely on tools beyond Mantoux test and chest X-ray while witnessing these cases.

Take Home Message

- Next time a child presents with fever and an atypical rash, do not rush to the diagnosis before thorough history, investigation, and regular follow-up.
- Skin tuberculosis is not as rare an entity as we may think.
- Diagnosis tuberculosis does not end with a Montoux test and a chest X-ray. We need to be more aggressive in detecting various forms of tuberculosis including the cutaneous form.

SUGGESTED READING

1. Bravo FG1, Gotuzzo E. Cutaneous Tuberculosis. Clin Dermatol. 2007;25(2): 173-80.
2. Caminero J. Guia de la tuberculosis paramedicosespecialistas. Paris: International Union against Tuberculosis and Respiratory Diseases. 2003;35-7.
3. Kumar B, Kumar S. Pediatric cutaneous tuberculosis: Indian scenario. Indian J Pediatr Dermatol. 2018;19(3):202-11.

CHAPTER 24

Adolescent Immunization

Ashok Banga

INTRODUCTION

About 22% of the country's population is of adolescents. In absolute numbers, it becomes 250,000,000, bigger than the whole population of many countries.

Adolescents are the biggest and strongest resource of any country and their health represents the country's true growth potential.

Unfortunately, the vaccination coverage for adolescents in our country is dismal in relation to early childhood immunization. In fact, so far, government does not even have a prescribed immunization card for adolescents.

Immunization is one of the most important preventive health services that can be provided for adolescents for following reasons:
- Adolescents are more vulnerable to a number of diseases and their complications because of their risk-taking behavior.
- Their falling sick jeopardize the growth of the entire family and the nation. Sickness during examination time may affect their academic achievements. Hence, it becomes imperative that they receive the recommended vaccines to prevent them from morbidity and mortality.
- With a better coverage of expanded program of immunization (EPI), the epidemiological trend of childhood diseases has seen a rightward shift leading to a surge of vaccine preventable diseases such as diphtheria, pertussis, measles, and mumps in adolescence and early adulthood.
- The susceptibility of the older population is also because of waning antibody levels induced by childhood immunization and lack of booster effect induced by subclinical natural infection. These are all the reasons there is so much buzz around "adolescent immunization" now.

Q1. Parents bring their 7-year-old daughter for treatment for fever. Second daughter, who was 10 years old, accompanied them. When asked about immunization status, they said, "they thought vaccination is over by 5 years". Is that true?

Ans. This is true that major part of vaccination is over by 5 years. This is also true that there are no vaccines to be given in next 5 years, except flu (every year) and if anything left of earlier schedule. But that is not the end.

At the age of 10 years (in fact 9 years for daughters), they need some more vaccines. That is called "adolescent immunization."

Q2. A bank manager came to me with his wife who is a teacher. Both are posted at different places. Their daughter, who is 10 years old, lives with mother in a small town and has come to father's place during vacations. They said that they have not given her any vaccine for last 5 years. Even by 5 years, some of the vaccines were missed. Which vaccines need to be given now?

Ans. Two vaccines are mandatory at this age: Tdap (tetanus, diphtheria, and acellular pertussis) and HPV (human papillomavirus vaccine). No HPV for boys as of now.

In addition, there are some vaccines for some of the adolescents under catch-up immunization and other categories.

Q3. They asked me, "What is catch-up immunization?" This term is new to parents.

Ans. Administration of vaccines at a later age, if due to any reason the vaccines have not been given at recommended age. I asked them, if their daughter received measles, mumps, and rubella (MMR), hepatitis A (Hep A), hepatitis B (Hep B), varicella, and typhoid till the age of 5 years? If missed any, is to be given now under this category.

Q4. Parents understood what they are supposed to do now but wanted to know more about "adolescent immunization"?

Ans. Adolescent immunization can be divided into the following four categories:
1. *Mandatory vaccines*: Tdap or Td, and HPV
2. *Catch-up vaccines*: MMR, Hep A, Hep B, and varicella and typhoid vaccine
3. *Vaccines to be given under special circumstances*: Flu, Japanese encephalitis (JE), pneumococcal polysaccharide vaccine (PPSV23), and rabies—postexposure
4. *Traveler's recommendations*: Meningococcal polysaccharide vaccine/meningococcal conjugate vaccine (MPSV/MCV), cholera-O, yellow fever, JE, and rabies—pre-exposure.

Q5. Teacher mother was eager to learn more about different vaccines because she wanted to help many more parents, who missed giving some vaccines to their children. I gave her a printout about the recommendations about each of these vaccines?

Ans. Following are the recommendations for individual vaccines:

Tdap (Tetanus, Diphtheria, and Acellular Pertussis Vaccine)/Td (Tetanus-diphtheria Vaccine)

Immunity has been shown to wane 5–10 years after primary immunization with whole cell or acellular pertussis vaccine. Because of this, more numbers of cases of pertussis have been reported in adolescents and adults worldwide. This is the reason, booster doses against pertussis are recommended at 10 years onward.

There is no data on the burden of pertussis in adolescents in India. What we have is data for tetanus vaccine only. India has attained >99% coverage for it by 2017 (WHO-UNICEF).

When to Administer

- All adolescents must take at least one dose of Tdap at 10 years or later. Then, Tdap or Td every 10 years.
- During every pregnancy, between 27 and 36 weeks. Tdap vaccine can be administered regardless of the interval since the last tetanus and diphtheria toxoid-containing vaccine.
- To all adolescents and adults in a house where they will come in contact with a newborn.

Weak Points

- Recent studies have shown that Tdap vaccine effectiveness decreases with the passage of time and protection wanes rapidly after 1–2 years.
- Also, there is no sufficient data on the efficacy/effectiveness of the Tdap from India and other South Asian countries.

Tdap or Td?

It is better to take Tdap. If not possible due to higher cost, go for Td. No tetanus toxoid stand-alone.

Human Papillomavirus Vaccine

Human Papillomavirus-related Diseases

Cervical cancer and precancerous dysplasia:
- Nearly 100% of cervical cancers are caused by HPV infection.
- Cervical cancer is the second most common cancer in women worldwide.
- India has very high burden of cervical cancer (nearly 25% of global cervical cancer deaths).
- *Year 2012*: 123,000 new cases of cervical cancer and 67,000 deaths.

Noncervical human papillomavirus disease:
- Infection with HPV is also associated with anal, vulvar, vaginal, and penile cancers.
- These HPV-related diseases are much less frequent than cervical cancer, but taken together, they represent a significant human health and economic burden. Of particular concern, the incidence of anal cancer has been increasing in both men and women over the past several decades.

It is estimated that present HPV vaccines may prevent 70% of cervical cancer, 80% of anal cancer, 60% of vaginal cancer, 40% of vulvar cancer and possibly some mouth cancer. They additionally prevent some genital warts.

Routine Vaccination

Minimum age for vaccination: 9 years
- *HPV2 (Cervarix)*: It protects from strains 16 and 18 that are mainly responsible for cervical cancer.
- *HPV4 (Gardasil)*: It protects from strains 6, 11, 16, and 18. Strains 6 and 11 are mainly responsible for anogenital warts.
- Both these are licensed and available in India.
- Recommended in a two-dose series for females 9 to 14 years at 0 and 6 months and three-dose series from 15 to 45 years (Cervarix at 0, 1, and 6 months) (Gardasil at 0, 2, and 6 months).
- Immunocompromised need three-dose schedule at any age.
- *HPV9 (Gardasil-9)*: It is not yet available in India.
- The 9vHPV vaccine targets HPV types 6, 11, 16, and 18 (also targeted by HPV4 vaccine) as well as HPV types 31, 33, 45, 52, and 58.
- HPV4 or HPV9 can also be given for males aged 11 or 12 years but not yet licensed for use in males in India.

Catch-up Vaccination

Administer the vaccine to females up to the age of 45 years, if not previously vaccinated.

In India, Gardasil 9 may prove better as:
- HPV types 16 and 18 account for about 83% cases of cervical cancers, while majority of the remaining 15–20% of the cases are said to be caused by the other five HPV types, HPV 31, 33, 45, 52, and 58 contained in Gardasil 9 vaccine.
- Overall Gardasil 9 is expected to protect from almost 98% of cervical cancers and about 73% of anal cancers in India.

Early administration (ideally before they indulge in sexual activity) is important for two reasons:
1. HPV vaccines are inactive against previously acquired infection.
2. Antibody response is highest in age group 9–15 years.

As of 2018, 81 countries include it in their routine vaccinations, at least for girls. India too needs it.

Meningococcal Vaccine

Recommended for:
- Certain high-risk group of children
- During outbreaks
- To international travelers, including students going for study abroad and travelers to Hajj and sub-Saharan Africa.

Vaccines: Either of these:
- Meningococcal conjugate vaccines (quadrivalent MenACWY-D, Menactra by Sanofi Pasteur)
- Polysaccharide vaccines (quadrivalent and bivalent). Both are licensed in India.

- PsA-TT is monovalent group A, (MenAfriVac by Serum Institute of India) is made for African countries only and is not available in India.

For high-risk children: Administer MCV4 to children aged 2 years through 10 years with persistent complement component deficiency, anatomic or functional asplenia, or certain other conditions placing them at high risk. Administer to children previously vaccinated with MCV4 or MPSV4 who remain at increased risk after 3 years (if first dose administered at age 2 years through 6 years) or after 5 years (if first dose administered at age 7 years or older).

Conjugate vaccines are preferred over polysaccharide vaccines due to their increased immunogenicity and their potential for herd protection. Moreover, only this can be used in children younger than 2 years of age.

Influenza Vaccine

Routine Vaccination

Routine vaccination should be given yearly to high-risk children and anyone who desires it. At risk, individuals include congenital or acquired immunodeficiency, chronic systemic illness, on long-term aspirin therapy, and elderly aged >65 years.

First Time Vaccination

- *6 months to <9 years*: Two doses 1 month apart
- *9 years and above*: Single dose

Annual Revaccination

With single dose at all ages.

Dosage (Trivalent Inactivated)

- *Aged 6 months till 3 years*: 0.25 mL
- *3 years and above*: 0.5 mL

All the currently available trivalent inactivated (TIVs) and quadrivalent vaccines in the country contain the "*Swine flu*" or "A(H1N1)"antigen; no need to vaccinate separately.

Best Time to Vaccinate

- As soon as the new vaccine is released and is available in the market, preferably before the onset of rainy season.
- The most appropriate composition for India is the one formulated as "Southern Hemisphere (SH)".

Pneumococcal Vaccines (PCVs)

- Incidence of pneumococcal diseases varies from place to place and children below the age of 2 years are at highest risk everywhere.
- High-risk population of every age and all elderly do need this vaccine.

Routine Vaccination
- *Vaccines*: PCV10 and PCV13
- *Minimum age*: 6 weeks; three doses at 1 month interval and then one booster at 18 months
- *Those with late start after 1 year*: Two doses of PCV10 or single dose of PCV13
- PCV13 is also licensed for the prevention of pneumococcal diseases in adults older than 50 years.

Vaccination of Persons with High-risk Conditions

Children aged 6 years through 18 years having anatomic or functional asplenia (including sickle cell disease), human immunodeficiency virus (HIV) infection or an immunocompromising condition, cochlear implant, or cerebrospinal fluid leak.

Pneumococcal Polysaccharide Vaccine (PPSV23)
- *Minimum age of administration*: 2 years
- Not recommended for routine use in healthy individuals. Recommended only for the vaccination of persons with certain high-risk conditions as mentioned above.
- Administer PPSV at least 8 weeks after the last dose of PCV13 to children or elderly.
- An additional dose of PPSV should be administered after 5 years to these children.
- PPSV should never be used alone for prevention of pneumococcal diseases amongst high-risk individuals.

Typhoid Vaccines

Typhoid is a disease of developing countries associated with poor public health and low socioeconomic indices. It is a big cause of morbidity and school absenteeism among adolescents.
- India and few other South-East Asian countries have very high incidence of typhoid (499 cases per 100,000 population in 2016).
- Children 5–15 years and adolescents are at greatest risk.
- In India, incidence is quite high at lower age also (in 2–4 years 340.1 cases per 100,000/year).

Routine Vaccination

Either of following two vaccines:
1. *Vi PS (polysaccharide) vaccines*: First dose at 2 years; revaccination every 3 years
2. *Vi-PS (conjugate) vaccine*: First dose at 9–12 months and a booster during second year of life. Single dose when administered for the first time after the age of 2 years.
   Booster dose not needed (at present).

Conjugate vaccine is preferred over polysaccharide vaccines due to increased immunogenicity and longer protection. Moreover, only this can be used in children younger than 2 years.

Oral typhoid vaccine: In form of three capsules, one per day. Not available in India.

Catch-up Vaccination

It is recommended throughout the adolescent period, i.e., 18 years.

Indian Academy of Pediatrics-Advisory Committee on Vaccines and Immunization Practices (IAP-ACVIP) considers typhoid as major public health problem with huge burden of disease in every part of the country and strongly urges the government to include typhoid vaccine in routine immunization.

Till then, protect the youth at least.

Hepatitis A Vaccine

With improving hygiene, safer water supply and immunization, incidence of Hep A virus infection is reducing in India. It has resulted in pushing the average age of infection upward. Problem with this is that Hep A is more severe when adolescents and adults suffer from it.

Due to their tendency or need of frequent eating outside home, adolescents are more vulnerable to acquire Hep A virus infection. Hep A vaccination therefore need to be given a high priority for catch-up immunization of adolescents.

Vaccines

- *Killed vaccine*: Two doses, at least 6 months apart
- *Live vaccine*: Single dose. This is not recommended during pregnancy and in immunocompromised.

Vaccine can be given 1 year onward and dose remains the same for all age groups.

It is effective in around 95% of cases and immunity lasts for at least 15 years and possibly throughout life.

Hepatitis B Vaccine

Hepatitis B virus is the major cause of chronic liver disease and hepatocellular carcinoma. Widespread immunization with Hep B vaccine has vastly reduced incidence of these conditions:
- Adolescents are more vulnerable to get Hep B infection through indulgence in sexual activities.
- India has prevalence of 2–7% (average of 4% are in chronic carrier state) of Hep B and is now in category of intermediate endemicity.
- Chronic Hep B virus infection in India is mostly acquired during childhood, before 5 years of age (horizontal transmission).

- Mother-to-child transmission (vertical transmission) is another major chunk.
- Up to 25% of chronic carriers die of chronic liver disease as adults.
- Thus, vaccination of adolescents against Hep B becomes imperative, if they missed it earlier.
- Administer a three-dose series to those not previously vaccinated at 0, 2, and 6 months' schedule.
- Immunity is life-long in all responders. No booster needed.
- Nonresponders need antibody level estimation and then higher doses of vaccine and booster dose.
- Safe during pregnancy and breastfeeding.
- It is genetically engineered, very economic, and can be combined with many vaccines.

Measles, Mumps, and Rubella Vaccine

Mumps vaccine: Available as combination only as measles, mumps, and rubella (MMR).

The highest incidence of mumps in India is seen in children above 5 years of age, mostly in the adolescent age group. Since the first dose of MMR is now offered before 12 months of age when a robust immune response may not be elicited, the need for additional doses becomes all the more important.

Rubella vaccine: Aim is to prevent congenital rubella syndrome (CRS) and not to prevent rubella infection per se, as it is usually benign and inconsequential.

Routine Vaccination

Minimum age: 9 months. First dose of MMR vaccine at age 9 months and second at 15 months.

If not MMR, then MR as in government setup. No measles vaccine stands alone.

At least, a single-dose of MMR is a must for every adolescent irrespective of their past vaccination status as there is a considerable waning of immunity following mumps vaccination. But whether the third dose of the vaccine be given to adolescents is a debatable issue so far.

Government replacing MMR with MR in national programs is also a debatable issue and IAP was not in favor of that.

American universities require MMR vaccination certificate from students coming from India because measles still continues to be a problem in some parts of the United States. Mumps and rubella infection, although under control in the United States, if emerges in a foreign student, can be of epidemiological concern.

Contraindications: Pregnancy and severe immunodeficiency.

Varicella Vaccine

The varicella disease is far more severe with greater morbidity and mortality in adolescents and adults than in early childhood. Furthermore, this infection during pregnancy may have serious health hazards for the fetus and newborn infant.

Routine Vaccination
Two doses at 15 and 18 months.

Catch-up Immunization
- For children up to 13 years without evidence of immunity, administer two doses at 3 months' interval.
- For any age >13 years, the minimum interval between two doses is 1–2 months.

Postexposure Prophylaxis
Vaccinating healthy children within 3–5 days after exposure (earlier the better) is effective in preventing or modifying varicella and therefore recommended postexposure also.

To be avoided to immunocompromised and during pregnancy.

Japanese Encephalitis Vaccine

Routine Vaccination
- Recommended only for individuals living in endemic areas, till 18 years of age.
- The vaccine should be offered to the children residing in rural areas only and those planning to visit endemic areas (depending upon the duration of stay)

Vaccines
Three types of new generation JE vaccines are licensed in India:
1. *Live-attenuated, cell culture-derived SA-14-14-2*:
   - *Minimum age*: 8 months; two-dose schedule, at 9 months and at 16–18 months.
   - Not available in private market.
2. *Inactivated cell culture-derived SA-14-14-2 (JEEV by BE India)*:
   - *Minimum age*: 1 year (US-FDA: 2 months)
   - *Primary immunization schedule*: Two doses of 0.25 mL each IM on days 0 and 28 for children aged ≥1 to ≤3 years.
   - Two doses of 0.5 ml for children >3 years and adults aged ≥18 years
   - Need of boosters still undetermined
3. *Inactivated Vero cell culture-derived Kolar strain, 821564XY, JE vaccine (JENVAC by Bharat Biotech)*:
   - *Minimum age*: 1 year
   - *Primary schedule*: Two doses of 0.5 mL each IM at 4 weeks' interval
   - Need of boosters still undetermined.

Catch-up Vaccination

All susceptible children up to 18 years should be administered during disease outbreak/ahead of anticipated outbreak in campaigns and traveler's to JE endemic regions.

Dengue Vaccine

Top concern for India and entire South-East Asia (SEA) region is dengue, which used to be the fastest spreading viral infection in the world (now COVID-19).

Though dengue affects all age groups, it is primarily a disease of adolescents and adults. Majority of dengue cases occur in the age group of 14-45 years with highest burden seen in the 15-24 years' subgroup.

Vaccine

Live-recombinant tetravalent dengue vaccine known as CYD-TDV (Dengvaxia). World Health Organization (WHO) has approved its use in the highly endemic countries but so far this is not available in India.

It is given as 3 doses.

Severe side effects may include anaphylaxis. Use is not recommended in people with poor immune function.

Cost was $207 in Indonesia in 2016 (= ₹ 160,000).

Two more robust vaccines are in pipeline.

Present vaccine has certain limitations:

The vaccine is only recommended in those who have previously had dengue fever or populations in which most people have been previously infected.

As of 2016, the dengue vaccine had been approved for medical use in 11 countries and in 2019, was approved for medical use in the United States.

Q6. When many vaccines are to be given, we may give two or more vaccines on every date. She asked, can MMR and chickenpox vaccine be given at the same time?

Ans. Yes, but at different sites. One combination preparation is also available with the name MMRV.

Q7. That teacher of girls' school understood the importance of rubella vaccine and wanted to know if she can motivate girls for this vaccination. Her query was, "Do we recommend MMR or rubella vaccine alone to adolescent girls"?

Ans. MMR is the ideal recommendation for both adolescent boys and girls, if not received earlier. When one dose is received earlier, give one more dose. Better to give MMR than only rubella, as for almost the same cost, you are protecting three illnesses.

Ideally, every girl must have protection against rubella before marriage.

Q8. I gave them interesting information that "Rubella vaccination certificate" is insisted by temple authorities at Tiruvannamalai, Tamil Nadu, India for performance of marriage in Arunachalesvara Temple. They asked with concern and curiosity, then why is this not practiced everywhere?

Ans. Yes, it would be ideal, if temple and school authorities everywhere insist on such a certificate for MMR (rather than rubella alone).

Q9. A boy, B. Tech from IIT, got admission in University of North Carolina, USA for masters. His admission formalities included producing his vaccination record. They wanted all entrants to have immunity against meningococcal meningitis, measles, and chickenpox. He was not vaccinated against hepatitis A and typhoid also.

Why should they insist for all these vaccinations?

Ans. Universities insist foreign students to be fully protected against certain diseases before they enter their country for two reasons. One is that individual must be safe when living in hostels far away from home (such as from meningitis) and second that they do not want diseases to be brought to their country, that are almost eliminated, such as measles.

Parents wished him to be safe and healthy in foreign land and were ready for all required vaccinations.

Q10. A family going for World tour approaches me for guidance regarding vaccinations.

Ans. It depends on where you are going and what you will be doing.
- Routine vaccines for review before traveling (that we already discussed)
- *Selective use for travelers*: These vaccines are recommended to provide protection against diseases endemic to the country of origin or of destination. They are intended to protect travelers and to prevent disease spread within and between countries.

Some countries require proof of vaccination for travelers wishing to enter or exit the country.
- Cholera
- Hep A
- Hep B
- Japanese encephalitis
- Meningococcal disease
- Oral polio (adult booster dose)
- Rabies
- Tick-borne encephalitis
- Typhoid fever
- Yellow fever

Quadrivalent meningococcal vaccine for those traveling to the US and bivalent (A+C) or quadrivalent for those traveling to the UK.

Yellow fever vaccine is mandatory for all travelers to yellow fever endemic zones (the yellow fever virus is found mainly in tropical and subtropical regions of Africa and South America) as per International Health Regulations. This is currently available only at select government-controlled centers in India.

Q11. People going for Hajj pilgrimage are asked for certain mandatory vaccinations. What are those vaccines?

Ans. All the persons, including adults, going to Saudi Arabia for Hajj pilgrimage are required to take one dose of oral poliovirus vaccine (OPV) in addition to quadrivalent meningococcal vaccine.

Q12. In school health program, a teacher asks, "if adolescent immunization is so important, why was it so much ignored? What are the barriers to adolescent vaccination?"

Ans.
- Most important barrier is the lack of knowledge of adolescent vaccines and their long-term benefits among providers as well as public.
- Fewer adolescent health maintenance visits
- Adolescents unaware of the need for immunization
- Adolescents/parents underestimate risk of vaccine-preventable disease
- Noncompliance with multiple vaccine doses
- Misperceptions about vaccine safety

Q13. Do you have any government prescribed immunization card for my children?

Ans. Government of India has not prescribed any schedule for adolescent immunization so far.

But IAP-ACVIP devised a card for this purpose in 2014 which is shown in Figures 1 and 2.

Vaccine ▼ Age ►	7–10 years	11–12 years	13–18 years
Tdap	1 dose (if indicated)	1 dose	1 dose (if indicated)
HPV		2 doses	Complete 2/3–dose series
MMR		Complete 2–dose series	
Varicella		Complete 2–dose series	
Hepatitis B		Complete 3–dose series	
Hepatitis A		Complete 1/2–dose series	
Typhoid		1 dose every 3 years	
Influenza vaccine		One dose every year	
Japanese encephalitis vaccine		Catch–up up to 15 years	
Pneumococcal vaccine			
Meningococcal vaccine			

☐ For all children/Pre-adolescents   ☐ For catch–up immunization   ☐ For high–risk group

Fig. 1: Adolescent immunization schedule card. Indian Academy of Pediatrics–Advisory Committee on Vaccines and Immunization Practices (IAP–ACVIP) immunization schedule for persons aged 7 years through 18 years, 2014 (with range).
(HPV: human papillomavirus; MMR: measles, mumps, and rubella; Tdap: tetanus, diphtheria, and acellular pertussis)

	Birth	6 weeks	10 weeks	14 weeks	6 months	9 months	12 months	13 months	15 months	16–18 months	2–3 years	4–6 years	9–14 years	15–18 years
BCG	BCG													
Hepatitis B	HB 1	HB 2	HB 3	HB* 4										
Polio	OPV 0	IPV** 1	IPV** 2	IPV** 3						IPV***B1				
DTwP/DTaP		DTP 1	DTP 2	DTP 3						DTP B1		DTPB2		
HiB		HiB 1	HiB 2	HiB 3						HiB B1				
Pneumococcal		PCV 1	PCV 2	PCV 3					PCV B1				PCV	
Rotavirus		Rota 1	Rota 2	Rota 3****										
MMR						MMR1			MMR2			MMR3/MMRV		
Varicella									Varicella 1			Varicella 2		
Hepatitis A							Hep A1			Hep A2*****				
Typhoid					TCV#									
Influenza							Influenza (yearly)******							
Meningococcal						MCV1	MCV 2				MCV			
JE							JE 1	JE 2						
Tdap													Tdap	Td
HPV##													HPV 1 and 2	HPV 1, 2, 3
Cholera									Cholera 1 and 2					

Range of recommended age for all children
Range of recommended age for high-risk children/area
Range of recommended age for catch-up immunization
Not recommended

*Fourth dose of hepatitis B permissible for combination vaccines only
**In case IPV is not available or feasible, the child should be offered bOPV (3 doses). In such cases, give two fractional doses of IPV at 6 weeks and 14 weeks
***b-OPV, if IPV booster (standalone or combination) not feasible
****Third dose not required for RV1. Catch-up up to 1 year of age in UIP schedule
*****Live attenuated hepatitis A vaccine: single dose only
******Begin influenza vaccination after 6 months of age, about 2–1 weeks before season; give 2 doses at the interval of 4 weeks during first year and then single dose yearly till 5 years of age
#TCV=Typhoid conjugate vaccine, ## HPV = human papilloma virus
Meningococcal vaccine (MCV): 9 months through 23 months; 2 doses, at least 3 months apart; 2 years through 55 years; single dose only
Japanese encephalitis (JE): For individuals living an endemic areas and for travelers to JE endemic areas provided their expected stay is for a minimum period of 4 weeks
HPV: 2 doses at 6 months interval 9–14 years age; 3 dose (at 0, 1–2 and 6 months) 15 years or older and immunocompromised
Cholera vaccine: Two doses 2 weeks apart for >1 year old; for individuals living in high endemic areas and travelling to areas with risk of transmission is very high
(BCG: Bacillus Calmette-Guerin; DTaP: diphtheria, tetanus, acellular pertussis vaccine; DTwP: diphtheria, tetanus, whole cell pertussis; Hib: Haemophilus influenzae type b; HPV: human papillomavirus; IPV: inactivated poliovirus vaccine; MMR: measles-mumps-rubella; OPV0: oral poliovirus vaccine at birth; PCV: pneumococcal conjugate vaccine; Td: tetanus, reduced dose diphtheria toxoid; Tdap: tetanus, reduced dose diphtheria and acellular pertussis vaccine)
Source: Balasubramanian S, Shah A, Pemde HK, et al. Indian Academy of Pediatrics (IAP) Advisory Committee on Vaccines and Immunization Practices (ACVIP) Recommended Immunization Schedule (2018-19) and Update on Immunization for Children Aged 0 Through 18 Years. Indian Pediatr. 2018;55(12):1066-74.

Fig. 2: Indian Academy of Pediatrics (IAP) recommended immunization schedule for children aged 0–18 years (with range), 2014.

Q14. If someone has not taken most of the vaccines or has lost all records and wants to repeat full vaccination, is it advisable?

Ans. Yes, he can take all age-appropriate vaccines.

Take Home Message

- Youth is precious human resource of every country.
- More than 21% of our population is of adolescents.
- Their perfect health should be our priority.
- Vaccination is the most cost-effective way of prevention.
- We have so far not given enough attention to adolescents.
- Time has come to focus on adolescent immunization.
- This is cost-effective, available, and doable.

SUGGESTED READING

1. Centers for Disease Control and Prevention. Recommended Child and Adolescent Immunization Schedule for ages 18 years or younger. [online] Available from: https://www.cdc.gov/vaccines/schedules/downloads/child/0-18yrs-child-combined-schedule.pdf [Last accessed June, 2020].
2. D'Addario M, Scott P, Redmond S, Lowet N. HPV vaccines: Review of alternative Vaccination Schedules: Preliminary Overview of the Literature. University of Bern, Bern, Switzerland. Report to WHO 3rd March 2014 (unpublished). [online] Available from: https://www.who.int/immunization/sage/meetings/2014/april/1_HPV_Evidence_based_recommendationsWHO_with_Appendices2_3.pdf?ua=1 [Last accessed June, 2020].
3. For more information on travelers vaccination, visit: http://wwwnc.cdc.gov/travel/default.aspx.
4. Indian Academy of Pediatrics Committee on Immunization (IAPCOI). Consensus recommendations on immunization and IAP immunization timetable 2012. Indian Pediatr. 2012;49(7):549-64.
5. Indian Academy of Pediatrics, Advisory Committee on Vaccines and Immunization Practices (ACVIP), Vashishtha VM, Kalra A, Bose A, Choudhury P, Yewale VN, et al. Indian Academy of Pediatrics (IAP) recommended immunization schedule for children aged 0 through 18 years, India, 2013 and updates on immunization. Indian Pediatr. 2013;50(12):1095-108.
6. Indian Academy of Pediatrics. Indian Academy of Pediatrics (IAP) Recommended Immunization Schedule for Children Aged 0 through 18 years – India, 2014 and Updates on Immunization. [online]Available from: http://www.indianpediatrics.net/oct2014/oct-785-803.htm [Last accessed June, 2020].
7. Recommended Adult Immunization Schedule/oct-78 States 2010. MMWR. [online] Available from: http://www.cdc.gov/mmwr/PDF/wk/mm5901-Immunization.pdf [Last accessed June, 2020].
8. Recommended Immunization Schedule for Persons Aged 7 through 18 Yearsfor Children A 2010. [online] Available from: http://www.cdc.gov/vaccines/recs/schedules/downloads/ child/2010/10_7-18yrs-schedule-pr.pdf [Last accessed June, 2020].
9. Sankaranarayanan R, Evaluation of fewer than three doses of HPV vaccination in India, in WHO Consultation Meeting. Geneva: WHO; 2013.

10. Sankaranarayanan R. Trial of two versus three doses of Human Papillomavirus (HPV) vaccine in India (2013). [online] Available from: http://clinicaltrials.gov/show/NCT00923702 [Last accessed June, 2020].
11. Sankaranarayanan R. Two vs. three doses HPV vaccine schedule: low- and middle-income countries, in Europe in 2013. Florence, Italy; International Multidisciplinary Congress; 2013.
12. Vashishtha VM, Bansal CP, Gupta SG. Pertussis vaccines: Position paper of Indian Academy of Pediatrics (IAP). Indian Pediatr. 2013;50(11):1001-9.
13. Vashishtha VM, Choudhury P, Bansal CP, Yewale VN, Agarwal R. (Eds). IAP Guidebook on Immunization 2013-2014. Gwalior: National Publication House, Indian Academy of Pediatrics; 2014.
14. Vashishtha VM, Yewale VN, Bansal CP, Mehta PJ, Indian Academy of Pediatrics, Advisory Committee on Vaccines and Immunization Practices (ACVIP). IAP perspectives on measles and rubella elimination strategies. Indian Pediatr. 2014;51(9):719-22.
15. World Health Organization (2007). WHO Technical Report Series No 941, 2007. Annex 6 Recommendations for whole-cell pertussis vaccine. [online] Available from: http://www.who.int/biologicals/publications/trs/areas/vaccines/whole_cell_pertussis/Annex%206%20whole%20cell%20pertussis.pdf [Last accessed June, 2020].
16. World Health Organization. Evidence Based Recommendations on Human Papillomavirus (HPV) Vaccines Schedules. Background paper for SAGE discussions, March 11, 2014. [online] Available from: http://www.who.int/immunization/sage/meetings/2014/april/1_HPV_Evidence_based_recommendationsWHO_with_ Appendices2_3.pdf?ua=1 [Last accessed June, 2020].
17. World Health Organization. Summary of the SAGE April 2014 Meeting. [online] Available from: http://www.who.int/immunization/sage/meetings/2014/april/report_ summary_april_2014/en/ [Last accessed June, 2020].
18. World Health Organization. Summary of the SAGE April 2014 Meeting. [online] Available from: http://www.who.int/immunization/sage/meetings/2014/april/report_ summary_april_2014/en/. [Last accessed June, 2020].
19. World Health Organization. Vaccines and biologicals: Recommendations from the Strategic Advisory Group of Experts. Wkly Epidemiol Rec. 2002;77(37): 305-11.
20. World Health Organization. WHO prequalified vaccines. [online] Available from: http://www.who.int/immunization_standards/vaccine_quality/PQ_vaccine_list_en/en/ [Last accessed June, 2020].
21. World Health Organization. WHO prequalified vaccines. [online] Available from: http://www.who.int/immunization. [Last accessed June, 2020].

Index

Page numbers followed by b refer to box, f refer to figure, fc refer to flowchart, and t refer to table.

A

Abdomen
 ultrasonography of 51, 162
 ultrasound of 42
Abdominal distension, mild 122
Abdominal pain 37, 163
ABM *See* Acute bacterial meningitis
Abscess 144
 pneumatocele 69
Absolute lymphocyte count 110
Acellular pertussis vaccine 217
Acetazolamide 32
Acholic stools 97
Acid-fast bacilli 46, 63, 215
Acidic pH 124
Acinetobacter 180
Acquired disease, history of 95
Actinomyces species 62
Activated partial thromboplastin time 57
Acute disseminated encephalomyelitis 10, 16, 26f
Acute fever, causes of 35
Acute kidney injury, staging of 191
Acyclovir 27, 28, 86
ADEM *See* Acute disseminated encephalomyelitis
Adenovirus 108
Adequate analgesia 71
Adrenaline 205
AES *See* Acute encephalitis syndrome
Aflatoxins 16
Alagille syndrome 104, 105
Alanine aminotransferase 59
Albendazole 147, 148
Albumin globulin 165
Alkaline phosphatase 41
Amatoxins 16
Amikacin 82
Anasarca 80f
Anemia 53, 118
 cause for 90
 severe 8, 90
Anorexia, symptoms of 161
Antenatal infections 134
Antibiotic 122, 202
 course, duration of 72
 dose 184
 misuse of 177
 prophylaxis 115
 resistance 177
 therapy 5, 72
Anti-endomysial antibodies 127
Antiepileptic
 drug 143
 valparin 86
Antimalarial drugs 7, 8
Antimotility agents 122
Antinuclear antibody test 51
Antiparasitic drugs 122
Anti-tetanus antibodies 38
Anti-tissue transglutaminase antibodies 127
Antitubercular drugs 214
Antitubercular therapy 161, 185
Antitubercular treatment 210
Artemether-lumefantrine 184
Arterial blood gas 201, 207
Arteriovenous malformation 141
Arthralgia 42
Arthritis 42, 48, 77
Aspergillus 114
 pneumonia 38, 113
Aspiration 152
 syndromes 108
Autoimmune hepatitis 165
Autoinflammatory diseases 44
AVM *See* Arteriovenous malformation
Azithromycin 28
 with steroids 27

B

Babinski's sign 172
Bacillus Calmette-Guérin
 infection 47
 vaccine 47
Bacterial diseases 43
Bacterial endocarditis 7
Bacterial infection 1, 7
 self-limiting 122
Bacterial meningitis 11, 32
Bacterial pneumonia 177
Bacterial strain 6
Bacteriostatic drug 182
Behçet's disease 43
BERA *See* Brainstem evoked response audiometry
Bile duct
 plugging of 99
 proliferation 99
Biliary atresia 99, 100
Biliary ducts, lymphocytic proliferation of 99
Biliary system, congenital defects in 164
Biliary tract, normal 101
Bladder, ultrasound of 105
Blastomycosis 36
Blood 206
 ammonia 136
 culture 77
 glucose 27, 136
 pressure 6, 200
Body ache 58
Body mass index 42
Body temperature, normal 35
Bone marrow 93, 96
 biopsy 96
 disorder 8
Borrelia recurrentis 43
Bowel movements, normal 127
BP *See* Blood pressure
Bradycardia 26
Brain
 damage 30
 herniation 30
 histopathology 15f
 magnetic resonance imaging 131

parenchyma,
    inflammation of 15f
Brain herniation syndromes
    signs of 31
    symptoms of 31
    types of 30f
Brainstem
    evoked response
        audiometry 132
    neurocysticercosis 145
Breathing
    irregular 26
    work of 200
Bronchiectasis 112
Bronchoalveolar lavage 157
Brucella 3, 77, 79
    antibody 36
Brucellosis 1, 88
    diagnosis of 79
    treatment for 36
Budd-Chiari syndrome 165
Burkholderia cepacia 114
Burkholderia pseudomallei 43
Burst suppression 132

C

Cachexia 94
Campylobacter 123
Capillary filling time 200
Cardiac abnormality 135
Cardiovascular disease 51
Cardiovascular dysfunction 199
Cardiovascular system 104
Cataract 117
    causes of 121
    etiology for 117
    with rubella 119
Catecholamine refractory 205
Causative organisms 181
Cefepime 71
Cefpodoxime 168
Ceftriaxone 82
    injection 84
Celiac disease 126
    diagnosis of 127
Central nervous system 200
    infections 10, 12
Central venous pressure 203
Cephalosporins 86
Cerebral cortex 131
Cerebral decongestants 173
Cerebral edema 141f, 143
Cerebral hemisphere, right 140

Cerebral ischemia 29, 30
Cerebral malaria 16, 28
Cerebral perfusion pressure 25, 29
Cerebrospinal fluid 5, 84, 139
Cervarix 219
Cervical cancer 218
Cervical lymph node 212, 213f
    enlargement of 93
Cervical lymphadenopathy 37, 40, 185
CFT *See* Capillary filling time
Chandipura 19
Chikungunya 19, 81
Chills 185
Cholangiogram,
    intraoperative 98
Cholangitis 43, 60
Cholecystitis 60
Choledochal cyst 100, 163
    prognosis of 100
Choledocholithiasis 163
Cholestasis 104, 105
    cause of neonatal 98, 100, 104
Chromosomal disorder 118, 130, 133
Chromosomal microarray 134
Chylothorax 65
Ciprofloxacin 125
Clarithromycin 28, 71
Clean-catch sample 182
Clindamycin 28
CMV *See* Cytomegalovirus
CNS *See* Central nervous system
Coccidioidomycosis 36
Coenzyme A 13
Cold 202
    shock 203, 205
Collagen disorders 82
Collagen vascular diseases 51
Coma 25
    diabetic 10
    fever with 10
Common metabolic
    syndrome 23b
Community-acquired
    empyema 71
Complete blood count 36, 38, 77, 89, 90, 92, 110, 111, 118, 201
Conjugate vaccine 221

Conjugated
    hyperbilirubinemia 97
Consanguineous marriage 104, 157
Consanguinity, absence of 131
Cotrimoxazole 114
Cough 185
    chronic 113, 157
Craniosynostosis 130
Crohn's disease 43
CRS *See* Congenital rubella syndrome
Cryptosporidium 115
Cushing's triad 26
Cutaneous tuberculosis,
    treatment for 212
CVP *See* Central venous pressure
Cystic fibrosis 127, 153
Cysticercosis 140
Cysticercotic encephalitis 146
Cysticercus encephalitis 146
Cysticidal therapy 147
    role of 146
Cytomegalovirus 1, 48, 77, 102, 106, 119, 129

D

Decompensated cirrhosis 99
Dehydrogenase deficiency 13
Dengue 19, 85, 211
    fever 50, 169
    hemorrhagic fever 17
    infection, normal in 89
    scrub typhus 56
    shock syndrome 17
    vaccine 225
Dengvaxia 225
Deoxyribonucleic acid 137
Deresuscitation 202
Diagnostic dilemma 10
Diagnostic pleural aspirate 70
Diarrhea 37
    acute 122
    prolonged 122
    worsening of 126
Diarrheal episode 122
Digestive enzymes,
    deficiencies of 126
DLC *See* Differential leukocyte count

Index

DNA *See* Deoxyribonucleic acid
Dopamine, dose of 205
Doxycycline 28, 36, 176
Drainage catheter placement 65
Drug hypersensitivity reaction 211
Drug rash 169
Drug-resistant *Streptococcus pneumoniae* 179
DSS *See* Dengue shock syndrome
Dysarthria 146
Dysfunctional bladder 197
Dysmorphic facies 105
Dysphasia 146

E

Ear 111
Ectodermal dysplasia 54
Ehrlich-Ziehl-Neelsen stain 215
ELISA *See* Enzyme-linked immunosorbent assay
Embryotoxon, posterior 105
Empirical antibiotic therapy 5
Empyema 69, 71-73
   antibiotic management of 71
   development of 67
   diagnosing 70
   management of 72
   thoracis 67
Encephalitis 11, 12, 12*t*, 26*f*, 172
   syndrome, acute 10, 11, 17, 25
Encephalopathy 11
   acute 22
   toxin-induced 16
Endocarditis, infective 43, 88
Endocrine disorders 117
Endoscopic retrograde cholangiopancreatography 163
Entamoeba 115
Enteric fever 56, 59
   complicated 57, 59
Enteroviruses 19
Enzyme
   assays 22
   immunoassays 119
Enzyme-linked immunosorbent assay 13, 144, 159
   immunotransfer blot 144

Eosinophils 49
Epilepsy 138
Epileptiform activity 141*f*
Epithelioid cells 212
Epstein-Barr virus 1, 16, 102, 119
Erythema multiforme 170
Erythematous rash, diffuse 169
Erythrocyte sedimentation rate 46, 183
Erythroderma 169
Erythromycin 71
Escalate antibiotic 179
Escherichia coli 114, 123, 182
Ethambutol 183
Exocrine pancreatic insufficiency 126
Extended-spectrum beta-lactamase 180
Extrahepatic cholestasis 103
Eyes
   watering of 170
   yellowness of 164

F

Falx cerebri 31*f*
Fatty acid oxidation 138
Febrile coma, management of 28
Febrile encephalopathy 11
   acute 11, 20, 23, 26, 28
   management of acute 25, 29
Feeding difficulties, absence of 113
Fever 1, 41, 50, 76, 163, 185
   confusing 76
   high-grade 79
   long duration 76
   low-grade 186
   of unknown origin 76
   prolonged 76
   recurrent 35
   short duration 76
   symptoms of 161
   types of 76
Fibrinolytic agents 72
Fibrinolytic therapy 72, 73
FIESTA *See* Fast-imaging employing steady-state acquisition sequence
Fine-needle aspiration cytology 41, 92
Fingers, gangrene of 80*f*

FISH *See* Fluorescence in situ hybridization
Fluid 28
   intolerance
      causes of 203
      management of 203
   management, basics of 193
   refractory shock 204
Fluorescence in situ hybridization 134
Fluorescent antibody, indirect 171
Foamy cells 15*f*
Focal deficits 146
Food protein sensitivity 126
Foreign body, chronic 46
Fosphenytoin 143
Fresh frozen plasma transfusion 84
Fungal granulomas 143
Fungal infections 113
Furosemide 32

G

Galactose-1-phosphate uridylyltransferase 101
Galactosemia 101, 102
Gamma-glutamyl transpeptidase 98, 106
Gardasil 219
Gas chromatography mass spectrometry 22
Gastroesophageal reflux disease 46, 109, 152
Gastrointestinal bleeding 91
Gastrointestinal tract 111
   upper 165
Gaze palsies 145
GCT *See* Glutaraldehyde coagulation test
Genetic syndromes 130
Genexpert mycobacterium tuberculosis 64
GERD *See* Gastroesophageal reflux disease
GGT *See* Gamma-glutamyl transpeptidase
Ghon's complex 213
Giardia 115
   cysts 111
   lamblia infestation 126
Glasgow coma scale 172
Glucose 207
Glucuronosyltransferase gene 164

Glutamic oxaloacetic transaminase 118
Glutaraldehyde coagulation test 106
Gluten-induced enteropathy 127
Glycerol 32
Glycosylation defects, congenital 138
Granulomatous disease, chronic 114, 159, 160
Granulomatous hepatitis 43
Gut diseases, chronic 112

H

Haemophilus influenzae 62, 74, 108, 178
Headache 89
Heart
  disease, congenital 46, 92, 95, 105
  rate 200
Hematological tests 82, 188
Hemiparesis 146
Hemoglobin 119
Hemolytic uremic syndrome 68, 170
Hemophagocytic lymphohistiocytosis 2, 77
Hemophagocytic syndromes 88
Hemorrhage 141
Hepatic duodenostomy 100
Hepatitis 57
  A 60, 217, 226
    vaccine 222
    virus 162
  acute 58, 162
  B 217
    vaccine 222
    virus 162
  jaundice in 2
Hepatobiliary iminodiacetic acid 98
Hepatocyte disease 35
Hepatojugular reflux 3
Hepatotoxic drugs 161
  history of 162
Herpes simplex virus 13, 26, 100, 106, 186
  encephalitis 18, 20*f*
Herpes virus 102
Herpes zoster 16
Hidden abscess 51
Histidine-rich protein 90

Histoplasmosis 36
HIV *See* Human immunodeficiency virus
Hodgkin's lymphoma 40, 186
Homogeneous opacity, left-sided 69*f*
Hospital-acquired empyema 71
HPV *See* Human papillomavirus
HSV *See* Herpes simplex virus
Human immunodeficiency virus 38, 46, 78, 100, 123, 137, 159
Human papillomavirus 227
  diseases 218
  vaccine 217, 218
Hydrogen breath test 125
Hyperammonemia 13
Hyperbilirubinemia 97
Hyperintense lesion 20*f*
Hyperkalemia 196
Hyperlactatemia 90
Hypernatremic dehydration, calculation for 193
Hyperphosphatemia 196
Hyperplasia, reactive 186
Hypertension 26, 194
Hyperthermia 33
Hypertonic saline 32
Hypoglycemia 90, 201
Hyponatremia 196
Hypoxic-ischemic encephalopathy 129, 131

I

Icterus 80*f*
Idiopathic neonatal hepatitis 100
IEM *See* Inborn errors of metabolism
Illness, severity of 179, 181
Immune thrombocytopenia 170
Immunization 216
Immunochromographic test 53
Immunodeficiency 39*t*, 40*t*
  diseases, primary 159
  disorder 37, 108, 159, 160
Inborn errors of metabolism, type of 21, 22, 23*b*, 130, 136

Indian Academy of Pediatrics 98
Infection
  chronic 2, 89
  congenital 102, 104, 137
  reports of 108
  severe 151
  site of 181
  unusual 108
Infectious mononucleosis 48, 175
Inflammatory disease, progressive 1
Inflammatory disorder 95
Influenza 108
  vaccine 220
Insecticides 16
Insulin 28
Internuclear ophthalmoplegias 145
Intestinal malabsorption 126
Intracranial pressure 25, 30
  management of raised 32
Intrapleural fibrinolytic therapy 65
Intrauterine growth restriction 102, 118
Intrauterine infection 117, 136
Intrauterine rubella infection 121
Intravenous immunoglobulin replacement therapy 112
Intraventricular cysticercosis 146
Invasive ventilation 204
Ionized calcium 207
Isoniazid 183, 184
Itch 163
Itraconazole 114, 115

J

Japanese encephalitis 11, 16, 18, 26*f*
  vaccine 224
Jaundice 56, 102, 163
  absence of 35
  infant with deep 97
  management of recurrent 161
  prolonged 97
  recurrent 161
  relapse of 162
JE *See* Japanese encephalitis

Joint pain 58
Juvenile chronic myeloid leukemia 40
Juvenile dermatomyositis 43
Juvenile idiopathic arthritis 42

K

Kala-azar 2, 8, 36, 51, 77, 88, 94*f*
Kasai portoenterostomy 99, 163
Kasai procedure 99
Kawasaki disease 169
Kidney
  disease, chronic 194
  injury, acute 191, 191*t*, 195
  ultrasound of 105
Killed vaccine 222
Klebsiella 180
Koch's disease, signs of 143
Koplik's spots 170

L

Lactate dehydrogenase 60, 173
Lactose tolerance test 125
Langhans giant cells 215
Left upper lobe 154*f*
Leishmania donovani 8
Leishmaniasis 8
Leptospirosis 50, 56, 57, 77, 175, 183
Lesion, skin biopsy of 212*f*
Leukemia 36
  lymphoproliferative disorder, acute 91*f*
Leukocyte
  adhesion deficiency 116
  count, differential 192, 195
Leukopenia 53
LFT *See* Liver function test
Lichen scrofulosorum, lesions of 213*f*
Liquid chromatography, high performance 14, 22
Live vaccine 222
Liver
  abscess 38
  biopsy 98, 99, 103, 104
  disease, chronic 166
  enzymes 56, 98
  function 41

function test 38, 78, 89, 161
  complete 98
  histopathology 14*f*, 15*f*
  transplantation, facility for 99
Lobar emphysema, congenital 154
Lorazepam 27, 33
  injection 173
Lower limb, gangrene of 80*f*
Lung 111
  congenital malformations of 46
  malformations, congenital 108, 109
Lupus vulgaris
  differential diagnosis of 214
  plaque 214*f*
Lymph node 92, 96
  biopsy 41
  classification of 187*t*
  group of 185
Lymphadenopathy 91*f*, 185, 186, 188, 188*fc*
Lymphogranuloma venereum 186
Lymphoma 36, 144
Lymphoreticular malignancy 41

M

Maculopapular rash 80*f*
Malaria 2, 56, 77, 85, 88, 175
  chloroquine-resistant 51
  complicated 89
  diagnosis of 90
Malarial parasite 42
Malnutrition
  acute 123, 125
  chronic 154, 155
Mantoux test 113, 214
Matted lymphadenopathy, etiology of 187*t*
Mean arterial pressure 201
Measles, mumps, and rubella 227
  vaccine 223
Mediterranean fever 43
Meningitis 11
  signs of 12
Meningococcal conjugate vaccines 219
Meningococcal septicaemia, acute 172

Meningococcal vaccine 219
Meningococcemia 43, 172
Meningoencephalitis 12, 16, 86, 146
Meropenem 82, 163, 180
Metabolic abnormalities 157
Metabolic acidosis 199
Metabolic disorders 102, 117
Metabolic encephalopathy 10
Metabolic syndrome 21-23, 23*b*
Metastasis 144
Methicillin-resistant *Staphylococcus aureus* 62, 74, 158, 179
Methylprednisolone
  injection 174
  pulse therapy 27
Metronidazole 71
Microcephaly 129
  with seizures, causes of 129*b*
Microdeletion syndrome 135
Micturating cystourethrogram 182
Midazolam 27, 33
  drip 84
Midbrain
  neurocysticercosis 145*f*
  tegmentum of 145
Middle lobe, right 154*f*
Milrinone 205
MMR *See* Measles, mumps, and rubella
Mouth ulcers 77
Multiorgan dysfunction syndrome 208
Multiple antibiotics 3
Mumps 16, 19
Mycobacteria 47
Mycobacterium tuberculosis 45, 93, 109, 113
Mycoplasma 16, 17, 28, 178
  pneumonia 67, 71, 180
Myeloid leukemia, chronic 94
Myocardial dysfunction 205
Myoclonic epilepsy, early 132

N

National Tuberculosis Control Program 45
Neonatal cholestasis 98*b*, 100-102, 106, 106*fc*

Neonatal hypoglycemia 129, 131
Neurocysticercosis 32, 140
Neurological disease, acute 11
Neurological disorders 133
Neurological symptoms 42
Neuropsychiatric reactions, risk of 28
Neutropenia 39
  syndromes, congenital 159
Neutrophilia 196
Neutrophilic leukocytosis 78
Nicotinamide adenine dinucleotide phosphate 114
Night sweats 41
Nipah 19
  virus 18
Nitroblue tetrazolium test 160
Nocardia 114
Noncervical human papillomavirus disease 218
Non-Hodgkin lymphoma 94, 186
Noninfective diseases 5
Nonrebreathing mask 200, 201
Nonresolving pneumonia 151, 153
Noradrenaline 205
Nucleic acid amplification test, cartridge-based 46, 93, 189

O

Ocular nerve palsies 145
Ohtahara syndrome 132
Oligohydramnios 194
Ophthalmological examination 105
Oral rehydration solution 122, 124
Oral typhoid vaccine 222
Organic acidemias 21
Organic acids, analysis of 22
Organic acidurias 21
Orientia tsutsugamushi 176
Osmotherapy 32
Otitis media, acute suppurative 37
Otoacoustic emissions 119

P

Packed cell volume 192, 195
Palate, high-arched 136

Pale stools 163
Pancreatic insufficiency 158
Papilledema 140
Parainfluenza viruses 108
Parapneumonic effusion 73
Parasites 88
Parasitic diseases 43
Parasitic tapeworm 140
Parenchymal cysticercosis 140
Parvovirus B19 119
Pathogenic bacterial infections 86
PCR *See* Polymerase chain reaction
PCV *See* Packed cell volume
Pediatric septic shock 198
Penicillin 28
Perinatal asphyxia, injury in 132*t*
Perinatal hypoxic-ischemic injury 131
Perinatal stroke 129, 131
Peripheral blood smear 38
Peripheral pulmonic stenosis 105
Peripheral smear 89
  examination 111
Persistent pneumonia 155
Pesticides 16
Petechiae, absence of 92
Pharyngitis, absence of 92
Phenytoin 143
  injection 173
PID *See* Primary immunodeficiency diseases
Piperacillin 71
Piperacillin tazobactam 82 plus 180
Plasmodium falciparum 90
Plasmodium vivax 90
  infection 91
Pleural biopsy 66
Pleural effusion 65, 67, 72
Pleural fluid 70
Pleural infection, management of 68*fc*
Pleurodesis 66
Pneumococcal polysaccharide vaccine 221
Pneumococcal vaccines 220
Pneumococcus 108
Pneumocystis 110
  carinii 110
  jirovecii pneumonia 39

Pneumonia 73, 108, 110, 155, 158, 179*f*
Pneumothorax 65
Polymerase chain reaction 19, 103, 184
Polysaccharide vaccines 219, 221
Pontine herniation syndromes, upper 30
Poor appetite 113
Portal fibrosis, lymphocytic proliferation of 99
Postexposure prophylaxis 224
Potassium hydroxide 110
Precancerous dysplasia 218
Prednisone 147
Preoxygenate 204
Prominent glabella 133
Proteinuria 194
Pseudomonas 180
  aeruginosa 67, 71
  bacteria 178
Pulmonary hypertension 205
Pulmonary plethora 156*f*
Pulmonary tuberculosis, sign of 214
Pulmonic stenosis 104
Pulse pressure 207
  low 205
PUO *See* Pyrexia of unknown origin
Purified protein derivative 47, 210
Purpura 92
  fulminans 172, 173
Pus discharge 85*f*
Putative toxin 14
Pyelonephritis 178
Pyrazinamide 183
Pyrexia 62
  of unknown origin 1
Pyuria 182

R

Rabies 19
Rash 89
  fever with 211
Rat-bite fever 43
Rational antibiotic usage 177
Refractory shock 208
Renal dysfunction and cataracts 102
Renal failure, acute 191
Renal function tests 41
Respiratory distress syndrome, acute 172, 198

Respiratory failure, acute 174
Respiratory symptoms 153
Respiratory syncytial virus 108
Respiratory system 67
  examination 172
Respiratory tract infections 151, 157
Retrognathia 136
Reye syndrome 13, 14, 15*f*, 23
  diagnosis of 13
Rheumatic diseases 1
Rheumatic heart disease 92
Rheumatoid arthritis 51
Rickettsia 169, 172, 176, 183
  conorii 168
Rickettsial diseases 77, 81, 83, 85, 87, 89, 168
  antibody titers for 86
  test for 79, 82, 84
Rickettsial fever 170
Rickettsial infection 50, 168
Rifampicin 64, 183, 184
Right lower lobe, collapse of 64*f*
Ring-enhancing lesions 142
Ringer's lactate 201
Rocky mountain, diagnosis of 82
Routine vaccination 219
Roux-en-Y hepaticojejunostomy 100
Roxithromycin 71
Rubella 16, 19, 129
  cytomegalovirus 100
  infection 120*fc*
  serology 119
    maternal 119
  syndrome, congenital 119
Rubeola 16

S

Salmonella 58, 123
  infection 58
    stage of 58
  liver abscess 60
  typhi 56
SAM *See* Severe acute malnutrition
Sanger's sequencing 138
Scarlet fever 169
Scrofuloderma 211
  diagnosis of 213
  lesions of 213*f*
Scrub typhus 94, 175

Seizures 146
  control 27
  recurrent 129
Sensorium, fever with altered 11*b*
Sepsis
  risk factors for 199
  screen 98
Septic shock 199, 200, 202, 206
  management of 198
  vasoactive drugs in 203*b*
Serological tests 57, 90
Serratia marcescens 114
Serum
  aminotransferase levels 60
  amylase and lipase 163
  bilirubin 99
  creatinine 191
  glutamic
    oxaloacetic trans aminase 192, 195
    pyruvic transaminase 52, 118, 192, 195
  immunoglobulins 38
  sodium 194
SGOT *See* Serum glutamic oxaloacetic transaminase
SGPT *See* Serum glutamic pyruvic transaminase
Shigella 123
Shock
  early recognition of 200*t*
  intubation in 204
  management 207
Single-enhancing lesions, causes of 142
Sinopulmonary infections 40
Sinus tenderness 37
Skin
  manifestations, unusual 210
  rash 48, 77
  tuberculosis 210
Skull, ultrasound of 103
Sore throat 185
Spina bifida occulta 104
Spine, X-ray 104
Spirillum minus 43
Spleen 88, 96
Splenic biopsy 96
Splenic enlargement 88
Splenomegaly
  fever with 88
  massive 94

Spongiosis, mild 15*f*
Spotted fever
  disease 174
  group 168
Staphylococcus 108
  aureus 62, 74, 114, 178
Step-ladder fever 175
Steroids 32, 147
Stevens-Johnson syndrome 170
Streptococcus
  pneumoniae 62, 74, 178
  species, group A 62
Subacute bacterial endocarditis 1, 6
Succinylcholine 204
SVR *See* Systemic vascular resistance
Swine flu 220
Systemic blood pressure 201
Systemic illness 65
Systemic inflammatory
  disease 2
  disorder 42, 48
Systemic lupus erythematosus 43, 88
Systemic vascular resistance 203
Systemic vasculitis 88

T

Tachycardia,
  disproportionate 4
Taenia solium 140
Tandem mass spectrometry 22, 136
Tazobactam 71
TBM *See* Tuberculous meningitis
T-cell defects 109
Td *See* Tetanus-diphtheria vaccine
Tdap *See* Tetanus, diphtheria, and acellular pertussis
Temperature 207
Temporal lobe, right 20*f*
Tentorium cerebelli 31*f*
Tetanus, diphtheria, and acellular pertussis 227
  vaccine 217
Tetanus-diphtheria vaccine 217
Tetracycline 176
Tetralogy of Fallot 105
Thalamic abnormalities 18

Therapeutic end goals 202
Therapeutic plasma exchange 208
Third-nerve palsy, acute 145
Thoracocentesis 65
Thoracoscopic surgery, video-assisted 63, 66
Throat swab 213
Thrombocytopenia 82, 118, 212
  renal impairment 90
Thrombotic thrombocytopenic purpura 172, 173
Thyroid function tests 98
Thyroid-stimulating hormone 100, 119
TMS *See* Tandem mass spectrometry
Todd's palsy 140
Toddler's diarrhea 126
Tolosa-Hunt syndrome 145
TORCH 100, 134
Total leukocyte count 89
Toxic epidermal necrolysis 211
Toxic injury, acute 14
Toxic shock 208
Toxoid-containing vaccine 218
Toxoplasma 143, 144
Toxoplasmosis 88, 100, 129
Tracheoesophageal fistula 152
Treponema pallidum 43
Triad of fever 89
TSH *See* Thyroid-stimulating hormone
TST *See* Tuberculin skin test
Tuberculin skin test 45
Tuberculin test 51
Tuberculomas 144
Tuberculosis 1, 35, 43, 77, 85, 88, 113, 183, 210
  diagnosis of 49

Tuberculous meningitis 10, 32
Typhoid 11, 175, 221, 226
  fever 56, 58, 59, 169, 170, 175
  hepatitis 58, 59
  vaccines 221
Typhus group 168

U

Uncal herniation 30
Upper respiratory tract infection 10, 112, 212
  symptoms of 37
Ureter, ultrasound of 105
Urethral valve, posterior 196
Urinary tract infection 77
  coexisting 124
  diagnosis of 78
Urine
  for glucose 136
  for ketones 136
  microscopy 51
  output 191

V

Vaginal delivery, vacuum-assisted 130
Vancomycin 71, 82
Varicella 16, 18, 85
  vaccine 223
Vasopressor-inotrope infusions 205
Ventricular septal defect 155
Vertebra 104, 105
Vertebral anomalies 105
Viral agents 18*b*
Viral diseases 43, 85
Viral encephalitis 11
  acute 13, 18*b*, 19, 28
  cause of 18
  etiology of 18
  types of acute 18*t*

Viral hepatitis 56, 59, 60, 89
  A, acute 162
  acute 60
Viral infections 1, 119
Viral meningitis 11, 12*t*
Viridans streptococci species 62
Viscera 14
Visceral abnormality 135
Visceral leishmaniasis 92
Visual acuity 144
Vital signs, normal pediatric 200*t*
Vitamin
  A 103, 105
  D 103, 105
  E 103, 105
  fat-soluble 105
  K 103, 105
Vomiting, symptoms of 161
Voriconazole 114, 115

W

Warm shock 199, 203
WBC *See* White blood cell
West-Nile virus 18, 19
Whipple's disease 43
White blood cell 192, 195
Widal titer 42
Wilson's disease 166
Wiskott-Aldrich syndrome 159

X

X-linked agammaglobulinemia 109, 112
  treatment of 112

Z

Zika
  fever 81
  virus 129